"You must sacrifice something on the altar of expediency if you wish to become successful," the American neurologist William A. Hammond, M.D., told his medical students in 1867. "Only take care that you preserve your love for science." In this first full-length biography of a major nineteenth-century American medical personality, Bonnie Ellen Blustein shows how Dr. Hammond developed his specialty practice in neurology as a vehicle on which to pursue broad scientific interests within the limits set by the solo-practitioner structure of the medicine of his day.

William Alexander Hammond, M.D. (1828–1900), one of the most successful American physicians of the nineteenth century, was first recognized in the 1850s as a natural history collector and as an original investigator in physiological chemistry. Appointed surgeon general of the United States Army in 1862, he supervised a sweeping reorganization of the Medical Department along lines of centralization and efficiency. Some of his more controversial projects, however, provided Hammond's political enemies with the opportunity to engineer his court-martial and dismissal from the army in 1864. He then established himself in New York as an exclusive specialist in neurology, one of the first in the country. Over the next decades, clinical neurology not only made him a rich man, but also proved to be the forum for a sustained expression of his scientific interests and his views on contemporary social problems, such as the "woman question." He wrote extensively for medical journals, for the popular press, and in a series of novels.

By the end of the century, Hammond's scientific work had already come to be seen not so much as mistaken as beside the point. The paths he followed were generally not those found on modern maps of scientific discovery. But William Alexander Hammond preserved his love for science, and the altars of expediency on which he felt compelled to sacrifice tell us a great deal about the social context of late nineteenth-century American medicine.

Cambridge History of Medicine

EDITORS: CHARLES WEBSTER AND
CHARLES ROSENBERG

Preserve Your Love for Science

OTHER BOOKS IN THIS SERIES

Charles Webster, ed.   *Health, medicine, and mortality in the sixteenth century*

Ian Maclean   *The Renaissance notion of woman*

Michael MacDonald   *Mystical Bedlam*

Robert E. Kohler   *From medical chemistry to biochemistry*

Walter Pagel   *Joan Baptista Van Helmont*

Nancy Tomes   *A generous confidence*

Roger Cooter   *The cultural meaning of popular science*

Anne Digby   *Madness, morality and medicine*

Roy Porter, ed.   *Patients and practitioners*

Guenter B. Risse   *Hospital life in Enlightenment Scotland*

Ann G. Carmichael   *Plague and the poor in Renaissance Florence*

S. E. D. Shortt   *Victorian lunacy*

Hilary Marland   *Medicine and society in Wakefield and Huddersfield 1780–1870*

Susan M. Reverby   *Ordered to care*

Russell C. Maulitz   *Morbid appearances*

Matthew Ramsey   *Professional and popular medicine in France, 1770–1830*

John Keown   *Abortion, doctors and the law*

Donald Denoon   *Public health in Papua New Guinea*

Paul Weindling   *Health, race and German politics between national unification and Nazism, 1870–1945*

Ornella Moscucci   *The science of woman*

Jack D. Ellis   *The physician-legislators of France*

William H. Schneider   *Quality and quantity*

John Farley   *Bilharzia*

Mary E. Fissell   *Patients, power, and the poor in eighteenth-century Bristol*

Preserve Your Love for Science

LIFE OF WILLIAM A. HAMMOND,
AMERICAN NEUROLOGIST

Bonnie Ellen Blustein
University of Wisconsin, Madison

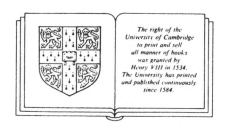

The right of the
University of Cambridge
to print and sell
all manner of books
was granted by
Henry VIII in 1534.
The University has printed
and published continuously
since 1584.

CAMBRIDGE UNIVERSITY PRESS

CAMBRIDGE

NEW YORK   PORT CHESTER   MELBOURNE   SYDNEY

PUBLISHED BY THE PRESS SYNDICATE OF THE UNIVERSITY OF CAMBRIDGE
The Pitt Building, Trumpington Street, Cambridge, United Kingdom

CAMBRIDGE UNIVERSITY PRESS
The Edinburgh Building, Cambridge CB2 2RU, UK
40 West 20th Street, New York NY 10011–4211, USA
477 Williamstown Road, Port Melbourne, VIC 3207, Australia
Ruiz de Alarcón 13, 28014 Madrid, Spain
Dock House, The Waterfront, Cape Town 8001, South Africa

http://www.cambridge.org

First published 1991
First paperback edition 2002

A catalogue record for this book is available from the British Library

Library of Congress Cataloguing in Publication data
Blustein, Bonnie Ellen.
Preserve your love for science: life of William A. Hammond, American
neurologist / Bonnie Ellen Blustein.
            p.   cm. – (Cambridge history of medicine)
ISBN 0 521 39262 4 (hardcover)
1. Hammond, William Alexander, 1828–1900.   2. Neurologists – United
States – Biography.   I. Title.   II. Series.
[DNLM: 1. Hammond, William Alexander, 1828–1900.   2. Neurology –
biography.   WZ 100 H227BA]
RC339.52.H35B58   1991
616.8′0092–dc20
[B]
DNLM/DLC
for Library of Congress   91-420   CIP

ISBN 0 521 39262 4 hardback
ISBN 0 521 52843 7 paperback

FOR HANNAH,
HER PARENTS
AND
HER GRANDPARENTS

Contents

List of illustrations   *page* viii
Acknowledgments   ix

1   Introduction   1
2   "I can make any post interesting"   18
3   "The first original Physiologist in the
     United States"   38
4   "The best friend the soldier has"   53
5   "Foggy with embarrassments"   76
6   "A New York medical man"   94
7   "A laborious and skilful observer"   115
8   "So great her science"   134
9   "Systems of cures and wonderful remedies"   151
10   "A positive mental science"   164
11   "All men are insane"   181
12   "I said that I would be back"   201
13   "Very near being a great man"   220

Notes   235
Note on sources   266
Bibliography of
     William Alexander Hammond, M.D.   269
Index   283

Illustrations

Drawing room of Hammond mansion.   *page* 14

Fort Riley, Kansas Territory, 1856.   29

Letter from Fort Riley, 1856.   30

"Urological Contributions" to the study of
    mind and brain.   42

Signed photograph of William A. Hammond,
    March 1859.   47

Surgeon General Hammond, 1863.   58

Apparatus for laboratory study of hygiene,
    ca. 1863.   64

Ground plan of the Hammond General
    Hospital, ca. 1863.   74

Patient with "glosso-labio-laryngeal paralysis,"
    ca. 1873.   117

Hand of patient with "athetosis," ca. 1869.   120

Patient with "spinal meningitis," ca. 1873.   122

Patient with "hystero-epilepsy," ca. 1880.   198

Advertisement for Hammond Sanitarium,
    1889.   202

Acknowledgments

The illustrations in this book are reproduced courtesy of the State Historical Society of Wisconsin, the American Philosophical Society, the College of Physicians of Philadelphia, and Dover Publications. I am especially grateful to Dorothy Whitcomb of the Middleton Library of the Health Sciences of the University of Wisconsin for her generous assistance in locating graphic materials and making them available to me. Parts of Chapters 9 and 10 were published earlier as "'A Hollow Square of Psychological Science': American Neurologists and Psychiatrists in Conflict," in *Madhouses, Mad-Doctors, and Madmen,* edited by Andrew T. Scull (Philadelphia: University of Pennsylvania Press, 1981), pp. 241–70; and as "The Brief Career of Cerebral Hyperaemia: William Hammond and His Insomniac Patients," *Journal of the History of Medicine and Allied Sciences* 41 (1986):24–51.

Many librarians and archivists helped me locate sources for this book from the Academy of Natural Sciences of Philadelphia, the American Neurological Association, the American Philosophical Society, the College of Physicians of Philadelphia, the National Archives, the New York Academy of Medicine, the New-York Historical Society, the Pennsylvania Hospital, and the libraries of the University of Pennsylvania and the University of Wisconsin. I am especially grateful to Ellen Gartrell, Caroline Morris, and Christine Ruggere for their personal support as well as for their professional assistance. Gert Brieger, Anne Millbrooke, Marc Rothenberg, Roy Selby, Jeffrey Sturchio, and Jack D. Key provided me with references, copies of manuscripts, and other material I might otherwise have overlooked. William Caref supplied computer facilities and expertise for the preparation of the final manuscript. I thank the American Philosophical Society for making possible a very important research trip in 1980, and the Department of History of Medicine of the University of Wisconsin, Madison, for the fellowship that supported the last stages of the work.

For less tangible but no less important help, in many different ways, at many different times, I am indebted to Mark B. Adams, Garland Allen, Rima Apple, P. Thomas Carroll, John T. Cumbler, Barbara C. Foley, Vanessa Northington Gamble, Diann Jacox, Barbara Kimmelman, Robert Joy, Judith W. Leavitt, Jonathan Liebenau, Marcia Livingston, Everett Mendelsohn, Russell C. Maulitz, Ronald L. Numbers, Kathryn Russell, Andrew Scull, Alan Spector, and especially to Charles E. Rosenberg.

1

Introduction

"You cannot afford to set yourselves above the world and to be utterly regardless of the demands of society," William A. Hammond told the medical students at Bellevue Hospital in 1867. "You must therefore sacrifice something on the altar of expediency if you wish to be successful in a material point of view. Only take care," he warned, "that you preserve your love for science, and that you pay no more tribute to the elegancies and the frivolities of life than will suffice to make society regard you as one of themselves, and show you the respect which you have right to claim."[1]

Hammond's own love for science developed early. He patterned his first original research, done in the 1850s, on French and German scientific traditions, notably Justus von Liebig's sweeping program for physiological chemistry. As surgeon general of the United States Army during the Civil War, Hammond did what he could to marshal his limited resources for the cause of scientific research. But, as historian Robert Kohler has noted, "particular scientific styles flourish only where intellectual priorities are congruent with institutional goals."[2] Physiology in the United States before the Civil War had virtually no institutional base. Among the physicians of Hammond's generation, only John Call Dalton (1825–89) could gratify his passion for scientific research in a university position that made medical practice unnecessary. But Dalton, America's "first professional physiologist," was a bachelor, and rather undemanding of the amenities of high society.[3] S. Weir Mitchell (1829–1914) struggled for years – with Hammond's support – to obtain a professional appointment that would afford him the leisure to pursue physiology. But the call never came, and Mitchell had to "work as hard as ever at practice," as he wrote to Jeffries Wyman in 1868, taking advantage as best he could of "the little time I can give to science."[4]

As a neurologist Hammond sacrificed a bit more on the altar of expediency than did Mitchell, whose roots were securely entrenched in Philadelphia medical society. Financial success counted for a great deal in Gilded Age New York society, and Hammond's high-toned and pricey specialty practice was indeed successful in a material point of view. And if laboratory physiology could not flourish within this institutional context, Hammond's widely read and original intellect easily imagined other scientific pursuits that could. His biography is, to a large extent, a story of one man's struggle to find a viable place for science in the medical context of nineteenth-century America, and to understand his society in terms of this scientific outlook.

THE EDUCATION OF AN AMERICAN MEDICAL SCIENTIST

On August 28, 1828, Sarah Pinckney and Dr. John Wesley Hammond of Annapolis, Maryland, produced baby William, their second son. The young family was not wealthy, although its lineage is well documented on both sides. William Alexander Hammond's great-grandfather had bought property in Anne Arundel County in 1764. His father had graduated in 1825 from the Medical College of the University of Maryland (at the age of twenty-one), but had not immediately settled down to establish a practice. Many Marylanders of the day were migrating northwest into the Susquehanna River valley and then west toward the Ohio. John Hammond, M.D., followed this route. He took his family in 1832 to Somerset County, Pennsylvania, south of Johnstown, then moved again two years later to the town of Williamsport (later Monongahela City), Washington County, in the southwestern corner of the state. After the gubernatorial election of 1836, William's father returned to Harrisburg as chief clerk of the state auditor general's office. He became one of the town's leading citizens, respected for his "urbanity, integrity, and intellectual ability." It is not clear to what extent he actually practiced medicine.[5] Half a century later, the coal country of Dauphin County provided the setting for a minor novel by William A. Hammond, *On the Susquehanna* (New York, 1887).

Like his father, William obtained much of his early education from private tutors. The most notable was a successful middle-aged Harrisburg physician, Edmund W. Roberts, who had studied at the prestigious medical school of the University of Pennsylvania.[6] William studied the classics with him, learning and liking them enough to retain interest and facility throughout his life. He also became interested in medicine. Still too young for medical school, however, he was sent back to Annapolis to pursue general studies at St. John's College. He thus arrived in New York City in 1844 with an intellectual background far surpassing that of the average medical student of his day.[7]

The tall, gangly sixteen-year-old, who stammered badly over his b's, p's, and t's, entered the New York medical office of William Holme Van Buren, his new preceptor.[8] Only nine years older than Hammond, Van Buren had himself just settled in the city after five years in Florida and on the Canadian frontier as an assistant surgeon in the United States Army. The slow pace of his small practice must have left his awkward young student with ample time to read and to attend lectures at the medical colleges. Van Buren only recorded about $50 per month in income between November 1844 and December 1846, and most of his early patients were apparently inmates of either an unnamed convent or a similarly anonymous "academy." An office practice probably supplemented this, but it is unlikely that he ever collected the full amounts recorded in his account book.

But Hammond was studying under one of the rising lights of New York medicine. Van Buren, who married the daughter of the eminent surgeon Valentine Mott, became Mott's protégé and assistant as well. By the spring of 1847, as Hammond was completing his first formal course of lectures at University Medical College, Van Buren was beginning to record receipts from students' fees as well as greatly increased receipts from his family practice. His total income – at least on paper – then approached $3,000 a year.[9] Van Buren was to exert a continuing influence over Hammond's professional career. It was widely reported that he was responsible for Hammond's appointment, fifteen years later, to the position of surgeon general of the United States Army.

University Medical College had been founded only five years before Hammond enrolled. Its *Annual Announcement* of 1846 pointed out that New York City was becoming a medical center for the entire nation. The faculty's goal was "the building up [of] a national school worthy of the country and the age." To this end, it had recently incurred the "heavy expense" of "a Chemical and Philosophical Apparatus of the best description." But pressures for reform in medical education were mounting from the new American Medical Association. The professors were thus somewhat sensitive about the shortcomings of their typical two-year ungraded curriculum. While clinical work was encouraged, for example, it was not required. The introduction to the *Annual Announcement* of 1848, in which Hammond's name was listed among the recent graduates, consisted mainly of a defense of the existing state of affairs. The school stressed the proximity of hospitals and dispensaries where "every facility is enjoyed for studying [diseases] collectively or as specialities."[10]

To Hammond, the most important of his teachers at University Medical College were probably Martyn Paine, the idiosyncratic professor of the "institutes of medicine and materia medica," and John William Draper, the professor of chemistry. Paine's influential textbook *Institutes of Medicine* first appeared in 1847. "Should you . . . be inclined to follow those inquirers who have been guided by the light of truth," he told Hammond and his classmates in his introductory lecture to the session of 1847–48, "you will find . . . that physiology, in its connection with organization [i.e., anatomy], lies at the foundation of pathology and therapeutics."[11] Hammond was definitely so inclined. Paine touched on the ways in which the "effects of life" could be modified "by the mind itself," a notion Hammond would explore in his medical thesis (now lost) on "The Etiological and Therapeutical Influence of the Imagination." Paine also impressed on his students his fervent belief in the "vitalist" school of experimental physiology, which he counterposed to the physical and chemical orientations then more in vogue.[12]

The years 1847–48 were perhaps the high point of "organic physics," the reductionist physiology of the "1847 group" that centered around Carl Ludwig, Hermann von Helmholtz, Ernst von Brucke, and Emil Du Bois-Reymond.[13] At the same time, Justus von Liebig's books *Organic Chemistry in Its Applications to Physiology and Pathology* (1842) and *Familiar Letters on Chemistry* (1844) were popularizing a chemical approach to medical science.

University Medical College had as professor of chemistry the eminent scientist John William Draper. He tried earnestly to convey the excitement of the age to his students. "There is hardly a book of science that comes across the Ocean which does not bring with it new facts, the coordination of which with those that are known, remains to be made," Draper lectured. "The formative process is beginning; a few years will give us a science, which will bring more revolutions in medicine, than that changeable science has even yet witnessed." He promised to instruct them on all available applications "of physical science to medicine, – it matters not whether it be Hydraulics, Pneumatics, Astronomy, or any thing else." Draper made a special point of demonstrating experiments in such a way as to make them repeatable by the students themselves in the expensive new laboratory.[14] Hammond took full advantage of the opportunity, absorbing enough of the spirit and technique to be able to carry out original experiments on digestion a few years later, under far more primitive laboratory conditions.

Professor Paine, in contrast, was vehemently "against chemistry when hunting for laurels in the field of physiology, of pathology, and of therapeutics." He denounced "this interference of the laboratory which has shaken so extensively the foundations of medicine, and which so cruelly debases the science."[15] Chemistry in medicine tended, he said, "to the subversion of physiological science, and therefore of pathological and therapeutical principles and, as another necessary consequence, of rational practice."[16] Paine, influenced by the Naturphilosophie movement and a member of several German medical societies, struggled doggedly against chemical and physical reductionism. He considered these doctrines self-contradictory, heretical, materialistic, and (ironically) "old-fashioned."[17]

Like many followers of romantic biology, Paine attached great significance to the nervous system. Its ailments, he said, showed that disease was caused by altered "vital properties," not "altered functions," as he understood the doctrines of Xavier Bichat.[18] He also singled out the physiology of digestion as the arena where "the physiologist must raise his principal defense against the invasions of chemistry." There can be little doubt that Hammond chose his research problems in response to (and perhaps in reaction against) Paine's lectures on physiology.[19]

William A. Hammond, M.D., emerged from University Medical School in March 1848, in spite of a formal requirement that graduates be at least twenty-one years old. He immediately enrolled as a resident medical student at the Pennsylvania Hospital in Philadelphia. Here he performed a wide variety of tasks, honing his skills on the charity patients in the free beds. Such valuable clinical experience was an exceptional opportunity for a young physician. There was also the chance to mingle with Philadelphia's medical elite, many of whom were in close contact with outstanding European practitioners and researchers. Among the attending physicians and surgeons at the Pennsylvania Hospital were William Pepper, a student and friend of Pierre Louis; George W. Norris, whose Parisian teachers had included Guillaume Dupuytren, A.-A.-L.-M. Velpeau, and François Magendie; and W. W. Gerhard, the most distinguished of the American students of Louis and perhaps the most careful medical researcher of the United States in his time.[20] Hammond also had access to the best medical library in the country, although there is little indication that he used it often. Although Hammond did not refer explicitly in later years to his hospital experience, it clearly marked him as one of the most promising young physicians of his generation.[21]

MEDICAL SCIENCE AND THE U.S. ARMY

His formal medical training completed, Hammond spent the next few months in Saco, Maine, about twenty miles southwest of Portland. He may have been vacationing there, or avoiding the cholera, or he may have attempted to set up a medical practice, as older biographical accounts suggest. Meanwhile, the twenty-one-year-old doctor began the application process for a post as assistant surgeon in the United States Army. This was the course his preceptor Van Buren had followed, and suggests an early distaste for the prospects of traditional family medical practice.

In a letter to President Zachary Taylor dated March 8, 1849, William Johnston of Harrisburg, a friend and political contact of the Hammond family, requested the appointment. "Dr. Hammond is a graduate of the University of New York and has been employed in the Almshouses and Hospitals of New York and Philadelphia. He is an excellent and worthy man," Johnston wrote in conventional phrases, "free from all bad habits, and eminently deserving of the situation he solicits." Hammond received his commission on July 3 and married Helen Nisbet, daughter of a Philadelphia attorney, the following day. On July 8 the young couple left from Carlisle Barracks, near Harrisburg, heading southwest to remote New Mexico Territory.[22]

Hammond remained in the Army as an assistant surgeon for eleven years, spending most of this time at frontier posts in New Mexico and Kansas Territories. His position enabled him to participate in two of the major projects of contemporary American science, the natural history surveys of the Smithsonian Institution and of the Academy of Natural Sciences of Philadelphia. At the same time he began experimental research into problems of physiological chemistry. These were of less immediate interest to most of his countrymen but were consistent with the work being carried out in the German and French laboratories already so admired by the American medical elite.

Toward the end of his stint in the army, Hammond spent some time on sick leave in Philadelphia. There he associated with other scientifically inclined young physicians, including Joseph Leidy, Henry Hartshorne, and S. Weir Mitchell. Together they attempted to establish a "biological" society in which such medical science could be institutionalized and coordinated. These short-lived efforts are important to an understanding both of Hammond's conception of scientific medicine and of the social constraints under which the aspiring scientist worked. Hammond's military experiences and scientific experiments in the antebellum years are discussed in Chapters 2 and 3.

The chief constraint was Hammond's need to support his family, which by the fall of 1860 included two toddlers. He resigned then from the army to accept a position as professor of anatomy and physiology at the University of Maryland Medical School. Typical of the times, the medical school did not provide full-time support for its faculty, so Hammond started a practice in Baltimore. This arrangement lasted barely six months. When the Civil War began Hammond reenlisted as an assistant surgeon, returning to the bottom of the seniority list. His experience was recognized, however, in his assignment: the organization of desperately needed military hospitals in Baltimore, Hagerstown, and Frederick, Maryland, and at Chambersburg, Pennsylvania. He was promoted in March 1862 to the position of inspector of hospitals, but had barely undertaken these new responsibilities when, a month later, President Lincoln appointed him surgeon general of the Medical Department. It was an unprecedented honor for a man of his age (thirty-three) and previous rank (assistant surgeon). It was also an unprecedented task. Hammond's accomplishments in a year and a half as surgeon general were, by themselves, sufficient to ensure him a place in the history of American medicine. His innovations prefigured and served as a model for developments that, while rooted in prewar American medicine, would accelerate rapidly in the decades following the Civil War. These are examined in Chapters 4 and 5.

Hammond's departure from Washington officialdom was still more dramatic than his arrival. Secretary of War Edwin Stanton had opposed Hammond and his backers on the United States Sanitary Commission almost from the start. In August 1863 he sent the Surgeon General on a western tour of inspection, delaying his return until long after this task was accomplished. With Hammond safely away from his desk, Stanton initiated a special investigation of the Medical Department. Hammond naively demanded a formal court-martial to clear his name of the suspicion he felt had been cast upon it. And a court-martial he received, on charges based mainly on the violation of protocol in the purchase of a lot of blankets and in the assignment of several medical officers. But he was shocked to be found guilty of conduct unbecoming an officer and a gentleman, summarily dismissed from his post, and enjoined from again holding office under the United States government.

THE MAKING OF A NEUROLOGIST

Hammond's standing among prominent American and foreign physicians was not substantially injured by this verdict, which was eventually overturned by Congress after a special investigation in 1878–79. But his immediate attempts to vindicate himself exhausted his modest financial resources.

"When I was dismissed from the service," Hammond told a *New York Tribune* reporter in 1879, "I resolved to go to the biggest place in the world and live it down. . . . I had nothing and was obliged to borrow money from whosoever would loan it to me in order to support myself. There were times when I really did not know how I was to get my next meal."[23] "Nothing" meant less than $500 in assets, some household goods, and his precious books. Fortunately, Hammond – like the hero of his 1867 novel *Robert Severne* – had loyal and affluent friends. Dr. J. H. Douglas, with whom Hammond had become intimate through the Sanitary Commission, helped him find the house at 162 West 34th Street in New York from which he would launch his practice. Douglas and the publisher J. B. Lippincott each loaned the destitute physician $2,000 for the down payment, and Douglas provided another $3,500 over the next few months toward expenses. Edward Olmsted, Hammond's brother-in-law, took up a subscription among friends and raised $2,000 more as a Christmas gift "to aid him in his pecuniary embarrassment."[24]

Douglas also arranged for Hammond to earn at least small amounts by writing popular articles on scientific and medical topics for the new weekly magazine *Nation*. These essays appeared anonymously and reflected the author's interest in what he called "social science." "The Humors of the Anthropologists" defended Hammond's white countrymen from European charges of race degeneration. "Poisoning as a Science" promoted the science of toxicology. His "Few Words About Cholera" added little novelty to the spate of articles on the impending epidemic, while "Slaughterhouses and Health" decried the sickening miasmas of those enterprises.[25] Even with this supplementary income, added to a total of about $1,200 from his practice, the impatient and ambitious Hammond "began to think [he] should never get along."

In the fall of 1865, however, he received a commission to accompany Eugene Langdon, an ailing and undistinguished grandson of John Jacob Astor, on a six-month voyage to Europe, leaving his own family behind. The work was not onerous. Hammond was able to catch up on the latest developments in medicine and in hospital organization in London, Paris, Rome, and Florence, while enjoying neighboring resorts as well. For this he received the very generous sum of $10,000 in gold, in addition to $7,000 for his own travel expenses. When he returned to New York in June 1866 he had $9,000 remaining with which to pay off his debts and make a new start in private practice. It was probably at this time that he decided to limit his practice exclusively to "neurology." Although his receipts for the remainder of 1866 amounted, he later declared, to about $40, business soon improved. His annual income rose from $2,225 in 1867 to $9,600 in 1868, and soared to over $60,000 ten years later.[26] This was nothing short of phenomenal: a survey of physicians' income around 1900 found that the wealthiest fifty then averaged $45,000 annually.[27]

New York City was already the medical center of the country in the late 1860s, as the congested and unhealthy metropolis was also a financial, commercial, and cultural center. Physicians were numerous and unfettered by government control. There was one doctor (of some sort) for every five hundred inhabitants, and these physicians vied with pharmacists, lay advisers, and the continuing reliance of many on self-help. Competition among doctors was intense, and a large gap separated the most and the least successful. A small but powerful elite, centered on the Medical and Surgical Society, dominated the medical schools, the hospital and dispensary positions for attending staff, and most of the city's medical organizations. While many in this group interested themselves in the latest advances in medical science, even contributing to it themselves, there were many more physicians who knew little and probably cared less.

The family practice was still central to the work of nearly all physicians, organized around the home visit and the formal consultation. Office practice, conducted on a cash basis, was financially useful but professionally somewhat suspect. The flexible etiological and pathological theories that were still overwhelmingly employed underlined the importance of a physician's knowledge of the family and history of the patient, and fit well with the largely traditional methods of diagnosis and therapeutics. But instabilities already existed which would provide the basis for the sweeping changes in medicine that characterized the period of Hammond's New York practice.

Hammond's career in neurology, the subject of Chapters 6 through 11, balanced precariously on the crest of this new wave. He never belonged to the Medical and Surgical Society, nor even to the far more inclusive New York Academy of Medicine. However, he maintained close ties with such members of the "inner circle" as his preceptor Van Buren and his colleagues on the faculties of New York's three leading medical colleges. When he first arrived in New York, the impecunious scientist joined only the Medical Journal Association, probably to gain access to its large collection of contemporary medical literature. A few years later he joined and became active in the County Medical Society, which many other intellectual leaders of the profession did not.

Hammond also maintained contact with the rank and file of the profession through such groups as the O.AE. Society of Bellevue Medical College and his own Alumni Association of the Medical Department of the City of New York. He directed a much larger share of his seemingly inexhaustible energy, however, toward new specialty societies. He joined the Medico-Legal Society soon after its incorporation in 1869, and initiated the New York Neurological Society in the early 1870s. Hammond also played a central role in the foundation of the American Neurological Association. This organizational work earned him more lasting recognition than any other aspect of his career with the major exception of his surgeon generalcy.[28]

By far the most distinctive feature of Hammond's new practice was his decision to treat only patients suffering from diseases of the nervous system. By 1865 it was already fairly common for well-educated doctors to take a special interest in a particular class of diseases. In Europe, a few physicians had already become exclusive specialists. But in the United States, virtually every respectable physician maintained a general family practice, together with consulting work. It was rare to limit one's practice to a particular specialty or to emphasize office work. And neurology had not yet achieved even the recognition of separate attention in medical school lectures or separate hospital wards. By the turn of the century, the picture had changed considerably. Through Hammond's career it is possible to trace in detail the emergence of neurology as a specialty, and to gain a deeper understanding of the process of specialization in American medicine.[29]

Neurology, as it was defined by the work of New York physicians such as William A. Hammond, George Beard, and Edward C. Spitzka, represented the convergence of a complicated set of theoretical and practical considerations. For a time, the result fit rather neatly into the dominant trends of New York medicine. It was both scientific and profitable, "high-toned" in its reliance on the latest in medical knowledge and technology while offering welcome advice to the general practitioner. In later years, however, there were increasing tensions between Hammond's sort of neurology and the laboratory-oriented scientific medicine that was coming to define the self-consciousness and public image of the profession. Younger neurologists, especially, became less willing or less able to overlook the many weaknesses and inconsistencies of Hammond's work, which he had extended to include psychology, psychiatry, and even morality. Hammond gave up his New York neurological practice in 1888, none too soon in the eyes of many, and moved to Washington, D.C., with his second wife, Esther D. Chapin of Providence, Rhode Island.

Hammond had an elegant private sanatorium built to his specifications on Columbia Heights, overlooking the city that he had left in disgrace a quarter of a century earlier. He again plunged into his work with an enthusiasm undiminished by his sixty years. Here he made his last foray into scientific research: investigations of the effects of so-called animal extracts. He engaged, meanwhile, in the profitable business of their manufacture and sale. Hammond doubtless saw nothing wrong in this combination of activities. But to many of his contemporaries the implausibility of his scientific results, superadded to the outright commercialism of the sanatorium, provided a particularly graphic illustration of what medicine ought not to be. Chapters 12 and 13 explore this last phase of Hammond's long and varied career.

MEDICAL PRACTICE AND PUBLIC LIFE

In his prime, William A. Hammond, M.D., was an imposing figure. He was "of leonine appearance, tall and stout," and "confident and assertive in manner," recorded the New York diarist James H. Morse, who thought Hammond "the picture of good-natured self-confidence."[30] He stood six feet, two inches tall, carrying over two hundred pounds of weight with a military bearing. His receding hairline emphasized a high forehead, and the full beard and sideburns he sported could not conceal a strong-featured face. His opinions were tenaciously held and often idiosyncratic, issued forth in a booming voice. To subordinates and antagonists he sometimes appeared to be intolerably arrogant.

As a New Yorker, Hammond took an active part in civic affairs. He served on the "Citizens' Committee Upon the Nuisances of New York City" formed in the summer of 1877 to force action against the "stench-factories" responsible for "the sickening smells pervading the city."[31] He was a leading candidate for the post of health officer of the port of New York in 1870 and again in 1878. Despite his outstanding credentials, however, Senate confirmation would have been impossible for a proscribed ex–surgeon general.[32] This episode may have prompted the move to have his case reopened and the decision reversed.

A broad range of scientific organizations also drew his attention. He joined or spoke before the American Social Science Association, the American Anthropological Association, the American Geographical Society, and the American Academy of Arts and Letters. He helped to found a short-lived "National Institute for Letters, Arts and Sciences," based in New York, in 1868. The literary public knew him as the author of half a dozen novels, and, in his last year, a rather contrived and melodramatic play. All this activity served to publicize his name (generally but not always in a favorable context), extend his contacts, and promote his medical career. But there is no reason to doubt his sincere enthusiasm for these diverse pursuits.

Hammond was known among affluent New Yorkers as one who particularly enjoyed society and its amenities. His gala receptions, often held in honor of the participants in some scientific gathering, were frequently noted in the medical press and in the columns of the daily newspapers. He was especially fond of the pleasures of the table. We are told that "mottoes illustrative of gastronomic matters" in various languages were worked in amid other decorations along the ceiling and walls of his dining room.[33] He showed little patience with proposals for restrictive sumptuary laws or the "mischievous ice-pitcher," which he found to be ruinous of stomach and palate. On finding himself once in the "dry" state of Rhode Island, he wrote himself a prescription for *vini campaniae* to be taken *p.r.n.* In the midst of the depression of the 1880s he was openly scornful of those ignorant of haute cuisine. His own dinner parties were elaborate, correct, and enlivened by his wide-ranging and fluent conversation. They earned for him a reputation as an excellent host.[34]

Hammond's tastes were sufficiently idiosyncratic to draw attention even amid the excesses of the Gilded Age. His family moved in 1873 into a large house at 43 West 54th Street, which also served as his private office. The hallway contained a statue of the Buddha, which (he said) he had repainted whenever he needed extra good fortune. The study in which he received patients was lined with

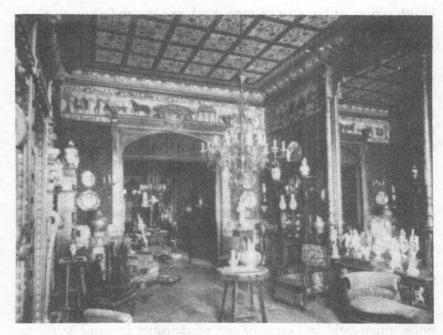

Drawing room of Hammond mansion. The drawing room of the Hammond family's New York mansion at 43 West 54th Street, reflecting the doctor's tastes, was considered one of the first and best of the new "artistic interiors" of the city. The Celtic designs on the ceiling were in turquoise and navy blue, and the frieze replicated portions of the Bayeux tapestry. The woodwork and most of the furniture were in satinwood and ebony, and the walls were covered in raw silk. Natural light filtered through two stained-glass windows depicting Saxon princesses. Hammond personally selected the many wall plaques from Limoges, Persia, North Africa, and the Far East, as well as the cloisonné chess sets, the Dresden china, the satsuma cup from the Mikado's collection, and the half-size copy of the Venus de Medici. He made one small brass table himself, covering it with velvet plush and reportedly telling a visitor that were he not a physician he should have liked to have been an upholsterer. ([George William Sheldon], *Artistic Houses,* vol. 1 [New York: Appleton, 1883–84], pp. 91–92. Plate reproduced from Arnold Lewis, James Turner, and Steven McQuillen, *The Opulent Interiors of the Gilded Age* [New York: Dover Publications, 1987], p. 126. Courtesy of Steenbock Library, University of Wisconsin, Madison.)

shelves containing a library of some 5,000 volumes, both contemporary medical works and older, rare books. It was adorned with exotic paintings and statuary "from Persia, Italy, Egypt and elsewhere," and with a "gorgeous polycolored chandelier." A musical clock struck the hours and half hours. In this sanctum sat the doctor in a "vast arm-chair" topped with "an image of an Egyptian female." Beside it stood a small table in the drawer of which he kept a pair of pistols with which to confront possibly dangerous insane clients. To many observers, however, the most conspicuous feature of the room was the pile of ten- and twenty-dollar bills on his desk. They testified to his large and lucrative consulting practice and to his taste for display as well.[35] When Hammond moved to Washington, D.C., in 1888 the house was sold to Mr. Chauncey DePew for the princely sum of $130,000.[36]

About Hammond's later family life little has been recorded. His mother died early in 1861. His father, after 1853 a resident of Philadelphia, survived until 1878. An older brother, the Reverend Jonathan Pinckney Hammond, was a respectable if undistinguished Episcopal minister who served as chaplain to the military hospital at Chester, Pennsylvania, during the Civil War. Of three other siblings, only the youngest, Nathaniel Hobart Hammond, reached maturity. He, too, served the Union Army, in the capacity of a hospital steward.

William A. Hammond married twice, and both his first and his second wife seem to have been overshadowed by the neurologist himself. William and Helen Hammond lost their first two infants, Helen and (probably) William, Jr., and little is known of them. Another son, Somerville P. Hammond, attended Bellevue Hospital Medical College between 1869 and 1871, but apparently died before 1883. But the son and daughter who lived to adulthood were both eminent in their own rights.

Graeme Monroe Hammond (1858–1944) pursued his father's interests in neurology and medico-legal affairs, after a preliminary education that included three years of scientific work at the Columbia School of Mines. He was for three decades the treasurer of the New York Neurological Society and for nearly twenty years an officer of the American Neurological Association, and he eventually added a doctorate of law to his medical degree. He also distinguished himself in athletics as an Olympic fencer – an exercise highly recommended by his father – and as sometime president of both the New York Athletic Association and the American Olympic Association. He was temperamentally quite different from his father, remembered for his "practical, sound, common sense point of view" and "never known to be aggressively sarcastic or vituperative."[37]

Graeme's "willful and romantic" sister Clara Hammond Lanza (1859–1939) was less conventional. She was also well-educated, and became a noted writer of realistic fiction and belles lettres and a correspondent of George Moore. She was married at the age of eighteen, in a fashionable Fifth Avenue wedding, to a genuine though impoverished Sicilian marquis, who had worked for a time as headwaiter at Delmonico's. The young marchioness remained unusually close to her father.[38] The two coauthored a volume of stories, *Tales of Eccentric Life* (1886), and frequently entertained guests together. She translated scientific papers for his journals, and her own fiction contains reflections on science and religion that suggest that she enjoyed philosophical discussions with her father as well. Clara's husband took an active part in Hammond's "animal extract" business. It is tempting to speculate that the neurologist's ties with his daughter mirrored the close father–daughter relationships often depicted in his fictional works.

* * * * *

William Alexander Hammond, M.D., was in many respects a rather unusual character. "Scheme after scheme, all laudable and promising (as he pictured them), would arise in his mind, for he was optimistic almost to the verge of the visionary," reflected a colleague, "but some defect that a more prudent man would have guarded against too often barred their fruition. His enthusiasm in these schemes was so manifestly the dominator of his thoughts that it was useless for his friends to argue against it."[39] But his eccentricities, however engaging, should not be allowed to obscure the central fact that his career represented – or perhaps caricatured – some of the major trends in mid-nineteenth-century medicine.

By the end of the century, science had come to play a vastly increased role in medical practice in the United States. American physicians had begun to play an increasingly important role in the advancement of medical science as well. But what counted as medical science, and how could it best be advanced? Who were the scientists, and how were they to be supported? Questions such as these engendered struggle, and sometimes open conflict, of which Hammond was not infrequently near the center: the furor over the calomel order, for example; smoldering resentments over "specialism"; more academic questions of the relation of physiology to clinical medicine. At the time these episodes were seen mainly in terms of factional squabbles. But they are more usefully viewed as conflicts motivating a series of profound and interconnected changes in the theory and practice of medicine. Tensions arising from these conflicts also marked the careers of individual physicians such as William Alexander Hammond. His biography is thus the story, not just of one man's life and work, but of the medical world that first supported his ascent to the height of his profession, and later consigned him to an undeserved obscurity.

2

"I can make any post interesting"

As he finished his stint at the Pennsylvania Hospital Dr. William A. Hammond, still not quite twenty-one years old, had to make a difficult decision about his future. The private practice of family medicine apparently never appealed to him. With his outstanding credentials, a European medical tour would have been the obvious way to pass the next year or so, but most likely the Hammond family could not afford this luxury. Another possibility presented itself: Hammond could follow the course of his preceptor Van Buren and try for one of the few positions available as assistant surgeon in the United States Army.

Military surgery in Europe was highly visible as a critical force in medical innovation. In the early nineteenth century, army veterans like Pierre Desault had helped to transform the Paris hospitals into leading research centers. Many outstanding French surgeons, internists, and researchers had army experiences under their belts. West of the Atlantic, William Beaumont had earned his reputation as the outstanding American physiologist of his time while an army medical officer.

Hammond was probably considering this option when he went to the Pennsylvania Hospital's famous medical library in May 1848 for books on military surgery by Dominique-Jean Larrey (in English translation) and John Hennen.[1] Perhaps he found these volumes encouraging. In fact, the U.S. Army Medical Department had significantly higher standards than the graduation requirements of even the best American medical schools. When a Medical Examining Board convened in New York in May 1849 to fill ten newly created positions for assistant surgeons, seventy-five candidates were invited to appear before it. The fifty-two who appeared were examined on their knowledge of Latin and physics or natural philosophy, as well as practical anatomy and clinical methods. Only Hammond and eight others were commissioned, a genuine testimonial to their abilities.[2]

FRONTIER MEDICINE IN NEW MEXICO, 1849–1852

Assistant Surgeon Hammond received immediate orders to report to the army base at Santa Fe, in New Mexico Territory. Colonel Stephen W. Kearny had taken the fort three years earlier in his Mexican-American War campaign. Then gold was discovered in California, increasing the demand for a transcontinental railroad. The areas severed from Mexico were still under U.S. military jurisdiction in 1849, but the new president, war hero Zachary Taylor, was encouraging statehood for both California and New Mexico. Thus Hammond's remote frontier post was at the center of the national controversy over the extension of slavery.

Meanwhile, Congress faced the related issue of choosing a railway route to the Pacific. A surveying expedition was dispatched to find out whether the only feasible southern route had been included in the territory acquired as a result of the war. It was not, and the result would be the Gadsden Purchase of 1853. Meanwhile, the Navaho people objected to these encroachments on their ancestral lands, as did the Apaches under the leadership of Mangus Colorado. U.S. Army forces were sent along with the surveyors to overcome the Native American resistance, and Hammond was sent along to doctor the soldiers.[3]

The journey to Santa Fe took over three months. The Hammonds probably traveled through Fort Leavenworth, Kansas, completing their trek over the southwestern plains and desert in late October. Dr. Hammond then accompanied a company of the Second Dragoons to a new post in Cebolleta, northeast of Zuñi, strategically situated at the intersection of two major Navaho trails. The base, second largest among the New Mexico garrisons with a population ranging between 110 and 160 men, became a center of troop movements. As an assistant surgeon, the young doctor (now legally of age) ranked second among the seven officers.[4]

Hammond's periodic reports to the Surgeon General say little about conditions at the post, but Inspector G. A. McCall found morale and efficiency low when he visited a year later. Commanding officers were young and inexperienced and frequently changed assignments. As a result, discipline was lax. Drill was neglected as soldiers occupied themselves in repairing their quarters, and livestock and weapons received little care. Penalties for infractions were harsh. A "favorite punishment of the commanding officer," Hammond remembered years later, required the offender to carry stones from one pile to another fifty feet away, then back again. The men dreaded this Sisyphean labor more than "bread and water for a week, deprivation of liberty, stoppage of pay, even 'bucking and gagging.' "[5]

But McCall was favorably impressed with Hammond's work. "The assistant surgeon appears to be very faithful in the discharge of his duties," he wrote. "His hospital is kept in very good order, and is well supplied . . . from New Orleans. The medicines, etc., have been very carefully and securely put up."[6]

Hammond's responsibilities included scientific work of a sort: the compilation of meteorological and medical statistics, to be sent to Surgeon General Lawson as regularly as the infrequent mails permitted. But practice at the base, and at smaller posts such as Abiquiu, demanded most of his professional attention. Occasionally he treated Mexican patients from the nearby village as well. Cebolleta was not a very healthy place. Usually at least half a dozen soldiers were on sick call. Between September 1850 and September 1851, only one man was reported "killed" but there were nine "ordinary" deaths. "Chronic diarrhea" was the leading cause, and Hammond also reported losing patients to "bronchitis" and "inflammation of the brain." He later reported that New Mexico had "had an unenviable reputation as a hotbed of syphilis."[7] Food supply posed a serious problem. Only mutton was to be had in abundance. Beef and vegetables were expensive, and the latter were in short supply. Corn was "always difficult, almost impossible, to obtain . . . from these Indians." When available, it was used mainly as fodder. The quartermaster had not enough mule teams and wagons available to haul beans, flour, and other staples.[8]

Dietary conditions in New Mexico furnished the basis for Hammond's first published paper, "On the Use of Potash in the Treatment of Scurvy," written in 1852 and appearing in print the following year. "During eight months of the year," he wrote, the disease "is exceedingly prevalent among the troops stationed in this territory, and from the scant vegetation of the country, it is impossible to obtain those vegetables generally esteemed most beneficial in the treatment." He observed that most of his scorbutic patients, including the worst cases, came from outside Cebolleta. Guessing that the comparatively low incidence at his own post was due to the potash he found in the water supply, he administered potash compounds to several patients and was gratified to see rapid cures.[9]

The inspiration for this clinical trial had come from a report of the work of the London physician Alfred Garrod, which Hammond had read in the *American Journal of the Medical Sciences.* Garrod had found scurvy still prevalent in the British navy in the 1840s. He viewed this not only as a practical problem to be overcome, but also as a promising field for the use of chemical methods in medical research. "As there is but little doubt that the disease arises from some alteration in the animal fluids and solids from error of diet," Garrod wrote, "I have always considered that it was in the power of chemistry to unravel the mystery."[10] Hammond probably did not read this passage, for it was omitted from the American excerpt of Garrod's article. But he too wrote of the importance to medicine of what has come to be called basic research. "The researches of animal chemistry have," he declared, "thrown some light upon the pathology of scurvy." If his anecdotal reports were confirmed by further research, "it will not be the least boon which that science has conferred upon the practice of medicine."[11]

Garrod's researches had been frustrated by a lack of patients on whom to test his theory. Hammond's isolated station was well suited to fill this gap. The shortage of vegetable food contributed to scurvy among the troops and also made it impossible to treat cases with the traditional dietary regimen. The assistant surgeon could experiment with potash as a remedy without subjecting his captive patients to undue deprivation. And while the research problem had been posed overseas, Hammond suggested that an American scurvy remedy was particularly appropriate. "In our own country especially will it prove a most valuable acquisition. Scurvy has been the scourge of the . . . overland emigrants to Oregon and California," he wrote, affecting more travelers than all other diseases combined. "Numbers have, in consequence, left their bones upon the plains."[12] Hammond's self-conscious rhetoric of 1853 belies the notion that basic medical research contradicted the imperatives of national development. For him, they were manifestly complementary.

Hammond would return to the problem of scurvy a decade later, during the Civil War, having retreated somewhat from this rather dogmatic faith in chemical explanations. While still identifying potash as a valid therapeutic agent, he no longer agreed with Garrod that potash deficiency caused scurvy. For one thing, "iron also effects a cure and with as much rapidity as potash." Rather, he said, the immediate cause of scurvy was "a morbid alteration in the constitution of the blood." Its exciting cause, he explained in the phrases of traditional etiology, was a concatenation of physical, moral, and dietetic conditions: darkness and cold, moisture, impure air, insufficient or excessive physical exercise; nostalgia, despondency, depression; salt meat and the lack of vegetable food.[13]

In New Mexico Hammond acquired a lively interest in anthropology. Not all Native Americans were hostile, and the curious young surgeon found time and opportunity to observe some of the customs of the Pueblo people. He was naive enough to be shocked at his discoveries, and conventional enough to refrain from publishing them until some fifteen years later. The "mujerados," as he finally described them to the American Neurological Association in 1882, were persons who were socially females and physically males with atrophied primary and secondary sex characteristics. He believed that they were forced deliberately into such a role for "the saturnalia" of the group and possibly for the private enjoyment of tribal leaders. Hammond's comments, made in the context of a discussion of sexual impotence, reveal far more about his own culture than that of the Pueblos. Even in the 1880s, when "sexual pathology" had become a more respectable topic among physicians, he made a point of defending the discussion of practices he found so abhorrent by ostentatiously invoking the values of disinterested scientific inquiry.[14]

The War Department spread its few forces thinly over New Mexico. Early in October 1851 Hammond left Cebolleta with Bvt. 2d Lt. Thomas Broker and the fifty-eight other young men of Company "H," Second Dragoons, to establish a new post at nearby Laguna. The place was described by a Dr. Kennerly two years later as "a dilapidated village, filthy, as all pueblos are, but differing from any other that we had seen, in containing many houses two stories high." The old adobe church contained a graveyard from which this scientifically minded physician admitted stealing a skull.[15]

After only a few months Hammond moved on to the Santa Rita copper mines, where the military escort for the United States–Mexico Boundary Commission had recently been based at Fort Webster. Apache resistance had prevented the profitable operation of the mines for some time. In the month of February 1852, two of Hammond's charges were killed in action and another died of wounds. That same month, Hammond wrote to Surgeon General Lawson requesting assignment to a less remote (and perhaps less dangerous) post. "By the time this request, if granted can take effect," he pleaded, "I will have been in New Mexico three years and . . . at five different posts and have perhaps been subjected to more changes than any other officer" in the Medical Department. Similar applications were made on his behalf by Pennsylvania congressmen. But Hammond was already on his way home when Lawson's reply reached New Mexico in June. He left "that benighted region," as he later described it, "in the mail coach without an escort through 1,500 Indians," with Major Grier, the future father-in-law of Hammond's friend John L. LeConte. "Though we did not lose one hair we might have met with this misfortune had it so pleased the redskins." He had suffered a crippling attack of what he believed to be a cardiac disorder, and spent the next six months with his family in Harrisburg, recuperating and writing his paper on scurvy.[16]

MEDICAL LEAVE AND MEDICAL STUDY, 1852–1854

It is possible that Hammond was well enough by the summer to visit Philadelphia, or even New York. If so, he would have had the opportunity to meet the French physiologist Charles Edouard Brown-Séquard, who in 1852 delivered the summer lecture series of the Philadelphia Association for Medical Instruction (known as the Summer Association). In October, Brown-Séquard wrote to a friend that "in New York and in Philadelphia, I have met with much more Medical Men strongly interested in that Science [physiology] than in Paris."[17] His acquaintances surely included many of Hammond's friends and teachers, and very likely Hammond himself.

In February 1853 Hammond reported himself fit for active duty and was ordered to Florida. A recurrence of his symptoms delayed his departure, but he was eager to be off. "I anticipate much benefit from the climate and situation of the section of the country," he wrote from Ocala, Florida, where he awaited transportation to Tampa. But when he finally reached Fort Meade at the end of March it did not measure up to his happy expectations. The isolated post had only about 130 inhabitants, and no other physician in the vicinity. The climate was not even healthful.

Within months Hammond's illness had returned so severely that he was frequently unable to work a full day. But the proud and ambitious young man was reluctant to apply again for sick leave so soon. "I did not wish to run the risk of having a character for inefficiency given me," he later wrote to the Surgeon General. "Moreover, I was seized with my present disease whilst on duty at an unpleasant post in New Mexico," he explained candidly, and did not wish to "lead persons unacquainted either with myself or the circumstances of the case to a misconception of the matter."[18]

By mid-June Hammond's disability could no longer be overlooked. Captain William F. Barry wrote directly to his superior at Fort Brooke that "although this determination does infinite credit to his self-devotion and high sense of official duty it is calculated to exert an injurious effect upon the public service." He reported that when Hammond had recently tried to reduce a soldier's dislocated leg, his illness had overcome him and "in a minute or two [he] was helpless, speechless, and . . . quite senseless." Reviving after half an hour, the young surgeon "insisted upon resuming his duties with his patient although still unable to stand alone, and supported by two men, he attempted to proceed." A second attack then rendered him "entirely insensible" for over an hour. When he again regained consciousness, only a direct order compelled him to instruct the attendants in completing the operation rather than trying again himself. Hammond, confined to his bed with "no prospect of speedy recovery," was at last persuaded to apply for leave "after the painful fact having been developed . . . that he was not equal to the crisis, his disease of the heart having rendered him powerless and senseless."[19]

He left Florida in the middle of July, arrived in Philadelphia, fatigued, by the end of the month, and spent his twenty-fifth birthday home again in Harrisburg. The nature of Hammond's recurrent illness remains a puzzle. The patient himself speculated that it might be "fatty degeneration of the heart or disease of the spinal cord." He added with some insight that "mental emotions and physical exertions both produce an attack." Dr. Richard Coolidge, writing to Surgeon General Lawson, referred to the condition as "Angina Pectoris" and thought it possibly related to his history of "rheumatism, superadded to an hereditary predisposition to gout."[20] There is no evidence that the condition bothered him later in life, although Hammond died at the age of seventy-two of a cardiac arrest.[21]

As his health improved, Hammond took up residence at 103 South 12th Street in the center of Philadelphia and attempted to further his medical education. He wrote to the Surgeon General in October requesting assignment as assistant to the surgeon on duty in Philadelphia. While he was not yet fit for active service, he said, his doctors had told him that such occupation would be beneficial. He also wished to prepare for his approaching examination for promotion. Active duty and ill health had prevented him from properly keeping up with professional developments, and he hoped to follow a course of lectures during the winter. His request was denied. If enough improved, he was told, he would be assigned to Boston or West Point. "I should . . . infinitely prefer to be assigned to Boston," he replied. The next day he was ordered to West Point.[22]

Hammond was probably pleasantly surprised to discover that other medical officers at West Point shared his growing interest in medical science. From Professor W. W. Bailey he could learn new microscopical techniques while reading up on the latest methods being used by Alfred Garrod, Albert Hassall, and Golding Bird in England and Charles Frick in Baltimore. Here, probably, he was also introduced to "the elegant work of Robin and Verdeil," their *Traité de chimie anatomique et physiologique* (Paris, 1853). There was also the opportunity to do research. While Hammond later claimed to have been interested in crystalline urinary deposits as early as 1850, his first original work (on previously undescribed dumbbell crystal forms) was begun early in 1854 and published shortly after he left West Point.[23]

Hammond was still anxious to resume formal medical studies and once again sought assignment to Boston. He was again refused. A new strategy occurred to him. He asked to be ordered to the brand-new Fort Riley in Kansas Territory, adding the request that he first be assigned for two or three months to "some one of the Atlantic cities," if compatible with the public interest. In this way he would be fully able to perform the arduous duties that would devolve on him as one of the two or three medical officers at the frontier post.[24] We can imagine Hammond's disappointment when he was ordered, in February 1854, directly to Kansas. He left Philadelphia on March 11, delayed by illness in his family, and reached Fort Leavenworth on April 7 after a difficult journey. He arrived at the site of Fort Riley – still under construction – with his wife Helen and her sister Clara on June 20, on the steamboat *Excel*. "We are very much pleased," he wrote to John L. LeConte, "the quarters are fine the situation and climate delightful and the officers very agreeable."[25]

LAND AND POLITICS IN KANSAS, 1854–1857

In the late spring of 1854, national attention was focused on Kansas, the front line of the struggle over the extension of slavery. The Kansas-Nebraska Act had narrowly passed into law on May 30, provoking an influx of pro- and antislavery settlers and promising imminent conflict in the newly organized territory. By the end of the year the region would be known as Bleeding Kansas. Meanwhile the land speculators swung into action. One project centered on Pawnee, a site that some anticipated to be the new state capital. The Pawnee Town Association was organized in October 1854, with Lt. Col. William Montgomery, commander of the fort, as president and Assistant Surgeon William A. Hammond as secretary. Andrew H. Reeder, a Pennsylvanian appointed by proslavery President Pierce to be the first governor of Kansas Territory, received eighty acres of land from the association, as did Robert Wilson, sutler of the post and another supporter of slavery. Hammond himself took forty acres from the Association. "Kansas is fast setting up," he wrote to LeConte a few months later. "Fort Riley is now in the midst of the inhabited portion of the territory and Pawnee situated a mile east of it is to be the seat of government. I am interested in this town," he confided, "and will probably make a handsome sum out of it. There is scarcely a country in the world so well adapted to cultivation as Kansas."[26]

The actual settlers of Pawnee were mostly free-soilers, but most of the Fort Riley officers supported slavery. Captain Nathaniel Lyon was an exception: his strong abolitionist sympathies would lead him, after secession, to take charge of a pro-Union Missouri home guard composed mainly of left-wing German immigrants.[27] Hammond was "born and brought up in a Southern state in the midst of slaves," as he put it, although his family had left Maryland for the free state of Pennsylvania when William was four years old. He even owned several slaves in Kansas, as did most of the officers. However, he soon came to oppose the extension of the slave system.

In the delegate election for the new state legislature in November 1854, Hammond was the only army man among the forty voters in the precinct, most of whom were civilian employees at the fort. Military personnel were not ordinarily entitled to vote. To cast his vote for the free-state ticket, Hammond had to swear that he considered himself a citizen of the territory and would give up his commission if posted elsewhere. Perhaps he meant it, for army life was rapidly losing its appeal. "I find so little congeniality of feeling among the great majority of officers and myself that I am pretty much dispirited," he told LeConte. "Their tastes and habits are entirely different from mine and though they are generally what the world calls 'good fellows' they are not exactly the kind of men I can make companions of."[28] At least he still had his wife and sister-in-law with him.

Local land politics occupied Hammond's immediate attention. Montgomery quickly took advantage of his position to redefine the territory originally claimed as a military reservation in a way that materially benefited the Pawnee Town Association. This (and probably political hostility) prompted Captain Lyon to prefer charges against him. In the ensuing court-martial, Montgomery was dismissed from the service largely on the basis of the testimony of Hammond, who apparently felt that the land development scheme had gotten out of hand. Charges were also brought against Governor Reeder for his part in the affair, and Hammond found himself with a powerful and vindictive enemy. Meanwhile, Secretary of War Jefferson Davis, acceding to the wishes of the proslavery "bogus" legislature elected in the spring of 1855, ordered the destruction of Pawnee.

"Kansas is pretty much of a humbug," Hammond confided to his friend Joseph Leidy in June 1855, "but people continue to pour

into it as if it were the garden spot of the earth."[29] But his hopes
for real-estate profits were not crushed in the rubble of Pawnee.
With his new friend Lyon and a few others he organized a company to develop the town of Chetolah, about six miles from the
fort. Nothing at all came of this venture, as the free-soilers chose
first Topeka and later Lawrence as the capital of their "shadow"
state government. Thirty years later, Hammond used Chetolah as
the setting for his popular second novel, *Lal* (New York, 1884).[30]
The whole episode illustrates his perennial difficulties in distinguishing between well-grounded and fanciful schemes, and his
apparently inextinguishable political naiveté. Reeder will reappear
in Hammond's story as the head of the investigatory commission
that was to engineer his dismissal from the office of surgeon general.

Hammond resisted and resented the increasingly hostile polarization of Kansas over the next few years. "We hear very little in
this region of the Kansas War," he wrote in June 1856, only weeks
after the destruction of free-state Lawrence by "border ruffians"
and the retaliatory raid by John Brown's group at Potawatomie
Creek. "Were it not for the lunatics on both sides the people would
take very little interest in the subject." He found the proslavery
Missourians "ten times worse than the most ultra northern man. I
came out here a moderate pro-slavery man," he admitted, yet
"because I am not in favor of hanging every man with free state
sentiments I am denounced as an abolitionist. If my mind was a
little weaker than I flatter myself it is," he continued, "I might
probably be drawn over to the abolitionists body and soul." But it
was more likely racism than strength of mind that kept him from
the radical Kansas abolitionists. He declared that "the whole contest is ridiculous," lamenting that "white men should set to work
and murder each other for the sake of the real or apparent benefit
of a set of miserable negroes little elevated in mental or physical
faculties above the monkey of an organ grinder." Hammond, who
was conscientiously searching for the brain of a dead Indian to
further Joseph Leidy's "ethnological" studies, probably meant this
literally.[31]

The anarchy of Bleeding Kansas also undermined Hammond's
confidence in democratic values generally. "I have lost my faith in
the capacity of the people for self-government," he proclaimed
with a touch of melodrama. "Republics are a miserable humbug

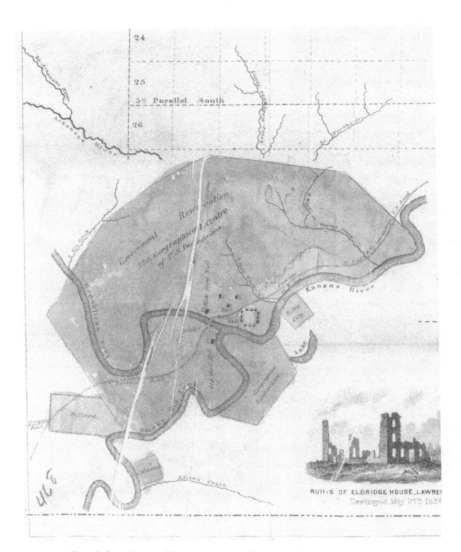

RUINS OF ELDRIDGE HOUSE, LAWRE

Destroyed May 21st 1856

Fort Riley, Kansas Territory, 1856. This was the scene of much of Hammond's work in natural history and experimental physiology, as well as the free-soil struggle and some ill-fated real-estate speculation. This 1856 map shows "Pawnee in ruins," destroyed by proslavery forces, and the designated site of Chetolah. The lake was probably the source of many of Hammond's zoological specimens. ("Map of Eastern Kansas by E. B. Whitman and A. D. Searl" [Boston: J. P. Jewett & Co., 1856], inset. Courtesy of the State Historical Society of Wisconsin.)

Fort Riley Kansas Ter.
June 2[9]th 1856

Dear Doctor

Your letter of the 29th ult. came safely to hand. I am very sorry those previously sent did not meet with the same good fortune, but as you intimate, the chances are very slim of a letter getting safely through the risk it runs in the west.

I shall anxiously await the publication of your reports. I am beginning to take quite an interest in the Coleoptera and your two memoirs on the Carabidae and Elateridae are certainly anything but favorable to Maine liquor laws and anti-tobacco using associations. As I use neither the one nor the other of these substances once in six months I can not be accused of working with interested motives. There is no doubt however that both alcoholic liquors and tobacco when employed in a decent and gentlemanly way exert a decidedly beneficial effect upon the system, especially when one can't get enough meat and bread to eat.

We hear very little in this region of the Kansas war. Were it not for the fanatics on either side the people would take very little interest in the sub[ject]

from General is disposed to do all in his power to oblige me but at present is so much in need of the services of the Medical officer that he is unable to grant me the indulgence. A bill has already passed the Senate increasing the Corps and if the House will only act upon it favorably it will be all right. In the event of my coming east I need not assure you how much pleasure it will give me to meet the Academicians in the way you propose.

I am busily engaged on a series of investigations relative to the effects of alcohol and tobacco upon the human system. My experiments so far millions of cattle interest either Prof Hammond and Prof Miller both desire to be remembered to you. I shall have an opportunity in a week or two of sending a large box of specimens to the Academy. I will let you know when it leaves here. Will you be kind enough to call at Rulison and Arnold's 6th and Arch streets and ask them to hurry off the last lot of chemicals &c I ordered? I am very much in need of them.

With my regards to Dr Leidy and other friends believe me

Yours sincerely
William A. Hammond

J. L. LeConte
Philadelphia

and the sooner some good and true man arises to subvert the most miserable of them all, the better." The twenty-eight-year-old surgeon announced himself a "sincere friend of true liberty," but had "yet to find out that we have more of it than the serfs of Russia. Our people do not respect the laws," he continued with perhaps more concern for order than for freedom, "and our officers are afraid to execute them. For my own part," he concluded, "I would rather be ruled by one man of education and intelligence than by twenty millions of rabble without either."[32] Six years later he would be chosen as that one man to rule over the Army Medical Department in much the same spirit.

SCIENCE AND FREE THOUGHT

At Fort Riley, Hammond's friendship with Nathaniel Lyon introduced him to controversial new ideas. It began with a quarrel over religion. "I well remember the horror I experienced," Hammond later reminisced, "when he . . . announced that he was an infidel, and perhaps even an atheist, and that Socrates was a nobler man than Jesus." The more conventional but equally dogmatic physician responded contentiously that "there was no morality in the world outside of the Christian religion." Lyon abruptly terminated the conversation, but the two became friends the next day. "I regarded him," Hammond later admitted, "not only as a bigoted ignoramus, but as one whose eccentricity was as near insanity as it ever is."[33] But their shared opposition to the extension of slavery and their mutual fascination with science drew them together.

Captain Lyon introduced Hammond to the notion of organic evolution in a similarly casual fashion. During his first months in Kansas, Hammond began a series of experiments on the chemistry of metabolism. In one he subjected black snakes to an oxygen-rich

---

Letter from Fort Riley, 1856. Hammond's Kansas letters to Philadelphia colleagues dealt mainly with scientific issues. Here he mentions his growing interest in the coleoptera (beetles), his desire "to meet the Academicians in the way of our profession," and experiments that had convinced him that the evils of alcohol and tobacco had been overstated. He also confides his conflicts over slavery and the "Kansas War," and conveys the regards of Mrs. Hammond and her sister Clara Nisbet. (John L. LeConte Papers. Courtesy of the Library of the American Philosophical Society, Philadelphia.)

atmosphere to increase their activity level. Lyon came daily to observe them, and was disappointed one morning to find that Hammond had finished his work and released the animals. "I was performing experiments of my own with the snakes," he told his new friend. "If you had kept them here a little longer I am very sure legs would have grown out of their bellies just as wings have developed on fishes that through the course of ages have been stranded on the shore and that are now birds." Hammond thought he was joking, but Lyon explained to him (as he later recollected it) that "organic beings owned [sic] their forms to the circumstances in which they were placed and the demands made upon them by the conditions of their existence." As Hammond told LeConte at the time, Lyon "builds his whole theory of nature on the 'Vestiges of Creation,' which in my opinion cannot stand the test of science." These were advanced ideas indeed for 1854.[34]

Hammond eventually became an enthusiastic if not very well informed supporter of Darwinism. In his 1884 novel *Lal,* the "doctress" Theodora Willis carries out a version of Lyon's experiment in which the black snakes are given electric shocks as well as an oxygen-rich atmosphere. A servant is assigned to watch the snakes and report any development. At a critical point in the narrative, this servant announces to the company that legs have begun to sprout. After convincing herself and several reliable observers that this is really the case, the young scientist goes off to write a letter to Darwin. She (like, presumably, the author) is sure he will be gratified by this confirmation of his theory. Hammond's confusion of Darwinian, Lamarckian, and more fanciful concepts of evolution was not uncommon even among well-educated Americans of his day.[35]

The presence at Fort Riley of Nathaniel Lyon, Richard Coolidge, and several other scientifically minded medical men made the Kansas post far more stimulating for Hammond than New Mexico and Florida had been. His medical duties there apparently left him with a great deal of freedom to pursue his own research interests. This scientific work was of two distinct types. One project was the collection of natural history specimens for American scientific institutions, mainly the Smithsonian and the Academy of Natural Sciences of Philadelphia. The other involved laboratory experimentation in what is now called basic medical science. While these pursuits were conceptually and methodologically divergent, they were linked through a network of Philadelphia friends, notably Joseph Leidy and John L. LeConte of the Academy.

Once the United States government had firmly established a claim to the vast western territories, the professional scientist played an increasingly important role in the "great scientific inventory of the natural and human resources of the new domain."[36] By the time of the Civil War, men with specialized formal scientific training in fields such as geology dominated this work.[37] But in the mid-1850s, army personnel were central to American natural history fieldwork. For example, Hammond was one of seventeen army surgeons who participated in the large-scale ornithological survey organized by Spencer Fullerton Baird of the Smithsonian, who had known the young physician "from boyhood." This project had begun in March 1853 when Congress appropriated funds for the Transcontinental Railway Survey. Each of the seven expeditions launched under this act included an army surgeon who was also to act as a naturalist, under Baird's direction. Hammond and his itinerant and iconoclastic Hungarian assistant John Xántus (traveling under the name Louis de Vesey) were among the ten additional medical men involved.[38]

Baird was in a certain sense an opportunist, for guidelines he established for his field workers reflected the interests of the American scientific community rather than narrower utilitarian goals. He called particular attention to birds, nests, and eggs, rather than geological formations, mineral resources, or other features of potential economic significance. Hammond was fairly typical of Baird's young naturalist-surgeons. Fourteen of them were born between 1820 and 1830, and thirteen of the sixteen with formal medical training had received their degrees between 1845 and 1855. All but one had attended one of the leading medical schools of New York City or Philadelphia. Hammond and six others had been commissioned within a year of graduation.[39] It was an exciting if somewhat daunting project. "I have endeavored to 'put up' the bird that we killed yesterday," Dr. Kennerly confided to his diary in June 1853, "but being a novice . . . I have illy succeeded." A month later, packing up specimens for shipment east, he was more confident: "I trust that the lot may afford my friends as much pleasure at the Smithsonian in looking over and classifying them as I have had in catching them."[40] Baird's survey was already in progress when Hammond sought assignment to

Fort Riley, and the possibility of scientific fieldwork may have inspired the request. It is likely that Professor Bailey of West Point had told him of his collaboration with such luminaries as Asa Gray of Harvard and John Torrey of Princeton on the classification and description of western specimens.[41]

Most of Hammond's bird specimens went to Washington, but he shipped nearly everything else he could find to Philadelphia. As he was beginning to explore Kansas Territory, his friends back east elected him a Corresponding Member of the Academy of Natural Sciences. "Nothing shall be wanting on my part to make the confidence of the Academy deserved," he assured LeConte. "My father shall hand you the diploma fee."[42] From his western post he deluged the Academy with crates of insects, mammals, fossils, and other curiosities. When Edward Hallowell requested reptiles, Hammond promised to start hunting them in a lake he knew of, once the weather improved and the foot-deep snow melted. Within the year, Hallowell could thank him for 480 specimens of forty different species. Hammond did his best to oblige the senior John LeConte as well, though "I have made as yet but small progress," he wrote to LeConte, junior, in January 1857, "(even with the assistance of quite a large corps of collectors here) in getting a series of mammals of this region for your father." The amateur taxidermist described how two of his hospital attendants had helped him gut a prairie fox "stuffed now and in fine order." He had also bagged "a few wood rats and field mice" and "expect[ed] soon to have a mink who has been making havoc with my chickens."[43]

Like many other field workers, Hammond had little idea of the technical aspects of the science to which he contributed materials for analysis. Rather, his collecting activities were guided by his secondhand knowledge of the interests of his Philadelphia colleagues. He pored over Leidy's *Ancient Fauna of Nebraska* and had books and journals sent out by his Philadelphia booksellers, Lindsay and Blakiston. The mails were uncertain and some letters were lost, but parcels generally arrived sooner or later. He was eager to receive copies of published papers. "Everything of the kind is doubly interesting from the fact of my being debarred opportunities of otherwise learning the discoveries made in science," he explained. He asked Leidy whether microscopical specimens were wanted, and sought LeConte's assistance in identifying a puzzling bird specimen. He was frustrated in his work with arachnids: "As I have not yet been able to acquaint myself with the principles of classification I have not made much progress in the science of the study." Perhaps LeConte could send him a reference; he had already sent for copies of the *Boston Journal of Natural History*.[44]

Another project deserves special notice in the light of Hammond's later neurological interests: the search for a brain specimen of a Native American, requested by Leidy for his study of comparative cerebral anatomy. Hammond had not yet found one in October 1854, but a chief of the Kansas Indians had promised him the head of the first Indian to die in the neighborhood. The technical problem he foresaw was that most local Indians "have more or less white blood in their veins and it will consequently be difficult to procure an absolutely pure specimen." Meanwhile, some of the officers embarking on the current Sioux expedition had promised to send him "Indian bodies preserved in whiskey," if they could find the Sioux and engage them in battle. Leidy, he urged, should persevere in his study. Hammond was "still on the lookout for Indian brains" in February. "I have several chiefs enlisted," he complained to LeConte, "but they are such confounded liars that you can't depend on them for anything." He still thought Leidy's study to be of "great importance to ethnology," despite – or perhaps because of – his own apparently firm prejudices.

Eight months later, Hammond informed Leidy that he had at last received an Indian head, but in impossibly decomposed condition. His friends were still trying to get him a better one. "I came very near getting you a hundred of them last year but was relieved from duty with the Sioux expedition and ordered back here to assist Dr. [James] Simons six days before a battle . . . in which large numbers of the Sioux were killed," Hammond wrote late in 1856. "Can't you come out to Fort Riley in the spring and join us in the Indian War? I will promise you any facility you could desire." He neglected to mention the cholera epidemic at the fort in which between seventy-five and a hundred persons had died and Assistant Surgeon Simons had deserted, and on account of which Hammond had been recalled to take charge and to collect facts pertaining to Simons's court-martial. Leidy declined in any case. "I was quite earnest in my invitation to you to join the Cheyenne expedition," Hammond urged him in a letter written a few days after Christmas. "I am sure you would enjoy the trip and advance the interests of science. . . . I should really be glad to have you along," he added.[45] Leidy did not go west, but the Academy resolved, on his motion, to tender Hammond a special vote of thanks.

The younger LeConte, like Charles Darwin, collected beetles. Hammond was happy to help out, but his first months in Kansas produced only a few good specimens. "Can't you come out and pay us a visit?" he suggested to his friend. "We will give the Coleoptera a thorough overhauling and if you are fond of sporting I can give you plenty of amusement." If LeConte could get to Fort Leavenworth, Hammond would meet him there with an ambulance. Six months later, Hammond renewed the invitation. His friend Lyon was probably to lead a spring expedition to open a road from Fort Riley "to Utah &tc. by way of Bridger's Pass in the Rocky Mountains," and Hammond was to accompany him. "Can't you join us?" he entreated LeConte. "Here is an entirely new field for observation." LeConte remained in the East but his reports reached Kansas, exciting Hammond's personal interest in the beetles. He could now identify some of them himself, and had adopted a plan of preserving them dry, rather than in alcohol, as it kept the hues better. In fact, he sent a box containing "about ten thousand" coleoptera to Philadelphia with Captain George Gibson in July 1856. "Capt. Gibson returns to New Mexico in a short time," Hammond told LeConte, "and will be happy to give you his services as bug-catcher general for that benighted region."[46]

Gibson was just one of the soldiers organized by Hammond into his informal network of collectors. He was "quite in the way of the business," he wrote to Leidy in December 1856, and "the soldiers here always bring me everything they find in their hunting expeditions, of any interest." Hammond was beginning to develop his administrative talents. "I am now organizing from among the best and most intelligent of the soldiers a corps of collectors and intend giving premiums to those who bring me the most specimens," he explained to LeConte. Foremost among Hammond's collectors was John Xántus (Louis de Vesey), whose "industry and perseverance" were "of great help." The assistant surgeon procured a two-month furlough for him in the spring, as well as election to the Academy of Natural Sciences. The Hungarian went off to

Philadelphia with a letter of introduction to Mrs. Hammond's sisters.[47]

Hammond's natural history work continued throughout his stay in the West, alongside the laboratory work that will be discussed in the next chapter. There is no evidence at all that he valued one over the other, nor that he sought intellectual links between the two distinct enterprises. Despite his reservations about Kansas and the army, the young scientist was even willing to postpone his trip to Europe to accompany the troops to the Rocky Mountains by way of the unexplored Arkansas River. He did not want to "miss such an excellent chance of procuring valuable specimens for the Academy." With Xántus along as his hospital steward, he intended "to bring home the most extensive collection yet made from the Plains." His "only regret," he told LeConte, was that "you or Dr. Leidy or Dr. Hallowell cannot join us."[48]

Hammond's usually cheerful missives to Leidy and LeConte convey little sense of the hardship, illness, and injuries that he saw and experienced. His wife is scarcely mentioned, and his toddler son Somerville Pinckney Hammond (probably born late in 1853) not at all. There is not a reflective word on the purpose or impact of the attempts to conquer Native American resistance to the army's march west. Hammond's attention seems to have been riveted – perhaps to a fault – on his science.

3

"The first original Physiologist in the United States"

Hammond had not yet, in 1854, enjoyed the privilege of studying science in Europe. But American scientific institutions and informal networks brought European science to him. These sources included his teachers in New York, his associates in Philadelphia and at West Point, and published excerpts and reviews in the *American Journal of Medical Sciences*. And by the time he reached Fort Riley he was using original European publications. For example, an early paper on urea and uric acid cited German data unavailable in the American secondary literature. Hammond's methods in this research were drawn, in part, from recent reports of Justus von Liebig.[1] Somehow he became the first American member of a large German scientific research association with a characteristically unwieldy title: the *Verein für die gemeinschaftlichen Arbeiten für Förderung der wissenschaftliche Heilkunde*.[2] Hammond was also personally in contact with John Xántus (Louis de Vesey) and possibly other European scholars and scientific adventurers who made the long journey to explore the natural wonders of the American West.[3]

A CHEMICAL LABORATORY IN KANSAS

In the summer of 1854, Fort Riley was little more than a collection of rough temporary shacks. Nonetheless, Hammond promptly set up a laboratory with equipment he had brought with him and began chemical experiments on "microscopical analysis of the urine," continuing work begun at West Point. He was enthusiastic about the project, intended as a monograph, and told John LeConte in July that he had already received an offer from a publisher. But the work proved difficult. "It takes every hour of my time and is a much more fatiguing task than I had any idea of," he confessed. "There are a great many drawings necessary for the complete elucidation of the subject all of which I am making from the microscope," he continued, "and not being much of a draughtsman I find it very troublesome."

He reported to Leidy in October that he had "succeeded in replacing the uric acid of the urine of serpents by urea" and was writing a report for Dr. Isaac Hays's *American Journal of the Medical Sciences*. His object was to test Liebig's theory that urea was formed from an intermediate substance, uric acid. While Liebig, Friedrich Wöhler, and their associates had generally conducted in vitro experiments, Hammond investigated metabolic processes in living animals: black snakes and himself. He believed his results confirmed those of Liebig and refuted J. Lehmann's challenge. "I intend continuing this investigation by submitting a number of animals to experiment," Hammond promised LeConte, "and will send the results to the Academy." He was "still at the book" in February 1855, although "forever much hampered by the want of chemical apparatus and other facilities which the country does not afford." He still expected to "get through with it," but never did. *Physiological Memoirs,* when it appeared in 1863, was a collection of essays rather than an illustrated treatise.[4]

This taste of the laboratory whetted the appetite of the young scientist for scientific work and study. By the middle of June 1855 Hammond was ready to come back east. He expected to be ordered home soon for examination for promotion, and was inclined to resign soon after. But once again he had misjudged the army bureaucracy – and possibly the political situation in Kansas – for no such orders materialized. Still, he was very anxious for a chance to study, with his sights now set on Europe. For this purpose he formally requested in February 1856 a one-year leave of absence. "My objects are of a purely professional character," he explained, "and it is my intention, should this indulgence be granted, to remain continuously at that place which, upon due consideration, shall be deemed most eligible for affording medical instruction."[5] "I think I shall get it," he told LeConte. "If I am not disappointed, it is my intention to go to Giessen and pass a year in the chemical laboratory there." Perhaps he realized that chemical studies would likely not impress his superiors as the most appropriate form of continuing medical education. The Surgeon General had just won a fight to increase the number of officers in the medical corps, and Hammond saw this as an opportunity. "I shall get my leave . . . if the Corps is increased," he predicted. "The Surgeon General is disposed to do all in his power to oblige me but at present is so much in need of the services of the medical officers that he is unable to grant me the indulgence." Hammond may have read too much meaning into the conventional phrases of his commander, for when the corps was increased his leave was denied. The irrepressible scientist asked that his application be kept on file. He told Leidy in November that he expected to make his voyage the following spring.[6]

In the meantime, Hammond spent much of his time during 1855 and 1856 "busily engaged" in his urological experiments. He was now interested in the effects on the urine (and implicitly on the metabolism) of tea, coffee, alcohol, tobacco, and changes in mental exertion.[7] Diet, regimen, and the lesser vices were popular topics of discussion in the United States in the 1850s, in the wake of the health crusades of Sylvester Graham and other advocates of vegetarianism and temperate habits.[8] Health reform often went hand in hand with hydropathy and other challenges to regular medicine. Hammond's decision to approach this issue with the latest European techniques represents an adaptation of the continental research tradition to the American context. He may have hoped that science would come to the defense of his somewhat beleaguered profession.

Snakes, being naturally abstemious, were inappropriate subjects for the new research. Thus Hammond's sole experimental subject was himself, although he was nearly as temperate as the snakes in those days. "As I use neither [tobacco nor alcohol] . . . once in six months I cannot be accused of working with interested motives," he wrote to LeConte. He used the most up-to-date methods available to assess the effects of each substance in turn on the chemical composition of his urine. The conclusions were reassuring, though "anything but favorable to Maine liquor laws and anti-tobacco-using associations." He found tea, coffee, and tobacco (all in moderation, of course) to be beneficial. Regarding alcohol he was more circumspect in print. Its use, he cautioned, "even in moderation, cannot . . . be either exclusively approved or condemned." Privately, however, he wrote that "no doubt . . . alcoholic liquors and tobacco when employed in a decent and gentlemanly way exert a decidedly beneficial effect upon the system especially when one can't get enough meat and bread to eat."[9]

Hammond elaborated on these findings a decade later, when the health crusades had abated, in an article for lay readers of the *North American Review*. Tobacco "lessens the destruction of the tissues as a whole, and especially diminishes the wear and tear of the nervous system," he declared. Thus it vitiates the unavoidable ill effects of high-pressured modern civilization. It also increases gastric secretions, promoting digestion. "To smoke after meals is," he concluded, "a perfectly orthodox physiological act, and is another happy example of the coincidence between instinct and science." His recent observations of the "tobacco manufactory of M. Pierre Lorillard," facilitated by the proprietor, reinforced his conviction that tobacco was benign.[10] Hammond's notion of physiological orthodoxy suggests the extent to which he would eventually come to see science as an alternative to religion, or perhaps even as an alternative religion. But this idea, and such a polemical tone, would have been discordant in Hammond's self-consciously objective papers of the 1850s.

Virtually all of Hammond's self-experiments included an investigation of the physiological effects of physical and mental exertion. His mental exercise was presumably obtained through reading scientific publications. The unaccustomed physical exercise consisted of "the lifting of a weight of one hundred pounds ten feet in a minute for three periods of fifteen minutes each at intervals of an hour." His resulting weight loss demonstrated, he said later, the "law that force results from decomposition of matter."[11]

Hammond said little in his early writings about his reasons for investigating the chemical effects of mental exertion, but he later cited them as evidence that mind was a function of the material brain. Brain substance, he argued, was consumed in mental exercise, leaving residues in the urine. It would have to be replenished constantly.[12] Most likely he was urged on in this line of work by his freethinking friend Lyon. Much of Hammond's later neurological practice, especially the treatment of patients diagnosed as suffering from "cerebral hyperaemia," would depend on the notion that mental pathology had a physical basis. This general idea had long been a part of the medical view of insanity. But the explicit materialism of Hammond's experimental results may have

	Quantity.	Urea.	Uric acid.	Chlorine.	Phosphoric acid.	Sulphuric acid.
1st day.......	40·10	741·53	12·30	168·22	62·08	47·18
2d day	43·67	748·55	10·35	171·94	65·89	48·91
3d day	44·59	749·67	11·06	175·18	69·85	54·17
4th day......	44·29	740·72	10·37	174·68	71·51	50·00
5th day......	43·17	747·56	10·93	170·85	66·99	48·79
6th day......	44·87	759·66	10·44	175·25	62·66	50·60
7th day......	45·18	754·23	9·82	166·83	68·73	50·78
8th day......	43·73	747·86	10·86	171·89	68·02	48·92
9th day......	42·13	755·69	11·01	179·75	66·27	42·23
10th day.....	43·90	747·92	10·38	172·24	60·04	49·00
Average...	43·56	749·33	10·75	172·62	66·15	49·05

B. The influence of *diminished* mental labor was next to be ascertained. I therefore omitted studying entirely, and passed the seven hours allotted to it in the standard experiments in reading light literature, and otherwise beguiling the time in amusements requiring but little mental exertion. As previously, this was continued for ten successive days. The food, exercise, etc. remained unaltered. The effects of this course upon the urine are shown in the following table. The mean temperature of the atmosphere during this series was 77.°

	Quantity.	Urea.	Uric acid.	Chlorine.	Phosphoric acid.	Sulphuric acid.
1st day........	33·36	590·90	14·70	144·70	28·79	37·01
2d day	33·39	581·65	15·81	148·11	25·17	37·12
3d day	30·12	591·77	15·00	143·40	28·21	39·23
4th day......	32·86	590·13	15·88	143·52	27·46	37·00
5th day......	32·73	586·55	17·58	141·18	25·80	35·36
6th day......	31·00	571·36	18·73	140·25	22·75	32·71
7th day......	35·47	583·22	18·28	139·15	23·84	35·16
8th day......	31·33	586·65	17·83	142·80	25·82	36·80
9th day......	31·60	570·84	19·14	140·69	20·58	33·18
10th day.....	30·59	582·43	18·27	140·17	22·60	34·62
Average...	32·24	588·55	17·12	142·34	25·10	35·81

"Urological Contributions" to the study of mind and brain. Hammond tried to identify experimentally a physiological basis for thought. The upper table gives results of his analysis of urine following increased mental exertion; the lower table shows effects of diminished mental labor. He concluded that intense thought accelerates the metamorphosis of brain tissue, requiring increased nutrition of that organ. (William A. Hammond, *Physiological Memoirs* [Philadelphia: Lippincott, 1863], p. 22. Courtesy of the Middleton Library of the Health Sciences, University of Wisconsin, Madison.)

seemed too controversial in the 1850s, in the view of a young researcher trying to establish himself and cognizant of the medical-philosophical debates that had raged during his school years. Then, too, he may not have been ready himself to draw such radical conclusions from his own work.

Hammond finished up these experiments in late August 1856. A congressional debate was dragging on over the new army appropriations bill, and the future of the Medical Department was uncertain. He wrote to Leidy that he was indifferent to the result as he did not intend to remain much longer in the service in any case. "I wish however they would come to a determination one way or the other," he confessed, "as when one does not know what one has to look forward to it interferes very much with all plans for study comfort or anything else." Hammond wanted to know whether the American Medical Association had recently offered any prizes for original research. If such a contest were open to nonmembers, he had thoughts of entering. He had already sent to his Philadelphia agents Lindsay and Blakiston for a better chemical balance, as his old one "although true is not sensitive enough." He had his eye on one advertised in the catalog of Bullock and Crenshaw, manufactured by Orthing and claiming accuracy to half a milligram. He asked John LeConte to get Dr. Bridges, Dr. Rand, or another member of the Academy of Natural Sciences to select a good one for him. "I should be glad if it can be done immediately," he urged, "as I am deterred from some investigations requiring delicacy for want of it." In mid-November, with another Kansas winter threatening to cut off the mails, the balance had not yet arrived. "When I shall get it," Hammond despaired, "the Lord only knows."[13] Eventually he did obtain the chemicals and equipment necessary to "get quite a laboratory established." The winter of 1856–57 was occupied in the new project.

The scientist was again his own subject, and his meticulous description of the research required a self-portrait. At the age of twenty-eight and a half years, Hammond was six feet, two inches tall, had a chest measuring thirty-eight and a half inches, and weighed a hefty 215–30 pounds, considerably more than a year or so earlier. The "habit of body is rather full," he confessed, "temperament sanguineo-nervous, I am of sedentary habits."[14] He would later describe persons of such a temperament as "brilliant, restless and impatient," a fairly apt characterization of himself.[15]

Throughout the snowy winter, with the mercury dropping to −23°F, he arose at 6:30 a.m. and retired at 10:30 p.m. Eight hours were spent in the laboratory and four more in "chemical and physiological studies." He squeezed everything else, including family responsibilities, meals, recreation, physical exercise, and professional duties, into the four remaining daytime hours. His normal diet consisted mostly of beef, potatoes, and bread and butter. Along with these came beets, chicken, cabbage, rice pudding, and occasional delicacies.[16]

Hammond began his A.M.A.-prize research project by establishing the chemical composition of his blood and urine under his normal regimen. Then for ten days he ingested only egg albumen (he does not mention water), carefully monitoring chemical changes in his bodily fluids. He used the methods of chemical analysis developed by Liebig for assays of urea, chlorine, and phosphoric acid in the urine, and those of Scherer for the blood. He also recorded variations associated with different levels of mental and physical activity. After a recovery period, he repeated the experiment with a diet of starch alone, and again with gelatin. A parallel attempt to study the effects of a gum-arabic diet was curtailed after four days because the investigator-subject was too ill to continue.[17]

Remote Fort Riley received no mail from the East for the first three weeks of February, so Dr. and Mrs. Hammond were "buried in darkness of all that is transpiring with you," he told LeConte. But the last post to arrive had brought the *Proceedings of the Academy of Natural Sciences* to 1856, with which the isolated scientist consoled himself. He assured LeConte that his father would pay his dues and subscription fee, and asked him to tell Leidy that about a month's work remained on his paper. He hoped it would not be too late. In March the diligent young researcher, a bit the worse for wear, did send his long essay to Leidy for submission to the American Medical Association. He had "taken a great deal of trouble with it," he told his friend, and the investigations had "been exceedingly laborious and [had] somewhat impaired my health." He thought the results important, and confessed he would be disappointed if the judges did not agree. The main problem had been getting up-to-date medical works in remote Kansas. "I have always consulted the original authorities in preference to getting the information at second hand," he reported with a touch of pride.[18]

Once the manuscript was in the mail, the usually decisive Hammond had second thoughts about it. He wrote to Leidy again the next day, asking him to read over the manuscript and not to submit it "if you do not think it is likely to gain the prize."[19] It was characteristic of Hammond to insist on first place, but he need not have worried. The essay not only won the competition but served to establish the author's credentials as a serious researcher in both American and European scientific circles.[20]

Hammond presented his results in spare, functional prose and data tables. He provided little in the way of interpretation, but did use the last pages to recommend experimental physiology, "the basis of all medical knowledge," to his countrymen. He hoped his inquiries would serve to "excite others throughout our land to investigate in living beings the operations of nature." Like his German colleagues, he expected much from "the united labors of those who seek by original investigations to build up a positive science," and looked forward confidently "to the perfect enlightenment of our minds in regard to the most obscure of the vital processes." Hammond referred often to this essay in later discussions of the physical basis of mind. He may well have been alluding to physiological psychology in particular when he concluded that only experimental research could "work out the sublime problems which the Great Creator of all has proposed for our solution."[21]

In April Hammond appealed once again to the Surgeon General to be sent east to study. He had been in the army eight years, almost entirely at frontier posts, and could be examined for promotion at any time. He had been studying on his own, but there were "branches of Medical science with which one cannot become thoroughly acquainted by mere reading." To refresh his knowledge of these he needed the "more extended advantages afforded by an eastern station."[22]

Hammond's friend and medical attendant Assistant Surgeon Richard H. Coolidge appended a novel suggestion. He had recently reported a case in which a patient had died from an impure tincture of chloroform. Perhaps the Surgeon General would "think it advisable to have the medicines purchased for the Army analyzed before being issued." If so, Coolidge could recommend Hammond as being specially qualified to perform that work, and to instruct newly appointed assistant surgeons in medical chemistry.[23] Hammond's request was taken under consideration, but

Coolidge's suggestion would have to wait for more progressive leadership of the Medical Department.

While awaiting a decision, Hammond began a new series of experiments "On the Injection of Urea and Other Substances into the Blood." They were designed principally to test Friedrich Theodore von Frerichs's theoretical explanation of uremic intoxication and Bright's disease.[24] It was an interesting choice, for it helps to locate Hammond more precisely within the spectrum of European medical science. Frerichs had already published important works on digestion and on liver disorders, including an 1851 book on Bright's disease. The first volume of his major treatise on liver disease was in press, and he was at the height of his research career. But his experimental work would soon be curtailed by a combination of circumstances including the hostility of the distinguished and powerful Rudolf Virchow. Frerichs would then turn to giving clinical lectures and building up an "enormous consulting practice." He became a key figure in the development of a scientific clinical medicine in Germany.[25] Hammond's career as a specialist after the Civil War paralleled that of Frerichs in many respects. While the option of a specialty practice that permitted clinical research was unusual in the United States, Hammond may well have been aware of the precedent Frerichs had helped to set in Germany.

Summer of 1857 found the normally sedentary scientist riding off to the Rocky Mountains on the long-anticipated Cheyenne expedition. He returned from this strenuous tour of duty on September 10 with a serious knee injury, possibly from an Indian bullet he was said to have carried to the grave. His cardiac-nervous episodes recurred.[26] Besides this, he wrote to Surgeon General Lawson, his father was in poor health and he had pressing family business in Philadelphia. At the end of October he was again officially found unable to perform his duties and ordered back to Philadelphia.[27]

BIOLOGY IN PHILADELPHIA

An extended leave from active duty allowed Hammond to stay in Philadelphia for two years that were probably among the happiest in his life. He settled into domestic life, fathering another son, named Graeme Monroe, in 1858, and a daughter, named after Mrs. Hammond's sister Clara, the following year. Opportunities

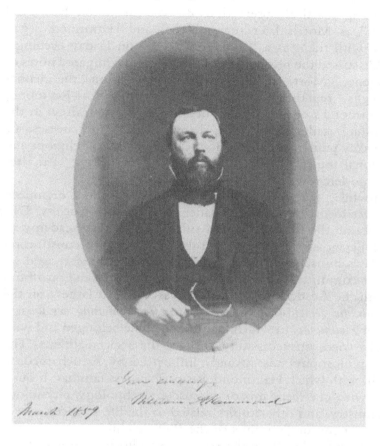

Signed photograph of William A. Hammond, March 1859. (Courtesy of the College of Physicians of Philadelphia.)

for scientific work and study abounded, and instead of a few isolated colleagues Hammond found himself amidst dozens of young physicians with similar interests. Some of the younger members of the Academy of Natural Sciences, including John L. LeConte, Joseph Leidy, S. Weir Mitchell, and J. Cheston Morris, had been meeting almost daily since early 1856 and "discussing men and things with the aid of cigars and pipes." When Hammond returned to Philadelphia he quickly fell in with this "Kapnological" group, also dubbed by LeConte the *Ewigsheitgesellschaft,* as its seemingly eternal sessions often ran into the early hours of the morning. Also, Morris and Charles S. Wurts had been "studying and making practical observations & experiments on Biological subjects," as Morris later remembered, and Hammond began meeting with them as a "Biological Club" on Friday evenings. They "discussed the physiology of that day and compared notes of experiments." Morris recalled particularly work on "the incubation of eggs," repetitions of the experiments of DuBois-Reymond, and Hammond's on nutrition. These meetings soon drew in the other young academicians, who shared crackers and cheeses, ale and whiskey punch, and discussions excluding only "religious and professional topics." They continued for many years, well after Hammond left town.[28]

Meanwhile, Hammond, Leidy, and a few others organized themselves formally into the Philadelphia Biological Society. This soon became the first specialized subsection of the Academy of Natural Sciences.[29] Hammond probably wrote the constitution and bylaws himself. He served officially as vice-director, and sat on major committees such as those on nominations and on affiliation with the Academy. The society was modeled largely on the *Verein für die gemeinschaftlichen Arbeiten für Förderung der wissenschaftliche Heilkunde,* to which Hammond alone belonged and with which he tried, unsuccessfully, to have the society affiliate. The group's philosophy was strongly influenced by French medical research, with which Hammond was perhaps less familiar. It busied itself with an eclectic mix of microscopy, ethnology, physiological chemistry, and other topics related to the life sciences.

Under Hammond's influence the Philadelphia group, like the *Verein,* committed itself to the method of collective investigation. It would choose research topics, draw up protocols for each, and encourage both members and nonmembers to collect data. The results were to be collated to produce solutions to important questions more efficiently than any individual could acting alone. Such methods had already been employed by the Army Medical Department in the collection of meteorological and epidemiological data. But the topics chosen by the new biological society reflected the latest efforts of the research institutes and universities of France and Germany.

Hammond took charge of the research on "the influence of the internal use of the alkaloids, quinia, cinchonia, morphia, and strychnia, upon tissue metamorphosis" and "the circumstances which determine the existence of sugar in the blood, and which

occasion its presence in the urine." Several of his proposals were
assigned to other members: "the physiological position of the
blood fibrin," "the illimination [*sic*] of ammonia from the lungs in
health and disease," "the variations in the amount of ozone in the
atmosphere and their connection with epidemics," and "the influence of ingesta upon the composition of the milk." George Read
Morehouse was to lead an investigation of "the minute anatomy of
the nerves and nerve-centers."[30] For the most part, these intelligently conceived but overly ambitious projects produced few
results, and by the time Hammond left Philadelphia in September
1859 the Biological Society was well on its way to extinction.

The Biological Society did provide Hammond and the others
with a much-appreciated forum for the active exchange of scientific ideas. For example, S. Weir Mitchell delivered an illustrated
lecture in March 1858 on the crystals he had found in sturgeon
blood. He explained why he thought these findings disproved
Lehmann's opinion that the "coloring-matter of the blood" was
essential to the "constitution of blood-crystals." A lively discussion followed, in which Hammond described his own attempts to
find similar crystals in turtle blood. He reported in September on
new findings "on the secondary formation of blood crystals." In
January it was Mitchell's turn again, and his comments on medicolegal aspects of blood-crystal analysis sparked an animated exchange. Hammond, inspired by a comment made by J. J. Woodward, went off to try some fresh experiments. He brought the
results to the next meeting, where they were discussed with great
interest.[31]

In 1858, also, Hammond finally made his long-awaited trip to
Europe, sailing from New York to Liverpool on May 8. He visited
Paris, Geneva, and probably other cities as well before returning to
Philadelphia in early August. This voyage was more likely recre-
ational than educational, but Hammond did find time to visit and
inspect a number of European hospitals.

Hammond had originally been elected to the Biological Society's committee on organic chemistry. In December 1858 he
switched to the committee on physiology and began to collaborate
more closely with Mitchell. First they examined the "contractile
element" they believed to exist in the skin. The results must have
been disappointing, because little more was said on the subject.
Instead, Hammond investigated the "hypothesis that the blood is

the excitor of contractility in the heart." His vivisection of a bat, he reported in March 1859, tended to disprove this idea.

By April, something new had come along. Through W. S. W. Ruschenberger of the Academy of Natural Sciences and Joseph Carson of the University of Pennsylvania, Hammond and Mitchell had obtained samples of two new varieties of a South American arrow poison that worked on the heart and nerves. Their preliminary findings, described to their colleagues on April 18, 1859, must have been particularly exciting since they contradicted the opinion of the distinguished Claude Bernard, who was working on similar problems. After "considerable labor" they produced a substantial paper on these poisons, called corroval and vao. This included a survey of the literature as well as Hammond and Mitchell's original experimental observations on the chemistry and physiological effects of the substances. The authors expressed their "regret that our engagements oblige us to defer the fuller consideration of this interesting subject to another occasion."[32]

The society did hear about the results of further collaboration between the two physiologists on nerve poisons, and each man later returned to the subject.[33] But Hammond was still in the army, and as his health improved he began to think of returning to active duty. In July Assistant Surgeon Hammond told the Surgeon General, to whom he had been reporting monthly, that he thought he could perform duties of a sedentary nature. This offer was apparently rejected. But, as he explained candidly, the situation was a delicate one. The dean of the University of Maryland had asked Hammond to apply for an assistant professorship in anatomy and physiology, with the understanding that a full professorship would be available in the spring. He could not support his family on the salary offered, but was sorely tempted by the prospect of the full professorship. He found it repugnant "to draw pay from the United States without rendering a return for the same," even though this was the "direct result of extraordinary overexertion in the discharge of my duty." He proposed to reside in Baltimore for the winter, and to resign his commission in the spring if not then fit for duty.[34] For once his request was granted.

THE BALTIMORE PROFESSORSHIP OF PHYSIOLOGY

Hammond was in Baltimore in September 1859, but only briefly. Perhaps the assistant professorship did not materialize, for on

Hammond's own application he was soon assigned to Fort Mack-inac, Michigan, the scene of William Beaumont's famous experiments some twenty-five years earlier. Hammond's routine duties at the small Michigan post, which he commenced on October 3, 1859, left him ample time for his own work. During the long winter months he conducted a series of twelve experiments on living animals to ascertain the effects of a supposed new species of the poison upas from the "Indian archipelago."[35] Meanwhile negotiations probably continued with the University of Maryland. In June 1860 Hammond requested six months' leave, to begin September 1 and after which he would resign. The leave was granted, but for two months only, and Hammond settled in at 36 Franklin Street in Baltimore at the beginning of September as a civilian and as a professor of anatomy and physiology. The examination for promotion had never come.

The editor of the *Charleston Medical Journal and Review* "congratulate[d] the University of Maryland on having secured the services of so distinguished and laborious a colleague, and our friend, Dr. Hammond, on his transfer to a position so suitable to his tastes and objects."[36] The university catalogue for 1860 advertised Dr. Hammond as a well-known contributor to medical literature who had "acquired a high position, both in this country and in Europe, by his anatomical and physiological investigations." The medical school at Maryland was open to the innovative scientific work that appealed to Hammond. Professor Frick, whose original work in urinary pathology Hammond had consulted for his own studies, had until recently taught materia medica there. A lectureship in experimental physiology and microscopy had been founded in 1854, and Hammond took this over from Christopher Johnson in 1861. He is credited with the introduction of histology into the regular curriculum. He obtained microscopes for the school's "museum" and began to build a collection of microscopical specimens that the school claimed as the first and largest in the country.[37]

Hammond was also appointed surgeon to the Baltimore Infirmary, which was under the immediate control of the medical faculty. Here he gave a series of clinical lectures on venereal disease.[38] He quickly began to establish a private practice, probably drawing on his family connections in the area. He joined the editorial staff of the *Maryland and Virginia Medical Journal* and contributed translations of French articles to the new *Baltimore Journal of Medicine*.[39]

These show that he was reading widely and still taking a special interest in medical chemistry.

At Maryland, Hammond also began a series of experiments on the physiology of sleep, a topic that would be central to the development of his neurological thought. He continued his work on uremic intoxication and vegetable diuretics. He published the results of therapeutic experiments with nitric acid in intermittent fever that he had conducted during an epidemic at Fort Riley.[40] His varied scientific achievements soon won him further international recognition. He was elected an honorary member of the British Medical Association. The Paris *Journal des Connaissances Médicales* commented that "the labors of this gentleman in the field of experimental physiology are widely known," and rejoiced that his new appointment allowed him more time for his "important researches."[41] No less a figure than Charles Edouard Brown-Séquard referred to him as the "first original Physiologist in the United States."[42] The thirty-two-year-old physician seemed securely established at last in a scientific career.

4

"The best friend the soldier has"

Hammond's native Baltimore was a southern town, but the outspoken scientist frankly disapproved of its secessionist leanings.
His "warm attachment to the National Flag" must have lifted a few
eyebrows. The winter session of 1861 at the University of Maryland ended amidst the secessionist riots of April 19. Hammond's
first taste of the Civil War came when Union troops of the Sixth
Massachusetts were attacked by a proslavery mob in the streets of
Baltimore. He found himself performing familiar surgery on the
wounded in the Baltimore Infirmary, and was offered a post as
surgeon of a Rebel militia regiment. This he reportedly "spurned
. . . with great warmth and no great fastidiousness in the choice of
his language." Instead he decided to give up his highly desirable
professorship and growing private practice to reenlist in the U.S.
Army. "The patriotism, which prompted this act on the part of a
man, whose great delight then was the pursuit of scientific investigation requiring the convenience of a fixed abode," recalled Lewis
H. Steiner years later, "and the pecuniary sacrifice it necessitated,
increased my respect for Dr. Hammond." The thirty-three-year-
old physician asked that the age limit for the post of assistant
surgeon be suspended in his case, and pledged to resign if his
"affection simulating a disease of the heart" again incapacitated
him. He passed the examination easily (before a board headed by
Clement A. Finley, soon to be surgeon general) at the head of the
class, and reported for duty at the end of May.[1]

The experienced army surgeon spent the summer organizing
military hospitals at Chambersburg, Pennsylvania, and Hagerstown and Frederick, Maryland. His exceptional experience as an
"intern" at the Pennsylvania Hospital here stood him in good
stead. He also began lobbying to be restored to the rank he had

acquired during his previous eleven years of service. "A number of
the most prominent physicians of Philadelphia and New York
have petitioned for my replacement [*sic*] and many officers of the
Army have informed me they would be pleased with my success,"
he told Senator J. C. Pomeroy.[2]

Hammond threw himself into the medical work with energy
and impatience, bombarding Medical Purveyor Richard S. Satterlee and the surgeon general's office with requisitions for supplies. When sent in September to organize the Army General Hospital in Baltimore, he inaugurated the employment of civilian
cooks and female nurses. This was a fairly innovative plan, as most
contemporary hospitals still relied on convalescent patients for
most of the necessary daily labor. He requisitioned additional
buildings and medical cadets to help staff them. He personally
attended to such details as the purchase of mattresses and comfort-
ers and the acquisition of a supply of smallpox vaccine.[3]

THE NEW SURGEON GENERAL

The outbreak of war had immediately conjured up, in the minds of
many, the horrifying specter of another Crimean disaster. The
small and tradition-bound Medical Department of the army was
manifestly incapable of organizing and policing the camps and
hospitals of massive numbers of volunteer as well as regular
troops. A group of New York civilians organized itself as the
United States Sanitary Commission in May 1861 to fill the breach.
They quickly found that the Medical Department needed not only
an auxiliary but an overhaul. Senator Henry Wilson's congressional bill "to increase the efficiency of the Medical Department" reflected the Sanitary Commission's nationalist viewpoint and its
almost industrial approach to discipline, accountability, and cost-
effectiveness.[4]

By the fall, the Sanitary Commission was seeking a promotion
for Hammond. Frederick Law Olmsted, general secretary of the
commission, wrote to George Bellows in September that he wanted Charles Tripler, medical director of the Army of the Potomac,
"shipped off to Missouri, Hammond put in his place, Van Buren
made S. Genl."[5] But Hammond, not his preceptor, soon became
the Commission's choice for the top job. "Dr. Hammond . . . is
in town," recorded the New York diarist George Templeton

Strong on October 13, 1861. "Only an Assistant Surgeon, but he has had intimations from the War Department that the last may be first, and that he may take Dr. Finley's place." Strong also noted that his fellow Sanitary Commissioner "Dr. [George] Bellows thinks well of him."[6] Hammond's scientific credentials, his decade of army service, his observations of European army hospitals in 1858, his long-standing friendship with Sanitary Commissioner William H. Van Buren, and his organizational work over the summer all recommended him for the top job.

But Hammond's confidence in the support of the War Department was misplaced. He was opposed not only by the acting surgeon general, Robert Wood (who wanted the position himself), but also by Secretary of War Simon Cameron. Cameron "pronounced against Hammond most emphatically the moment he was named," Strong reported. "Some official pique or personal grievance was evidently in his mind."[7] The War Secretary was already notorious for political machinations of doubtful legitimacy, and he virtually ran the Democratic Party in Harrisburg, Pennsylvania, where Hammond's father had been politically active. Perhaps Cameron's animosity to the younger Hammond stemmed from a local feud.[8]

In January 1862 Hammond was designated medical purveyor at Wheeling with General William Starke Rosecrans and the Army of Western Virginia. After a short leave of absence to attend his mother's funeral he began to make a nuisance of himself with unusually large orders for supplies. Satterlee was bothered enough to ask the Surgeon General whether he was required to "furnish all and every thing called for on all requisitions, which are approved by the Surgeon General and are ordered by him to be issued." He mentioned that "several items on Dr. Hammond's requisition seem extraordinary." Hammond wanted ten General Operating Sets of Instruments "which are not allowed since the Field Cases were ordered." He also wanted 500 "Hair Mattresses" and iron bedsteads to go with them. One request especially puzzled Satterlee: large quantities of books. Meanwhile Rosecrans sent Hammond to Washington and New York "to represent the great necessity which existed in this Department for Medical Supplies and to do all in my power," he reported to the Surgeon General, "to facilitate the early furnishing of the hospital stores for which I had made requisition." Hammond remained in Philadelphia to supervise the shipment of materials, returning to Wheeling at the end of February.[9]

His next assignment was the inspection of the military hospitals at Grafton, [West] Virginia, and Cumberland, Maryland, not far from his childhood home in southwestern Pennsylvania. He reported his findings in Sanitary Commission Document #41. Conditions at both locations were disgraceful. The buildings were filthy, undersupplied, and frightfully overcrowded. Patients were packed in with as little as 84 cubic feet of space apiece, although 1,200 cubic feet were generally considered necessary. Hammond praised the medical officer at Grafton but commented acidly that "it can hardly be expected that the proper sanitary measures will be enforced in this camp, so long as the field officers do not reside in it, and experience the discomfort which arises from their neglect." Of Cumberland he noted succinctly "police bad." The first building he visited "defie[d] description. It is simply disgusting." He emphasized that its terrible condition "*does not exist in any other hospital in the civilized world,* and that this hospital is altogether worse than any which were appropriate [*sic*] to the allies in the Crimean War." Supplies were scarce: medicines, hospital stores, bedding, and hospital furniture. The physicians were inexperienced, the chief surgeon "unfit to take charge," and one building was actually under the charge of an "*enlisted man!*" Records were imperfectly kept, many sick and dying men were not accounted for, no attention was paid to diet, and the "utmost confusion" had led to a "most disgusting want of cleanliness."[10]

Hammond recommended that most of the buildings in use be abandoned altogether. He detailed a plan for their replacement with a series of "huts" capable of holding fifty patients each. These would be arranged in "echelons" to allow proper ventilation, in a variation of the pavilion plan sanctioned by general medical opinion. The large civilian hospitals of the postwar decades would be built on this model.[11] Hammond's boldness and energy helped to win him an official appointment as inspector of hospitals and camps, effective at the end of March.

The Sanitary Commission had meanwhile won its legislative battle to reorganize the Army Medical Department from the top down.[12] Marveling at the procedure, Olmsted wrote to his father:

The Medical Bill after having been kicked about like a football, from House to Committee & Committee to House, and House to Committee

& Committee & Committee to subCommittee & back to House & thro' similar processes in Senate . . . until it was so thoroughly flabbergasted that nobody knew where or what it was, and a new one had to be started, . . . all of a sudden a bill which is just the thing we wanted quietly passes thro' both houses the same day, and before we know it is a law.[13]

Senator Henry Wilson's bill "to increase the efficiency of the Army" took effect on April 16, 1862, and the controversy over the appointment of a new surgeon general came to a head.

"The Commission has the best feeling toward Dr. Hammond," Wolcott Gibbs had assured John L. LeConte in March. "In fact he is our candidate for Surgeon General so far at least as we can have a candidate when there is no vacancy." The commissioners were powerless in the matter. "We can only advise & recommend & Finley pays no attention to our advice & scorns our recommendations." But once passage of the Wilson bill was assured, Hammond pushed his scientific friends into action. He wrote to the Philadelphians Henry Hartshorne and S. Weir Mitchell, asking them to organize a "memorial" on his behalf. He asked John LeConte to follow up on this, soliciting in particular the signatures of Judge Grier (LeConte's father-in-law) and Aubry Smith. LeConte was also to notify Gibbs of the Philadelphia effort "so that there may be concert of action." Hammond wrote exuberantly from Wheeling that "the old fellows will make every effort to defeat my nomination but Stanton says I shall have it."[14]

President Lincoln was sympathetic to Acting Surgeon General Robert Wood, but with Cameron out of the way Hammond "had it" indeed. The Senate confirmed his promotion to brigadier general, in charge of the Medical Department, on April 25, 1862. He was a popular choice – outside the War Department. "Men . . . like the newly appointed Surgeon General, are wanted," wrote Dr. Robert King Stone to his patient Abraham Lincoln, "men who combine energy, physical power, observation, experience and professional erudition. Of enlarged views," he continued, "they will soar above the miserable contracted policy of the past and render the new Medical Department entirely efficient and a model for the world."[15]

"No man could be selected," editorialized the *American Medical Times*, "who so happily combines in his professional relations the confidence and esteem of both the Medical Staff of the Army, and

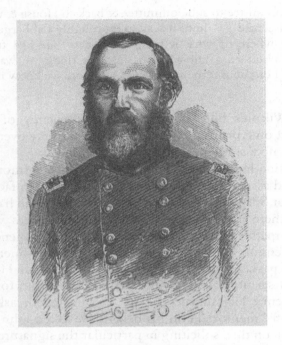

Surgeon General Hammond, 1863. The informality of this contemporary sketch suggests the young surgeon general's image as an energetic reformer. (*The Soldier in Our Civil War,* vol. 2 [New York, 1886], p. 387. Courtesy of the State Historical Society of Wisconsin.)

the profession of the country, as Dr. Hammond." The Philadelphia *Inquirer* favored the appointment but anticipated difficulties: "Dr. Hammond will have, although a dignified, yet a somewhat unenviable position. Those jealousies from which no profession or station is free will undoubtedly beset and surround him as they have others."[16] They did at once. The new secretary of war, Edwin Stanton, refused to confirm Hammond's choices for medical inspector, key positions created by the Wilson bill. Hammond plunged into his new work undeterred.

REORGANIZATION OF THE MEDICAL DEPARTMENT

Congress and the Sanitary Commission had debated the politics of reshaping the Medical Department and had settled on a general plan. Now it was Hammond's job to carry out the plan, and the question of organization was primary. This was no routine assignment: the vastly increased scale of the largely volunteer army had created qualitatively new medical problems requiring correspondingly new solutions.

Hammond acquiesced (against his friends' advice) in Stanton's plan of naming Robert Wood as his assistant. Then the War Secretary delayed signing the nomination papers. "Wood's appointment does not give unalloyed discomfort," Olmsted wrote to John Foster Jenkins, "though comfort hardly predominates. I would have preferred – someone else."[17] Perhaps Hammond was trying to be diplomatic, or perhaps he wanted to take advantage of the older man's experience. In any case it was a mistake. Hammond was more than a little arrogant and Wood more than a little conservative. The two did not work well together. Wood was soon replaced by Joseph R. Smith, a younger man recently returned from active duty and a stint as a prisoner of war in Texas. Much of the day-to-day work of the surgeon general's office involved paying bills and responding to inquiries about wounded soldiers. Smith took over most of this routine business, leaving Hammond free to travel to the front, handle emergencies, and develop special projects.

It is hard to reconcile twentieth-century images of Washington bureaucracy with the four-room office out of which Hammond was to reorganize a medical service responsible for the care of hundreds of thousands of troops. Samuel Ramsay, who apparently acted as a sort of office manager, reported problems in finding hospital stewards who met his standards for clerical duties. He tested their competence in "Spelling, English Grammar, Elementary Arithmetic, and Geography of the United States." Good penmanship was considered an asset, but surviving records demonstrate that it was not strictly necessary. Satisfactory workers were hard to keep. A Corporal Gibb had reported for duty one day and had done well, but had not been heard from since.

Ramsay wanted to rearrange the desks in accordance with a simple division of labor, but he consulted his superior first. "Our room is a small one," he wrote to Hammond in 1863, "and there are six of us in it, and a good many persons calling to see about their accounts. Mr. Watson and Mr. Kefferstein have entirely different work, and perhaps could be accommodated in some other room." The rapidly accumulating paperwork was also a problem. "I have no case for papers," he complained, "and a few pigeon-holes would be a great convenience." Ramsay suggested that "the settlement of private claims, and the keeping of the accounts of the Medical Department . . . will be best done by one experienced clerk with suitable assistants." He worried over the placement of Mr. Nichols in this work, as "neither his grade, as third class clerk, nor his turn of mind is suited to a subordinate position."[18] The Medical Department was rigid with encrusted tradition and entrenched senior officers, but it was scarcely a bureaucracy in the modern sense. That it became one was in large part a result of Hammond's efforts to render it "entirely efficient, and a model for the world."

Hammond had little time in the first few weeks to worry about office arrangements. In April and May 1862, General George B. McClellan was in the midst of the Virginia Peninsular campaign, an ill-fated attempt to capture Richmond by way of the peninsula between the James and York rivers. When Olmsted arrived in Washington to organize hospital transport ships under the auspices of the Sanitary Commission, he was nearly overwhelmed by the task of getting the wounded to Northern hospitals. He thought, with much justice, that Hammond did not fully appreciate the problem. "I confess . . . I can not understand the slowness of the Surgeon General," he wrote to John Foster Jenkins on May 29. Two weeks later, with battle expected in the evening, he expressed his frustration to Henry Bellows: "I think you & the Sgn General are made a little sick by the atmosphere of Washington. . . . the lion [i.e., Hammond] has been in his place these two months and I see that things are worse than they were before." He thought it urgent that "Hammond must be made to do something at once to revolutionize the policy of the Medical Department."[19]

Hammond probably had not thought of the Peninsula crisis as a policy issue. The new surgeon general had offered his support to the medical director of the Army of the Potomac, Dr. Charles S. Tripler. "You have the entire confidence of the Department," he wrote, "and its whole strength will be given to support you in the line of action you may determine to pursue." A similar missive went to Dr. Charles McDougall of the Army of the Tennessee, General Grant's command, which had recently suffered heavy losses in the battle of Shiloh. Hammond was accustomed to taking initiative, and he clearly expected his subordinates to do the same. "You have been given full powers to act altogether independently, and must be your own judge of what is best to be done," he telegraphed Tripler on May 19. He specifically authorized the Medical Director to assume entire control of all transports used by the Sanitary Commission or state agents, as well as those of the surgeon general's office.

Hammond was frustrated by the Peninsula situation, too. He had sent blankets down with Dr. Asch, from his own office staff, but the emissary found no one willing to receive them and brought them back. Tripler's views on ambulance transport were "eminently proper, but it is impossible to have the present system changed now," as the matter had to be put before the quartermaster general and the war secretary. Hammond thought, with an optimism that proved unjustified, that the ambulance problem would be solved within a month.[20]

The fifty-six-year-old Tripler was shaken by this "mild reproof," as Olmsted put it. "Now see how they misunderstand me," he complained to the Sanitary Commissioner. Olmsted took charge himself, realizing that Tripler was dependent on an already overtaxed quartermaster's department, and suspecting that he might not be the man for the job.[21] Hammond wrote again to Tripler a few days later sympathizing with his difficulties but insisting again that it was his job to solve them. "I do not blame you for this condition of affairs," he assured Tripler, "but I do blame those who, as I am given to understand, turned a deaf ear to your supplications." But if Tripler and General McClellan could not surmount the obstacles in their way on the Peninsula, it surely could not be done from afar. Hammond was exerting himself to establish new hospitals that would be ready in just ten days to receive 5,000 patients. "Like you," he hastened to assure Tripler, "I labor under much difficulty of the lack of physicians and nurses," but he would try to send thirty or forty doctors out from Philadelphia and New York, along with hospital supplies.[22]

Henry W. Bellows, the Sanitary Commission representative in Washington, had a broader view of the new surgeon general's work, and he was more satisfied than Olmsted. "I am more and more pleased with Dr. Hammond," he wrote his friend on June 9.

"His views are large, his mind active & prompt – his action at present embarrassed by almost insuperable difficulties. But he is cutting his way out." Hammond appointed a new medical director of the Army of the Potomac on June 19, replacing Tripler with the far more dynamic Jonathan Letterman. By the middle of July, even Olmsted was mollified.[23]

But the supply and transportation problems remained. In August Hammond came up with a new plan to create an ambulance corps controlled by the Medical Department and staffed entirely with trained noncombatants. In September he begged the War Secretary to adopt any plan, not necessarily his own, to remedy the "frightful state of disorder existing in the arrangements for removing the wounded from the field of battle."[24] A big part of the problem was the smoldering conflict between the Medical Department and Quartermaster General Montgomery C. Meigs, who had overall charge of transporting supplies and equipment. Meigs came from a medical family: his father, Charles Delucena Meigs, and his brother, John Forsyth Meigs, were well-known Philadelphia physicians. The sanitary commissioners thought well of his general efficiency and enforcement of discipline. But the Quartermaster General distrusted his energetic counterpart in the Medical Department. "There seems to be a desire in some quarters to make the Medical Department self-sustaining and independent of all aid or assistance from the Quartermaster's," Meigs complained to the Boston sanitary activist Dr. Henry I. Bowditch in October, "and indeed from all other departments. This is a mistake."[25]

George Templeton Strong had already begun to worry in August that "Dr. Hammond [was] working vigorously, but in danger of collision with Meigs, which would be a pity." A few weeks later he sided with the Surgeon General. "The fossil old [Medical] Bureau is not yet galvanized into life, with all Dr. Hammond's energy," he concluded. "Want of transportation seems its main difficulty. Hammond is paralyzed by dependence on the Quartermaster Department. We must mend this, even at the risk of alienating General Meigs."[26] The problem was never satisfactorily resolved, and Washington in-fighting delayed the implementation of a full-scale ambulance system until 1864. Nor did Hammond ever learn how to navigate successfully the stormy political seas of the capital.

Hammond interested himself personally in hospital planning. He visited the environs of several of the large Northern cities, helping to spot presumably salubrious sites. He sorted through offers of buildings for hospitals and suggestions for locations from Mattapoisett, Massachusetts, to Davenport, Iowa. Everyone seemed to want facilities for the wounded of their own town close at hand. Many were openly interested in the boom to local business and agriculture that a hospital might bring, so that the siting of hospitals was a political as well as a sanitary issue.[27] It was also a chance for Hammond to implement the recommendations he had made a few months earlier.

One of Hammond's first pet projects was the construction of a model hospital in West Philadelphia. He "draughted the plans, had a supervision of its construction, and personally selected its corps of physicians." The facilities originally consisted of "twenty-one one-story buildings, arranged in the form of a parallelogram," with a building for the surgeons in the middle. Each ward contained fifty beds. In the middle of May he promised Surgeon George E. Cooper he would "attend to the matter of the roof."[28] By the 24th he was in Philadelphia advising Cooper on the details of staffing. Perhaps Cooper resented the chief's apparent lack of confidence in him, because he soon added his name to the list of Hammond's enemies.

According to Hammond, there was to be one responsible medical officer in charge of each building. Unlike civilian hospitals, there would be no lay board of managers to meddle in his affairs. For each seventy-five beds there would be one medical officer (equivalent to an attending physician) having "the entire control of the patients assigned to him." To perform the duties of resident physicians there would be one medical cadet to each fifty beds. Hammond emphasized that the steward assigned to each hospital would be subordinate to all the medical officers. This hospital would be controlled by physicians; it would be a medical, not a charity, institution.[29]

Hammond put Dr. J. J. Hayes in charge, but continued to oversee operations. He telegraphed from Washington early in June to order the employment of fifty male nurses, each to receive $20 per month plus one ration. Hayes was also to see Hammond's friend

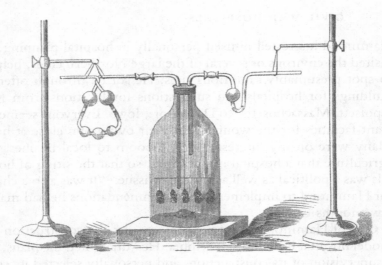

Apparatus for laboratory study of hygiene, ca. 1863. This experiment was to prove that diseases such as typhus fever resulted from "concentrated organic emanations from the bodies of those who have been confined in close and ill-ventilated places." The apparatus allowed the free flow of fresh air into the jar, while sponges saturated with "baryta-water" removed carbon dioxide. The enclosed mouse survived less than an hour, presumably poisoned by its own noxious exhalations. (William A. Hammond, *A Treatise on Hygiene, With Special Reference to the Military Service* [Philadelphia: Lippincott, 1863], p. 170. Courtesy of Middleton Library of the Health Sciences, University of Wisconsin, Madison.)

Dr. Atlee and have him obtain the services of fifty Catholic Sisters of Charity or Mercy, presumably at less cost to the army. Hammond expected to start sending patients almost immediately. Soon Hayes had assembled "a corps of Surgeons and nurses sufficient for nearly 2000 patients." He could have that many beds, or more, ready "as fast as patients can be loaded from ambulances." One of the seven resident surgeons under Hayes was Hammond's friend William Darrach, from the Philadelphia Biological Society. Nine "nonresident" (attending) physicians included some of the city's medical luminaries. By June 11 Hammond's assistant Dr. L. A. Edwards could recommend that Dr. Goddard, who was trying to organize the Master Street Hospital, consult Surgeon Cooper for guidance.[30]

It all looked good on paper, but the problems of the Medical

Department could not be solved simply by utopian model-building. "The expense of Surgeons and nurses is accumulating at a terrible rate," Hayes worried, but "I have less than *400* patients." Meanwhile "patients are being crowded into certain hospitals (for instance 4th & George St) while the carpenters are at work, and before the hospital was in any way ready to receive them." Hayes thought it would be "both unofficer like and insolent" to beg Dr. King, the medical director, for arriving boatloads of patients. Hammond had to intervene personally, instructing Joseph Smith to ask Dr. King to fill up the West Philadelphia hospital as soon as possible.[31]

The organization of a national military hospital system was a challenge as well as an opportunity for the new surgeon general. There were two levels of struggle involved. First was the conflict of national and local interests, not only as an underlying cause of the war but within the Union itself. This was played out in skirmishes for control of army hospitals. Second, leading American physicians had striven for over a century for increased control over the hospital as an institution. For the scientifically inclined physician, especially, the Civil War represented an almost unprecedented opening.

The Sanitary Commission had wanted Hammond as surgeon general because its members were convinced that science and efficiency went hand in hand. Hammond shared their goal of rationalizing the Army Medical Department as a national institution, transcending local interests. For him, this meant that the local sanitary committees should be "auxiliary & subordinate to the Medl. Department of the Army." In addition, "all Military Hospitals should be entirely within the control of this Bureau – outside the hands of this Department all responsibility ceases."[32]

Local authorities might agree in principle, but they often balked in practice. Dr. H. H. Smith, the surgeon general of Pennsylvania, did not seem to understand the arrangements Hammond had made with Governor Curtin. "If you supposed that my aim was simply to certify to the accounts, you have fallen into a grave error," Hammond warned Smith. "I intended to assume the entire control of these Hospitals, and to employ the medical officers on duty with them not as State officers but as United States officers." Smith's position entitled him to respect, Hammond conceded, but to "no authority over United States troops." The surgeon general of the United States Army would listen to the suggestions and views of his Pennsylvania counterpart as a matter of courtesy, but, he insisted, not as a matter of right.[33]

Issues of federalism also surfaced in Hammond's response a few days later to an offer from Surgeon General S. Oakley Vanderpoel of New York to turn over the public hospitals of that state to the Army Medical Department. Hammond had already begun arrangements "to bring all under the charge and control of the Federal authority." Vanderpoel was concerned that the doctors currently holding appointments at these hospitals might be replaced. Hammond appreciated the "embarrassment of your position" and reassured Vanderpoel that they shared a "harmony of intention." He would contract with the incumbents if they wanted to stay on the regular terms: $100 per month for the chief surgeon and "visiting physicians," and $80 for the hardworking young residents. Dressers (often medical students) had to be content with rations. The Medical Department and the quartermaster would divide the expenses for outfitting the hospital. The state hospitals' debts could not be liquidated as "the funds of this Department are all exhausted," and in any case that would be a matter for the Treasury Department. Hammond's new job was probably proving more complicated than he had anticipated.[34]

Other controversies than localism threatened the creation of an efficient national military hospital system. One of the most hotly debated was the question of hospital staffing. Nursing and housekeeping tasks were traditionally performed in antebellum American hospitals by convalescents or, in some cases, former patients who remained in the hospital for want of anywhere else to go. Military hospitals functioned in much the same way, although always under pressure from line officers to return their men to the ranks as quickly as possible. The employment of able-bodied male civilians was also considered suspect.

An earnest if poorly educated "Regular" poignantly expressed a "general complaint" about Northern contract doctors:

[They have] all their friends around them in some position if the[y] cannot have no other way the[y] will send for their friends to act as Contract Nurses but at the same time doing nothing of the work the first chance why they will have him appointed an Hospital Steward in the U.S.A. which has been a respectable position before these friends of Contract Doctors got there [sic] cowardly friend to escape Draft. . . . the

Doctors keeps some of their friends in Hospitals that there is nothing in the world the matter with them any more than Cowardice. Indeed it grieves a good many wounded soldiers lying from wound to see these friends of Doctors in charge of Store rooms and every thing around the building . . . and several old disabled men from wounds that could do in the [place] of these fancy men dressing in Citizens cloathes and going to town.[35]

Even if the corruption was exaggerated, the novelty of regular hospital personnel was not.

Hammond tried to alleviate the problem with his "Circular #7" of July 14, 1862, ordering the employment of female nurses under the supervision of Dorothea Dix. Those most readily available were the Catholic Sisters of Charity and of Mercy. But anti-Catholic prejudice immediately created embarrassments here too.[36] Two days later Hammond had to explain to President Lincoln why the Medical Department employed more Catholic than Protestant female nurses. "We found in the Sisters of Charity, a Corps of faithful, devoted and trained Nurses ready to administer to the sick and wounded," he wrote. "No such organization exists among the Protestants of this country, and those whom we have employed cannot compare in efficiency" – that magic word – "and faithfulness with the Sisters of Charity." The military surgeon was most impressed with the Sisters' training in obedience.

"I am a Protestant myself," he urged, "and therefore cannot be accused of partiality." He asked the President to be objective as well, and not demand the replacement of the Sisters with "others whose religious faith is different," but were less qualified. He would try to get more Protestants in the future, "but it will be a difficult task, as they will not submit to the same discipline, nor undergo the same hardships. I have a large experience with both kinds," Hammond emphasized, "and therefore speak what I know."[37]

The matter was not so easily resolved. Lucretia D. Mott wrote privately to Hammond, whom she knew personally, with a plea for "the protestant ladies of our city" who had established the Ladies' Home for Sick and Wounded Soldiers. She was distressed to hear that "Mr. Farley our old enemy" had "obtained an order for the Sisters of Charity to take possession" of it. "It cannot be possible that after cheerfully resigning the direction of it to the military authorities that we are to have our work made over to those who have thrown every obstacle in our way," she wrote, entreating him "most earnestly to spare us this mortification." And in August 1863 the Woolsey sisters arrived from New York at the Hammond General Hospital in Point Lookout, Maryland, to find it divided down the middle into a Catholic half and a Protestant half.[38]

But a number of physicians found secular female nurses even more objectionable. Many army men wondered openly why a respectable woman would want such a job. Others were more empirical – or more circumspect. E. J. Marsh wrote to his superior, R. O. Abbott, that his experience in the Judiciary Square Hospital in Washington, D.C., had convinced him that "female nurses are, as a rule, of slight benefit, and . . . not as useful as male attendants." He found that "men can much better perform all the duties required and do much more work, and occasion far less trouble." Apart from "one or two in the linen room & another to superintend the culinary department," he wished to discharge them. Abbott forwarded the letter to the surgeon general's office, and the request was approved apparently without question as to the nature of the "trouble." Hammond wanted female nurses, but he believed in giving medical officers broad authority over their hospitals.

Dr. G. A. McCall came to a similar conclusion after observing Miss Dix's nurses in the Mt. Pleasant General Hospital (also in Washington) for eight months. "Their duties can be performed by convalescent soldiers with infinitely greater efficiency and promptness," he explained, "their sex confining them entirely to a scope of action which would be widely extended were men to be employed in their stead." That is, the women's activities were restricted by convention and the women themselves blamed for the limitation of their work. McCall was allowed to dismiss the nurses, but his request to retain three as seamstresses was denied.[39]

Nurses were not necessarily enthusiastic about the Surgeon General, either. The worldly Hannah Ropes, a long-time abolitionist and reformer who served as a Civil War nurse, found Hammond to be arrogant and his office rigidly bureaucratic. "To help the oppressed did not seem at all the sphere of the place where we sat," she commented icily. "That broad built piece of humanity with gilded straps, with a stomach made extensively capacious by much good living – what had it in common with my poor, half-starving soldiers?" Ropes had been refused an audience with Hammond, and put off by his assistant. Outraged by the abuses she saw in the Union Hospital and by the lack of courtesy – much less sympathy – she found at the Medical Department, she took her case to Hammond's superior and enemy, War Secretary Stanton.[40]

SCIENTIFIC RESEARCH PROJECTS

Hammond was an administrator, but he was also a scientist with an agenda of his own for the Medical Department. As surgeon general he took responsibility for advancing the cause of medical research. Autopsies should be done on all cases of sudden death where the cause was not obvious, he informed Dr. J. A. Armstrong, "both as a source of satisfaction to the friends of the deceased as well as to the Attending Surgeon, and also as a matter of professional interest, and it may be of importance."[41] A circular issued May 21, 1862, called on surgeons to report all cases of fractures and gunshot wounds so that the information might be collected and analyzed. Three weeks later he announced plans for the publication of a multivolume medical and surgical history of the war. But his scientific vision went beyond the haphazard collection of medical statistics.

The best medical research of the first part of the century had come from the large hospitals of Paris. Such institutions were very marginal to American medical practice: many physicians, as well as patients, would see the inside (or even the outside) of a hospital for the first time during the Civil War. But for the elite physicians who worked within their walls, hospitals were at the center of medical science.[42] Civil War hospitals would provide concentrations of patients and therefore "clinical material" for systematic statistical and other studies. Thus Hammond promised the eminent Philadelphian Dr. Samuel D. Gross that "if at any time I can offer you the charge of a surgical Hospital, I shall certainly do so with great pleasure." Within a month, Gross was installed as the head of St. Joseph's Hospital.[43]

The most famous of the Civil War research hospitals was Turner's Lane in Philadelphia. In the spring of 1862 Hammond's physiological co-worker Weir Mitchell "began to take interest in cases of nervous diseases." No one else wanted such patients because "they were so little understood and so unsatisfactory in their results." On his own, Mitchell began to exchange cases of other types in the Filbert Street Hospital under his charge for neurological cases. Hammond soon found out, and in May 1862 gave Mitchell facilities in Moyamensing Hall on Christian Street in South Philadelphia for a special ward. By August construction was underway on the Turner's Lane Hospital at 22d and Oxford Streets in the northern part of the city. It was designed on the pavilion plan and reserved for soldiers with nervous injuries and illnesses.[44]

The significance of the work done by Mitchell with George Read Morehouse (another alumnus of the Philadelphia Biological Society) and W. W. Keen at Turner's Lane has been widely recognized.[45] Their works on *Gunshot Wounds and Other Injuries of Nerves* (1864) and on *Reflex Paralysis* (1864), based on their notes from this hospital, were regarded by European as well as American contemporaries as valuable scientific contributions. The wide range of well-defined injuries they encountered among the wounded soldiers offered unprecedented opportunities to study conditions that occurred rarely at other times and that were difficult or impossible to induce in laboratory animals.

For example, Mitchell discussed Brown-Séquard's contention that paraplegia could be brought about experimentally by ablation of the kidney or suprarenal capsules. Other researchers, including Hammond as well as Frederick W. Pavy and Arthur E. Durham, failed in their attempts to replicate Brown-Séquard's results. At Turner's Lane, Mitchell could test the theory clinically by observing his injured human patients, a procedure far more satisfactory in many respects than ambiguous laboratory experiments on dogs and rabbits.[46] The latter line of research would lead Brown-Séquard to his important theory of the "internal secretions," but Mitchell's clinical approach to neurological science would come to characterize the specialty in the United States.

Mitchell generously praised Hammond's indirect role in this enterprise. "The wisdom of the policy which founded special hospitals in Philadelphia was amply justified by the medical results," he wrote later, "while without such a classification . . . it was scarcely possible to look for any careful scientific study of rare instances of disease or wounds." He claimed that lost "notes on cases of acute exhaustion would have entirely anticipated the delineation of the condition we now accept as neurasthenia." It is certainly the case that J. M. DaCosta's classic work on "exhausted hearts" was based on his studies of the cases set aside for him at Turner's Lane.[47]

Hammond also ordered the establishment of other special hospitals, and in some cases specialized wards within larger hospitals. Early in 1863 a facility in Washington was set aside for diseases of the eye and ear. The West Philadelphia hospital also boasted a special department for eye injuries. John M. Cuyler suggested that special facilities be established in the New York area for "inveterate cases of chronic diarrhoea" and for diseases of the heart and nervous system. There was also an "Eye and Ear Infirmary" in St. Louis.[48]

All this came at a time when only a few subdivisions existed in even the largest civilian hospitals. The New York Commission of Charities and Corrections, for example, made a difficult decision against special wards for Bellevue Hospital in 1863 since "a census of the hospital shows too few diseases of the kind referable to the several proposed specialties, and the Board prefers to retain those in their present positions."[49] Even where institutions had enough patients to make specialized wards feasible, "specialism" was still suspect and attending physicians were under the watchful eyes of lay managers usually suspicious of research. The Civil War hospitals thus offered a few American physicians an opportunity for clinical research almost unprecedented in their own country. While they did not last long, they contributed in a significant way to the new clinical specialism that Hammond himself adopted when he moved into the private practice of neurology.

"There are few things in my professional career in which I take more pride," wrote Hammond in 1878, "than that the ideas of the Army Medical Museum and of the Medical and Surgical History of the Rebellion were conceived by me, and that both were in successful operation when Dr. Barnes succeeded to the office of Surgeon General." Hammond "duly saw and grasped a great opportunity," in the words of S. Weir Mitchell.[50] His authority as surgeon general in command of a huge corps of surgeons gave him the chance to realize the sort of large-scale collective research project that the Philadelphia Biological Society had tried unsuccessfully to organize a few years earlier.

For example, Mitchell had proposed an ethnological survey of the vital statistics of native-born white Americans. It was the only suggestion for formal collective investigation that the Society had seriously attempted to implement and the effort had died quickly. The young biologists could only raise $25 for the project, and they were unable to mobilize the necessary corps of investigators. In contrast, the careful examination of tens of thousands of Civil War recruits provided data for a study far larger and more thorough than even Mitchell had envisioned. Army physicians did the work, acting under standardized protocols, and the government picked up the tab.[51]

Other examples illustrate the same point. George Read Morehouse, encouraged by Hammond, had already interested himself in the minute anatomy of the nerves. He could research this at Turner's Lane. Joseph J. Woodward, another member of the defunct Biological Society, had been interested in microscopy. Now he could pursue it as a career officer in the Medical Department, and the Surgeon General did his best to recruit others to the field as well. "Applications for microscopes by medical officers in charge of general hospitals will be favorably considered," he announced, "provided the evidence is satisfactory that the officer will use the instrument for the benefit of science, and will report the results to the Surgeon General." A circular "on the care and use of the Army microscope" provided detailed instructions. And some surgeons did request microscopes from Washington. Among them was Elliot Coues, like Hammond an amateur ornithologist, later to be recognized as one of America's foremost naturalists.[52]

Instruments of clinical investigation were also available to army surgeons: new tools such as the stethoscope, the stomach pump, the aural speculum and even the vaginal speculum were listed in the Standard Supply Table issued by Hammond's office. Books were issued in quantity. "It is contemplated," Hammond wrote to Surgeon George Cooper in his fourth week on the job, "to place Sargeant's Minor Surgery in the hands of all the Hospital Stewards in the Army." He wanted Cooper to buy 800 copies from the publishers, and a like number of "Longmore on Gunshot Wounds; 200 of Guthrie's Commentaries on the Surgery of War & 200 of McLeeds Notes on the Surgery of the Crimean War."[53]

A general hospital or the medical officer of a regiment at a permanent post was entitled under Hammond's rules to a library of two dozen titles, including dictionaries, handbooks, textbooks in basic and clinical medical sciences, and even texts on the special diseases of the eye, the ear, and the skin, and on venereal diseases.

Not all army surgeons were interested, but some placed orders for Joseph Leidy's recent *Elementary Treatise on Human Anatomy* (1861) and current issues of the *American Journal of the Medical Sciences,* the *Medical News,* the *Boston Medical and Surgical Journal,* and the *American Medical Times.*[54]

The most persistent problem plaguing the Medical Department was the hygiene of the camps. On this subject no comprehensive English-language work existed, and the Surgeon General took it on himself to fill the gap. His *Treatise on Hygiene With Special Reference to the Military Service* (Philadelphia, 1863) received excellent reviews in the medical press and immediately became a standard work, although it went out of print shortly after the war.[55] A large part of the book concerned hospital construction, developing in practical detail the pavilion system he advocated. Hammond's recommendations were hardly novel to any medical man who kept abreast of scientific developments – but such men formed only a minority of his intended audience.

* * * * *

Hammond's work had a direct impact on the health of the troops in the field. Dr. Thomas T. Ellis was not a wholly reliable individual, but there is no reason to doubt his 1863 declaration that there had been a "marked improvement in the surgeons attached to the army in contrast with their inefficiency at the commencement of the rebellion." Sir William Muir, deputy inspector general of the British army, visited the battlefield at Antietam with Hammond and reportedly remarked afterward that "no battlefield was ever as quickly and abundantly provided with every necessary for the wounded." Henry Bellows wrote privately that "the sick and wounded owe a hundred times over more to the government and the Medical Department than to all the outside influences and benevolence of the country combined, including the Sanitary Commission. *The Surgeon-General,*" he emphasized, "*is the best friend the soldier has in this country.*"[56]

A recent study of the *Medical and Surgical History of the War* identifies four specific areas in which policies implemented by Hammond saved soldiers' lives. First, the "prompt evacuation and rapid treatment of wounded soldiers" appears to have limited infection and decreased wound mortality from over 25 percent in the first year of the war to under 10 percent in the third year. Second,

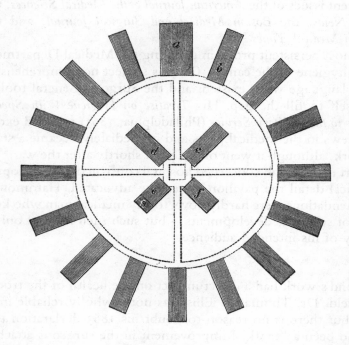

Ground plan of the Hammond General Hospital, ca. 1863. Surgeon General Hammond considered this 780-bed hospital, at the junction of the Potomac River and Chesapeake Bay (Point Lookout, Maryland), to be "one of the best, in every respect, belonging to the army." The circular arrangement of wards, linked by open corridors, allowed free circulation of the fresh sea air and encouraged efficient management. Buildings: (a) administration; (b) ward for fifty-two patients, at least twelve yards from the next ward and ventilated by twenty-four windows and two side doors and along the full 145-foot ridge of the roof; (c) kitchen; (d) mechanized laundry; (e) guard house; (f) knapsack room; (g) deadhouse. About 1,000 additional patients and some 200 medical officers and attendants resided in nearby cottages and a former hotel. (William A. Hammond, *A Treatise on Hygiene, With Special Reference to the Military Service* [Philadelphia: Lippincott, 1863], p. 378. Courtesy of Middleton Library of the Health Sciences, University of Wisconsin, Madison.)

epidemics of contagious diseases were curtailed by requiring troops to stay in training camps until "seasoned" by surviving attacks of self-limited diseases such as measles and mumps. Third, the extensive use of quinine tended to reduce the mortality from malaria. Perhaps most important, improvements in camp and hospital hygiene decreased the incidence (but not the mortality rate) of contamination disorders characterized by severe diarrhea.[57]

The policies pursued and the measures inaugurated by Hammond, with the support of medical friends such as William Van Buren, Jonathan Letterman, and Weir Mitchell, as well as the lay reformers of the Sanitary Commission, played a decisive role (by all accounts) in transforming the Medical Department of the United States Army during the Civil War. The effects on civilian medical and sanitary practices were also profound, if less direct. Mitchell wrote, for example, that "the war so trained vast numbers of country doctors that for a long time the cases for grave operations ceased to be sent to the cities as had been usual." He also saw value in "the constant mingling of men of high medical culture with the less educated." Daniel B. St. John Roosa, arguing later for physician control of hospitals, cited the Civil War institutions as a model. "These, . . . when they were upon a scale seldom equalled in any country, were entirely under the management of medical men. There was no added financial wisdom from gentlemen learned in commercial pursuits. . . In them," he stressed, "the medical profession not only exhibited its skill, but also vindicated its ability to assume the control of its own affairs." The full measure of the postbellum influence of Civil War medicine has yet to be taken.[58]

And Hammond's Civil War experiences had a crucial influence on his own career. Specialism as a scientific mode of practice became intellectually more plausible, and an empirical basis for neurology came within reach. Further, his close contact with leading physicians of the major Northern cities, especially Philadelphia and New York, established connections that would prove invaluable when he began to define himself as a full-time specialty consultant after the war. His scientific interests were thereby directed decisively toward clinical, rather than laboratory, work. And he developed a far better understanding of the limits on medical reform imposed by the nature of the profession and of American society.

5

"Foggy with embarrassments"

Shortly after Hammond took over the Medical Department he received a letter from Surgeon George Suckley, his replacement as medical director of the Army of the Cumberland, suggesting bluntly that some of the brigade surgeons be "weeded out" as incompetents. The problem was widely recognized, not the least by the soldiers in the field. Regular army physicians had all proved their qualifications through examination, but the volunteer regiments had been allowed to bring with them the practitioners of their choice. This made good medical sense in the light of traditional practice that emphasized the physician's familiarity with the family and personal history of the patient. But it conflicted with principles of national authority and scientific rigor emphasized by the Medical Department. Contract surgeons, who generally served in army hospitals, had also been employed haphazardly.

MEDICAL CREDENTIALS AND PROFESSIONAL CONFLICTS

Hammond tackled the issue boldly. "The best professional talent has not in every instance been secured in appointing the Medical Officers of the several hospitals," he wrote to Surgeon Cooper in Philadelphia on May 15, 1862. Hammond asked for the names of the incompetents so he could annul their contracts.[1] He soon instituted a system of stringent examinations for all physicians who wished to doctor the Union troops. The post of regimental physician was abolished, and all medical personnel were brought under the direct supervision of his department. For this Hammond was generally applauded. The Ohio State Medical Society, for example, offered its assistance through a communication from Governor David Tod to the War Secretary. Dr. L. A. Edwards, answering for the Surgeon General, was "happy to see such zeal . . . to promote the efficiency of the Corps of Army Surgeons," and appreciated all efforts to "secure high professional qualifications."[2]

But the idea of a standardized examination was so new that it had to be explained even to those who were to administer it. Dr J. J. Hayes wrote to Surgeon General Hammond on September 4, 1862, to report that his examining board had met that morning and organized for business. But the new members had not received detailed instructions and were "therefore quite ignorant of how to proceed, or what is required of us."[3] The surgeon general's office had to provide more guidance. "It is desirable, as far as possible, for the different examining Boards assembled for the same purposes, to adopt a uniform plan of examination and standard of proficiency," Joseph R. Smith wrote in July 1862 to Dr. T. R. Azpell, president of the St. Louis board of examiners. He enclosed a plan of examination and requested monthly reports on the outcomes.

The test began with a short written medical autobiography. Next came a written examination on anatomy, surgery, and practice of medicine, consisting of four "well-selected" questions on each, followed by an oral examination on the same subjects and on general pathology. The candidate then faced an oral examination on chemistry, physiology, hygiene, toxicology, and materia medica, and a clinical examination on medicine and surgery conducted at a hospital. Where practicable, the examination concluded with a demonstration of surgical operations on a cadaver. Obviously the examiners were allowed a great deal of leeway, but the test must have been a daunting experience for most of the candidates.[4]

Dozens, perhaps hundreds, of letters addressed to the surgeon general on the subject of examinations attest to the magnitude of the attempt by ordinary doctors to comprehend and come to terms with the new standards. For example, Dr. Griffith of Louisville, Kentucky, explained that "a constant field duty for eighteen months" had left him without "sufficient opportunity for preparing . . . for so critical an examination." He withdrew halfway through the week-long ordeal, asking that the papers he had already written on anatomy be referred to the surgeon general, apparently hoping for his personal approval. Charles R. Reber of Reading, Pennsylvania, wrote to complain that "the time allowed me, from Monday Ap. 20 to Saturday Ap. 25th [1863], with nearly the entire day of the 24th in the dissecting room was too short to do justice to the questions submitted." He could have used three more days, but the examinations were cut off on Saturday so that the results might be taken to Washington. He, too, wanted another chance.[5]

The system was, in practice, subject to political pressures and personal evasion. Stanton occasionally ordered the surgeon general's office to reexamine particular candidates who had previously failed, with the unmistakable hint that they ought to pass. Weir Mitchell, as recorder of the board of medical examiners of Philadelphia, notified Hammond formally of the problems encountered there. A Dr. J. C. Fox of that city, recommended by the eminent Dr. R. J. Levis as "a respectable medical practitioner . . . and a regular graduate in Medicine," had been examined and "marked Zero throughout. We did not consider him as fit to be a nurse," amplified Mitchell, "certainly not a cadet." But Dr. King had apparently awarded him a contract as acting assistant surgeon. Cases of this sort were so well known, Mitchell alleged, that "some of the candidates have withdrawn their names during the progress of the examination in order to secure contracts at once by direct appointment." Others complained bitterly that they lacked the influence to obtain a post. The board suggested that the test "should either be rigidly exacted or in all cases dispensed with," as the existing arrangements brought only ridicule and charges of inconsistency.[6]

Even those entrusted with enforcing the new standards seem to have had their doubts about the policy. Dr. A. P. Meylert, chairman of the Louisville examining board, wrote to ask what he should do about regimental physicians who were "well informed in the practical portion of Surgery and Medical Practice – who are men of sound mind – good judgment and who have become perfectly familiar with the routine of duty . . . and have always given satisfaction . . . but are not well informed in Chemistry, Minute Anatomy, Physiology and Pathology, and perhaps not fully informed in Materia Medica." He clearly felt he needed such men.

Meylert was also confused about the grading policy. He noticed that on the blank record forms "in some instances the maximum is 100 and the minimum 80, in others the maximum is 80 and the minimum 50, and in one instance the maximum is 50 and the minimum 30." He wanted to know whether "100 shall represent a perfect knowledge of the subject or is the standard of perfection in the one case 100, in the other 80 and in the other 50." In cases of examination for promotion, was there "any fixed minimum for the candidate to be recommended for the position of Surgeon?"[7]

Dr. Meylert was not the only puzzled correspondent. Questions poured in from across the country. Were those found unfit for the position of surgeon of volunteers automatically ineligible for the post of assistant surgeon? Were females eligible for examination? Were black physicians eligible? Should all applicants be examined, or only those who were graduates in medicine? Was examination necessary for applicants as surgeon to the U.S. Colored Troops?[8] A picture emerges from the correspondence of the surgeon general's office of an extremely heterogeneous medical profession lacking consensus even on minimum standards of eligibility.

The men chosen to serve on the examining boards were among the leaders of the profession. From the point of view of the medical elite, it could scarcely have been otherwise. Yet the weeding-out process highlighted and even exacerbated tensions between this elite and their earnest though poorly educated professional colleagues. The hardworking physician who may have already served in the army for a year or more in the field surely resented the arrival of a curt letter requesting his resignation on the basis of a poor showing on what may have seemed an unreasonable test. Women physicians, unorthodox healers, and others denied even the privilege of examination must have been equally resentful. The issue of physicians' qualifications probably contributed more to the voluminous correspondence of the surgeon general's office than any other.

On the surface, the profession seemed to stand behind Hammond's policy. Medical editors generally belonged to the well-educated elite, or at least identified with it, and supported the more restrictive standards. Those who failed the tests may have been disgruntled, but they were probably also at least a little ashamed. While there was little open opposition to the concept of qualifying examinations, they generated considerable hostility toward Hammond, the tinder that would ignite with his famous "calomel order." Weir Mitchell later recollected that, "as the Surgeon General said, there was not an aspect of his work which was not foggy with embarrassments."[9] Here was a prime example.

Apparently Hammond was not satisfied with the quality even of

the physicians who passed the entrance examinations, for he proposed the establishment of a special school to instruct them in
military medicine and hygiene. It was modeled on the medical
schools of the English and French armies, and the students were to
be graduate physicians already accepted into the Army Medical
Corps. In a sense it foreshadowed the postgraduate schools organized (by Hammond, among others) twenty years later.

Classes were to be held in a room specially fitted up for this
purpose in the basement of the building housing the Army Medical Museum that Hammond had organized in his first months on
the job.[10] The museum collection would thus be readily available
to illustrate lectures to be given by some of the outstanding American physicians belonging to the Medical Department. John H.
Brinton would teach "gunshot injuries" and Richard H. Coolidge,
"customs of the service and military medical ethics." William
Thomas and Joseph J. Woodward were responsible for "military
medicine." Dr. J. J. Sidell would provide instruction in "chemical
surgery," probably anesthesia and antisepsis. Other prominent
physicians, such as Roberts Bartholow, would also be on hand.

The only thing lacking was the approval of the Secretary of War.
But Stanton was not interested. The students, he said, would
simply go to the theater and neglect their official duties. He delayed formal denial of permission until the end of the war, and no
army medical school would exist until the 1890s. Hammond was,
however, able to encourage medical schools to provide formal
instruction in hygiene and military surgery by ordering in December 1862 that all candidates for appointment to the medical
staff of the regular army must have attended such a course.[11] He
was also able to grant permission to medical cadets and assistant
surgeons to attend medical lectures in order to further their education and to prepare for the examinations. Such permission was
generously bestowed by the young surgeon general who had tried
so hard and so unsuccessfully to obtain it himself.[12]

THERAPEUTIC CONTROVERSIES

One of the trickiest personnel issues concerned homeopathic doctors. Many Americans were favorably disposed to this medical
sect, and its practitioners were frequently at least as well educated
as their "allopathic," or regular, counterparts. Illinois Governor

Richard Yates, for example, complained to the War Department that the Medical Examining Board was composed entirely of "Allopathists who refuse to examine homeopathists and thereby turned away many valuable physicians." This was indeed the policy. Homeopaths "are not considered by this Department eligible or fit to be entrusted with the great responsibility of the health and lives of our brave soldiers," Joseph Smith explained to Yates. "This Department, while straining every nerve to make every proper provision for the care of the sick and wounded, is clear in its conviction that rather than employ an incompetent officer it is preferable to employ none."

But such a rigid – dogmatic, some might have said – policy was difficult to enforce. The two systems were virtually identical in many respects, including anatomy, physiology, and surgery. Some "homeopathists have been examined and passed on the supposition that they were allopathists." The questions that would distinguish between the schools might not be asked unless the candidate were suspected of homeopathic leanings. And then there seemed to be nothing to prevent a physician from practicing on the homeopathic system once in the service. For example, Dr. William T. Collins, formerly assistant surgeon to the Sixth Delaware Volunteers, complained that Captain Newberry was employing the homeopath C. L. Mahan to tend the troops, in violation of Collins's contract. But Collins was clearly an interested party.[13]

And if the surgeon general's office did not sympathize with homeopathy, other friends could be found in the army hierarchy. For example, J. M. Howard of Detroit transmitted directly to Stanton a memorial of the Michigan Homeopathic Institute, requesting equal privileges. These physicians declared themselves "*without exception* loyal and patriotic men." Comparing their situation to that of chaplains, they argued that "a Republican government cannot with propriety have a national system of Religion or, legitimately, a national practice of medicine." Howard himself had "great confidence in the homeopathic style of practice in cases of individual ailment, tho' not so much where the disease has attacked a whole nation." He feared that "our excellent Surgeon General Dr. Hammond wont [*sic*] agree" but expected that both he and Stanton "will do what is honest & right." "[I]f you won't," he added ominously, "I avow I will appeal to *McClellan,* who believes in and practices the homeopathic system."[14]

Mid-century America abounded in therapeutic systems and empirical cures. Whether because of philanthropy or avarice or a
combination of both, the surgeon general's office was flooded
with offers of service, complaints of discrimination, and gra-
tuitous advice from all quarters. Two New York chiropodists and
another from Philadelphia wanted positions, and I. Zacharias suggested the creation of a whole corps of chiropodists to treat the
foot soldiers of the republic. W. H. Cook of Cincinnati wanted to
treat cases by the Botanic method, if the patients wanted such care.
Sherman B. Lum of Boscobel, Wisconsin, wanted to take charge
of a hospital where he could treat diseases on "principles of his
own." New England hydropaths offered their establishments for
use as military hospitals. Albert Borchard was "a curer of Rheumatism," J. F. Terry of Detroit an "oculist," and A. Williams of
Albany, New York, was a "medical Electrician." The well-known
water-cure advocate R. T. Trall of Harrisburg, Pennsylvania,
wanted to practice the "Hygienic Plan" on the battlefield itself,
while Ruth C. Thompson offered to serve for six months without
pay in a military hospital established on the same principle.[15]

The most notorious of the irregulars was surely "a certain quack
named Forsha," in the words of Sanitary Commissioner George
Templeton Strong, "proprietor of a certain oil which acts like
magic on all wounds and contusions." Forsha had convinced President Lincoln, as well as half a dozen cabinet members, to intercede
on his behalf. Hammond stood firm, insisting that Forsha was "an
ignorant pretender, and that if he wants his panacea used by the
Medical Bureau he must reveal its ingredients." "I have met with
Dr. Forsha before and am satisfied that he is an ignorant quack," he
wrote to Lincoln.[16]

It was not always easy in mid-century America to distinguish
quackish remedies from potentially useful items. Suggestions
poured into the surgeon general's office for products the army
might wish to purchase: Frederic Brown's "essence of ginger";
Piercey's Piles Pipes; Condy's Disinfecting Fluid; a prescription
from Circleville, Ohio, for the prevention of lockjaw; Champlin &
Co.'s "Golden Treasure"; and the "Anti-Rheumatic Bands" of G.
Smith & Co., to name a few. The State Department forwarded
suggestions from abroad: the U.S. consul at Manchester offered
the timely suggestion of carbolic acid as an antiseptic and disinfectant, the minister at Paris sent a box of chemicals (the gift of a local

manufacturer), and the consul at Malta passed along news of the recent discovery of inoculation with quinine.[17]

Some of these ideas could, perhaps, be disregarded, but the Medical Department was loath to reject anything that might lessen the terrible mortality among the troops. Systematic tests were often ordered. Warren Webster, assistant surgeon at the Douglas Hospital in Washington, conducted trials of Minthon's Disinfecting Fluid and tested "chloride of propylamin" for rheumatism. R. S. Satterlee found the "Blistering Tissue" of Messrs. E. and S. Fougera to be "a convenient article, and not very expensive." The "Powdre Corne" recommended by Elisha Harris was found useful for general disinfection and as a dressing for "foetid ulcers," but the surgeon general's office was unable to locate a supplier.

Eventually facilities were established in Astoria, Queens, and in Philadelphia for the analysis of samples of chemical and pharmaceutical supplies, and the production of expensive or unobtainable substances. Coolidge had suggested such an army laboratory seven years earlier, recommending that Hammond be put in charge. Now Hammond was in the position to establish the lab himself. America's leading pharmaceutical manufacturer, Edward R. Squibb, generously allowed army personnel to examine his premises and methods, although the government enterprise clearly represented serious competition.[18]

At first Hammond thought the official pharmacopoeia too limited. He had Surgeon Edwards send Richard Satterlee, the medical purveyor for New York, a list of preparations that should be added to the supplies or ordered in greater quantities: gum acacia, opium, and powdered gum to make paregoric and laudanum; and colchicum, zinc carbonate, bicarbonate and nitrate of potash, expectorants, and vegetable tonics. More instruments were wanted for the hospitals, beyond the personal cases issued to individual surgeons. Satterlee had complained that Hammond's requests were excessive; now Hammond was complaining that Satterlee's were deficient. He also directed Satterlee to enlist the help of Drs. Abbott and Squibb in enlarging the supply tables.[19]

The Surgeon General issued a series of circulars on therapeutics to supplement the periodic revisions of the supply table. For example, Circular #12 (July 29, 1863) called the attention of medical officers to "the virtues of Permanganate of Potassa as a disinfectant and deodorizer." Circular #13, two weeks later, permitted the substitution of Tarragona wine for port wine, which was unavailable. Distribution of the circulars was irregular and their filing haphazard. For example, S. H. Melcher requested a complete file of the circulars for the Army of Southwestern Missouri and the Army of the Frontier, as he could not obtain one in St. Louis. "No. 20 is being copied by the Medical Officers in this Army," he wrote in November 1862, "not one fourth of whom had ever heard of them before last week and not one in 20 seen a single number you have issued."[20] One circular, however, became known to almost everyone: Hammond's famous "calomel order," Circular #6, issued on May 4, 1863.

Motivated by reports of widespread overuse of calomel and tartar emetic, Hammond announced the removal of these staples of heroic practice from the supply table. That meant they would no longer be made available routinely, although surgeons could order them by special request. To many physicians this order seemed not only wrongheaded but inconceivable. Surgeon H. S. Hendee of the 153d Regiment, New York Volunteers, stationed in Alexandria, Virginia, read incredulously a newspaper report that Hammond had prohibited the use of calomel and tartar emetic, and dashed off an indignant letter to the editor. "I have received no such order or circular," he wrote, thinking the report mistaken. "If not a mistake, then is the circular breathing an unmittigated [*sic*] wrong (however unintended by the General) to the Medical profession of the Union Army. And not only to us," he added, "but to the Fathers of the profession for four thousand years past."

Hendee conceded that "the use of Calomel & Tar. Emetic has been abused in the Army in individual instances," but felt strongly that "to place two thousand Surgeons & Asst. Surgeons of our Army under the ban of incompitancy [*sic*] to prescribe those articles when actually indicated . . . is more than the good natured forbearance & intelligence of the profession can cheerfully endure." He believed that "our Surgeon-in-chief is far from desiring in word or deed to place the Surgeons of the Army under such lasting disgrace both at home and abroad," and asked the editor of the *Chronicle* to give his missive "the same publicity that you have the *Sensation* article" that had prompted him to write.[21]

The Surgeon General had spent most of his professional life in the company of the medical elite of the country. For the most part, the order was supported enthusiastically by this segment of the profession. The calomel order may have even been instigated by one of the medical members of the Sanitary Commission, most likely William H. Van Buren or Cornelius R. Agnew. About a year before his death Hammond was planning to tell the whole story in print, but the manuscript, if it ever existed, was never found.[22]

In wider medical circles, however, the order was roundly condemned. The Ohio Medical Society, which had supported Hammond less than a year earlier, passed and publicized a resolution against the new policy. Ohio Governor David Tod wrote personally to the War Department to urge that the order be rescinded. A large portion of the annual meeting of the American Medical Association was devoted to a heated and largely critical discussion of Hammond's move. In the face of this pressure, Hammond issued a belated and rather one-sided questionnaire to physicians across the country. It surveyed the extent to which they used the disputed remedies in their own practices, and their opinion as to the possibilities of misuse under the stressful and often unsupervised conditions of army medicine.

The debate raged for years. Surgeon John R. McClurg of the Army General Hospital in Cleveland, Ohio, kept Hammond abreast of developments there. A Dr. Weber, who had recently been "expelled from the faculty" of the Cleveland Medical College, had "been using all his efforts against the Surgeon General on account of his order against Calomel & Tart Emetic. He is an ambitious man," McClurg warned, "& will do all in his power in this respect but I *now well know*," he emphasized, "that public sentiment among Physicians & surgeons is turning strongly in favor of the Order."[23] The Baltimore Medical Association was still debating the issue in 1867.[24]

Hammond had not completely proscribed the medications. Other mercurials were still listed in the supply table, and calomel could be had by special order. But unlike Hendee he felt that the abuse of calomel did outweigh its beneficial effects. His order was, as John Harley Warner has explained, "a singularly publicized and institutionally powerful criticism of the kind American physicians since the 1820s had been bringing against therapeutic excesses engendered by mechanical adherence to theory and habit." But the publicity and force of the decree were perhaps its most offensive features. Physicians feared that its newspaper notoriety would encourage sectarian healers and discourage public confidence in the medical profession. It was seen as restrictive and illiberal, revoking the practitioner's time-honored freedom of clinical judgment. Whatever the Surgeon General's original intention – and it is hard to tell whether he had foreseen the clamor his order would provoke – he had in effect "launched a frontal attack on the therapeutic tradition." As Hendee suggested, Hammond's order was seen as "indicting both past and current practice."[25]

Hammond had intended to use the surgeon generalcy to advance the interests of the medical profession, but he seems not to have taken into account that this profession was itself deeply divided. His "inconsiderate action," in the words of S. Weir Mitchell, served mainly to deepen already existing rifts.[26] The examination policies had already alienated many physicians who had been told they were not qualified to serve under the brash young surgeon general. Now even those who had been certified as competent felt insulted. Hammond's base of support was narrowing rapidly, leaving him increasingly vulnerable to attacks by politically motivated or vindictive enemies.

COURT-MARTIAL

Hammond exercised the authority of the surgeon general's office for only sixteen months. By February 1863, less than a year after his appointment, the Sanitary Commission was already worried about his position. "The Surgeon-General has brought order out of chaos in his department," wrote Henry Bellows to Henry Wilson, "and efficiency out of imbecility. . . . For God's sake don't thwart his zeal and wisdom!" In March George T. Strong recorded in his diary, "Talked mostly of the feud between Stanton and the Surgeon General, and of measures to restore harmony between them, or to bring the case before the President or before the people." A month later Strong reported a conversation that was said to have taken place between the War Secretary and Mr. Whiting, solicitor for the War Department. "'Well,' said the Secretary, 'the fact is the Commission wanted Hammond to be Surgeon General and I did not. I did my best with the President and with the Military Committee of the Senate, but the Commission beat me and got Hammond appointed. I'm not used to being beaten, and don't like it, and therefore I am hostile to the Commission.'"[27]

Hammond suspected trouble in August when he was ordered

on a tour of inspection of the western posts, which Stanton had previously refused to authorize. Shortly before he left, the Surgeon General told Strong, Agnew, and Van Buren that, as Strong reported it, Hammond thought it "the first step in a scheme of Stanton's to supersede him." Strong confided to his diary that "he is probably right. Stanton shook him by both hands when he bade him good-bye, and it is generally understood at Washington that that mark of cordiality is the invariable precursor of some stab or blow at its recipient."[28]

Hammond was a bit more reticent with his scientific friends, but they soon learned of his troubles and began to rally support. F. J. Hayden suggested to Joseph Leidy in September that they should begin a scientists' letter-writing campaign on Hammond's behalf, and outlined the contents of the letter Leidy was to write to the President. "Will his friends suffer him to be deposed without a severe struggle –," he asked rhetorically. "Write to [our] friends who may need working up somewhat in the matter," he urged; "I would like to be called to Washington in the winter and then I might work [harder] for him among certain friends who would regard my wishes."

"I am ready to do all in my power," responded Leidy. "We were as much surprised as you to learn of his virtual displacement, and even now are at a loss to know the cause." He and Weir Mitchell were at work on a plan of action. Their motives extended beyond personal loyalty to Hammond: Leidy feared that "all his plans for the establishment of an Army Medical and Surgical Museum, etc., would be broken up."[29]

In fact, Stanton had appointed a special commission in mid-July with a broad mandate to look into the affairs of the Medical Department. This fishing expedition was headed by Hammond's old enemy, ex-Governor Andrew H. Reeder of Kansas. In August Stanton had demanded a compilation of all the reports of all medical inspectors and all other medical officers from the beginning of the war to date. The patently biased investigatory commission used as an agent one Silas H. Swetland, who had gotten the endorsements of several members of Congress for his appeal to Hammond for an appointment as inspector of liquors for the Medical Department. When Hammond turned him down, saying that no such position existed or was needed, Swetland complained to Stanton – and got a job with the Reeder commission instead.[30]

Almost nobody was surprised when rumors began circulating

that Reeder's investigators had found irregularities and improprieties in Hammond's office. But Strong and the other Sanitary Commissioners saw no immediate reason to intervene. Hammond's reform efforts had many supporters as well as detractors, and the rumored charges must have seemed trivial amid the bloody war news. "The Surgeon General deserves special commendation," editorialized the *Medical Times,* for he had "set an example which other departments may follow to advantage."[31] Besides, for what it was worth, the War Secretary had personally assured Helen Hammond that "he never dreamed of ousting her husband from the Surgeon Generalship." Strong thought optimistically in September that "perhaps Stanton has been a little enlightened within the last month." A letter that had been planted in the *Herald,* supposedly written by a surgeon of volunteers, in fact written by Col. Charles G. Halpine, had "made a sensation in the medico-military circles of Washington." It appeared to have convinced the War Secretary that "his manipulation of the Medical Bureau was watched."[32] Besides, the Sanitary Commission, weakened by internal strife and the resignation of Frederick Law Olmsted as general secretary, had enough problems of its own.

Hammond finished up his western inspection tour, but Stanton would not issue the orders to return him to Washington. Christmas 1863 found him languishing in Tennessee. The Sanitary Commission finally decided to act. "We propose to open the campaign with an address to the President by the Sanitary Commission," wrote Strong on December 23, "and perhaps to follow this up by a circular to a few leading Congressmen which is already in type and has been signed by Agassiz, Peirce, Hill, and Longfellow of Harvard, and by a lot of eminent New York and Boston doctors." The Commission could also be devious. "The first gun will be fired in the next (fifth) number of the [Sanitary Commission] *Bulletin,*" Strong confided. "It is an anonymous letter purporting to come from an outsider, asking information as to the meaning of the Surgeon General's banishment to Knoxville, which letter I concocted last night." He rather enjoyed the maneuver. "Agnew read it to Van Buren and Bellows this evening, and they heartily approved it without knowing who wrote it."[33] The letter, signed "Republican," appeared on the first of the year with an editorial comment expressing confidence that the American people would not allow Hammond to be "officially garroted."[34]

Hammond, still in Tennessee, had meanwhile fallen down a flight of stairs, injuring his spinal cord. Both legs were partially paralyzed below the knees. Characteristically, Strong noted, the patient was "profoundly interested in the minute scientific observations and experiments he is making in his own case and diligently recording."[35] He recovered without much difficulty, to find legal troubles staring him in the face.

Hammond returned to Washington in mid-January on crutches. The War Secretary was hesitating in the face of the swirl of disapproval generated by the Sanitary Commission. An editorial in the *Medical Times* portrayed the investigation as having "an appearance of a secret and deliberate conspiracy against the Surgeon General directly, and against the medical department indirectly." Physicians were urged to lay aside "whatever prejudices may have been created by any of [Hammond's] official acts." The calomel order was still fresh in the minds of many. But "a united effort [must] be made to restore him to his legitimate position, or secure him a fair and impartial hearing."[36] Foreign representatives of the medical profession were already taking his side.[37]

Stanton hinted that he might be willing to drop the affair. Strong noted that "being politic as well as arbitrary, he told a Senator to tell a surgeon to tell Hammond that he would abandon the persecution if H. would consent to let bygones be bygones." But Hammond was as stubborn as he was proud. "He would be glad to do so if the Secretary would apologize, but . . . if the Secretary wouldn't, he must have a court-martial" to clear his name. It was a serious misjudgment, as his friends tried to convince him. "The Surgeon General gave me an outline of the case," Strong continued, "and on *his* showing it is plain enough, of course. He proposed to try his own case, without counsel, against which preposterous course I gave him advice gratis, most emphatically."

Behind-the-scenes machinations continued. Now Louis Agassiz and Benjamin Peirce, two of the original signers of the circular, denied any connection with it. They left a widespread impression that Hammond's defense had perpetrated a fraud. Strong was bitter. "They were at Washington last week attending a session of the National Academy of Sciences." Stanton refused to meet them at dinner, and "when the Wise Men heard this, their hearts failed them and their knees became as water, because they had given offense to a great mandarin and a Cabinet member; so they declared it was all a forgery and a fabrication. They never signed the circular," continued Strong, "or did anything else that could be displeasing unto so sweet a prince – God forbid they should presume to take on themselves to do this thing! Did the Honorable Secretary suppose they didn't know their place? Of course they knowed their place! Were they not even as dead dogs before our Honorable Secretary? Of course, they were," Strong wound up, "and that's my opinion too."[38]

Strong's judgment may have been excessively harsh. The fledgling National Academy and the Permanent Commission of the Navy with which it was connected were both in a precarious position early in 1864, and the scientists had good reason to avoid antagonizing military authorities. And the scientific community was itself divided over the National Academy. Leidy had written to Hayden in June 1863 that he expected it to be a "grand humbug" and intended to have nothing to do with it. "A society of the kind that leaves out such men as Baird, Draper, Hammond, Lea, Cassin, yourself," he scoffed, "and appropriates a number who never turned a pen or did a thing for science, certainly can't be of much value."[39] In any case, Hammond's own naiveté hurt him far more than the defection of a few scientific leaders who had difficulty making their own claims heard.

Hammond demanded a court-martial, and he got one. But it was officially designated as being at the request of the government, a fact of which the defendant was ignorant and which worked against his interests. The specific charges now seem almost ridiculously insignificant in the context of the daily tragedies of the war years, but to the military mind they could well have appeared to be significant breaches of discipline. It was claimed, first, that he had exceeded his legal authority by personally ordering a quantity of blankets, rather than following the normal procedure of ordering a medical purveyor to make the purchase. The blankets were said to have been overpriced and of poor quality.

Reeder's report had not accused Hammond of corrupt intent, but Judge Advocate General John A. Bingham, who prosecuted the case himself, did make that claim a part of the legal charges. Hammond argued that it was absurd to suppose that he could not legally do himself what he was allowed to authorize a subordinate to do. Comparison shopping was not feasible in a wartime mar-

ket, and it was never alleged that the Surgeon General had personally profited from the transactions, although in Bingham's version
Hammond was guilty of favoring his friends.[40]

The remaining charges revolved around alleged conduct unbecoming an officer and a gentleman. Hammond had told Surgeon George E. Cooper that he had been replaced at Philadelphia
by Surgeon Robert Murray at the request of General Hallack. As
Hallack failed to recollect this request, Hammond was accused of
lying to Cooper. Hammond claimed that documents that would
have exonerated him had disappeared from his desk during his
absence in the West. The evidence thus came down to one man's
word against another's. To many at the time and since, the alleged
transgressions, even if proved, scarcely warranted the removal of a
man who had so successfully conducted the main business of his
office.[41]

When Stanton finally moved, he moved quickly. The trial began
on January 19, 1864, the court refusing the defendant's request for
a postponement. Hammond wanted time to prepare his case and
to bring his former assistant and star witness, Joseph R. Smith,
back from Little Rock to testify. He was still optimistic, saying
privately that he thought well of the court and detected "no symptom of prejudice or partiality." Strong was less so. Although he
believed Hammond's case "honest and good," he did not expect an
acquittal. "Some impulsive blunder of his will probably spoil it,
and Stanton is an ugly adversary."[42]

In retrospect, the outcome of the trial was probably never in
doubt. Reeder had done his work carefully, and Judge Advocate
General Bingham proved increasingly hostile to the defendant.
Although the proceedings dragged on for months, producing a
voluminous manuscript record, the court recessed for less than
two hours before reaching a verdict of guilty. President Lincoln
confirmed the sentence of dismissal, and Hammond left the service in official disgrace on August 18, 1864, just ten days before his
thirty-sixth birthday.[43]

Throughout the trial Hammond had expected an acquittal, or at
worst a minor reprimand. Just days before the verdict he told
Joseph Henry that "the court-martial could find nothing against
him of any consequence." In this he was not alone. Samuel Jackson, one of the most prominent of the older generation of American physicians, had written to him in mid-May that he had "read

your defence and vindication with great pleasure. . . . [Y]ou have not only silenced your detractors but have exposed their malice and folly." He was gratified that "the wiles of the envious, the jealous and malicious are defeated and the evil intended for others recoils on the inventors." He fully expected that "a reputation, destined to be . . . the pride of the profession of the country" would emerge "without a stain."[44]

Shocked, hurt, angered, and disillusioned by the unexpected verdict of guilty, Hammond threw himself into the cause of vindicating himself before the public. He quickly exhausted his financial resources in the publication and distribution of a lengthy pamphlet telling his side of the story. Some American physicians, still angry about the calomel order, delighted in Hammond's embarrassment, but many medical men on both sides of the Atlantic supported their colleague. The *American Medical Times* expressed "profound regret" since Hammond had represented American medicine not just formally but "as a man of science" whose official career had not disappointed his friends. The *Archives Générales de Médecine* gave French physicians an account favorable to Hammond of what the editor called "un triste épisode." Joseph Henry told Alexander Dallas Bache in private that "I cannot believe that he has been guilty of a dishonest act although in his zeal for the service and the advance of the medical profession he may have been imprudent." Henry was "very sorry for him and his family" and thought he would yet have a chance to "vindicate his character."[45]

Henry did not suggest to Bache that they help Hammond to do so, and apparently neither the Sanitary Commissioners nor Hammond's other friends were prepared to help him continue his fight. The ex–surgeon general wrote immediately to George B. Moore, president of the College of Physicians of Philadelphia, to which he belonged, seeking assistance. If the "charges involving my personal honor . . . are true," he conceded, "I am unworthy to remain a member of a high-toned scientific society." But "if they are false it is I conceive the right and duty of the College of Physicians to vindicate the unjustly aspersed character of one of its fellows." Hammond therefore requested that the college "appoint a committee to examine the record . . . and determine whether or not it contains any evidence which reflects directly or indirectly upon my character as a physician and a gentleman."[46] Aid of this sort was not forthcoming, and Hammond's vindication was delayed fifteen years.[47] His friends were more interested in helping him get back on his feet than they were in fighting his battles for him.

Hammond's reputation sustained less damage from the court-martial than either his pride or his pocketbook. For example, the eminent surgeon D. J. Larrey addressed Hammond as "Sir and very honored confrere" only a few years later.[48] Only his bitterest enemies ever taunted him publicly with his dismissal, and his vindication, when it came, was welcomed by physicians across the country. But the affair obviously hurt him deeply. Hammond's first novel, *Robert Severne* (1867), concerned a gentleman preoccupied with philosophical studies who is falsely accused of the murder of his wife. The hero learns through his legal misadventures (as perhaps the author thought he himself did) who are his friends and who are his enemies.

Hammond tried hard not to bear a grudge, but he could not entirely hide his resentment. In a revealing eulogy of Abraham Lincoln he remarked in May 1865 that the dead president's character, unlike that of most persons, had not been misunderstood during his life. The president who had refused to grant Mrs. Hammond an interview was described less than a year later as honest, sincere, and even merciful. "If, during his administration, acts were done in his name not in themselves right," Hammond wrote, "if others were omitted which should have been performed; if wrongs were inflicted upon individuals for which full amendment can never be made, the responsibility cannot with justice be fastened upon him." These errors were the fault of his advisers, "in whom he trusted with the childlike confidence which formed so prominent a feature of his open and ingenuous disposition."[49] Hammond, still smarting from his own personal wrong, and perhaps somewhat less ingenuous than he had been a year earlier, embarked on a career almost unique among American physicians of his day: a full-time specialty consulting practice in the highly competitive medical world of New York.

6

"A New York medical man"

"Had any shadow of disgrace attached to [Hammond] in 1864," wrote Spencer Fullerton Baird fifteen years later, "we should not have witnessed his rapid ascent to the very height of the profession in his specialty, which has given him perhaps the most lucrative medical practice in the United States." According to the eminent naturalist, "the appreciation of Dr. Hammond's character is also shown by his social status in New York, associating as he does with the best people of that city, and being brought forward prominently on all public occasions." Professor Hammond, remarked a colleague in 1888, "has perhaps been among the busiest of active practitioners in America . . . and [his] investigations and records have established him as the father of, and *the* authority in American neurology."[1]

Hammond reached the summit of his specialty in part by building and promoting institutions in which neurology could be taught, discussed, and perpetuated. But his success was ultimately based on his neurological practice. Hammond had an almost uncanny ability to attract and generally to satisfy his clients. This talent is all the more noteworthy in view of the incurability of the conditions that characterized so many of his patients and the vagueness of the complaints of an even greater number. These two aspects of his work – the clinical and the organizational – were intimately related. The neurologist's reputation among his peers contributed to his practice directly through referrals and consultations, and indirectly through the publicity his scientific work attracted. At the same time, his practical success supplied him with case materials for study, and also made it difficult for other physicians to ignore his work, even when they thought him in error.

Clinical neurology proved to be the forum for the most sustained expression of Hammond's scientific interests. In common with the vast majority of physicians of his day, he organized his professional life mainly around seeing patients in the setting of an individual entrepreneurial private practice. The scientific ambition that inspired him to specialize in neurology set him apart from most of his contemporaries. But Hammond's neurology was quite different from the twentieth-century science bearing the same name, and bore the distinct imprint of the conditions of medical practice in Gilded Age America.

NEUROLOGY AND MEDICAL SPECIALISM

When Hammond arrived in New York in the winter of 1864–65, the idea of an exclusive specialty practice was almost unheard of in respectable American medical circles. A physician wishing to concentrate on a particular class of patients would most likely seek an appointment as professor of that branch of medicine in one of the leading medical schools. Any other route invited charges of quackery. Advertising one's specialty on calling cards, letterheads, or (still worse) in the newspapers would violate the code of ethics to which all respectable physicians subscribed. But professorships and affiliations with special hospital services or clinics could properly be made known.

Since a relatively small group of privileged physicians had access to these institutions, many others saw the situation as unjust. The letter columns of medical journals were filled with complaints. "Private doctors are not allowed to advertise by the code of ethics," bemoaned one especially noisy opponent of specialism, "but doctors who get themselves attached to public institutions are allowed full sway as to advertising, providing it is done in a certain way." He concluded that "what is sauce for the goose is *not* sauce for the gander."[2] Hammond was a star example of one who made the most out of this controversial opportunity.

Neurology was rarely taught as a separate branch of medicine before the Civil War, although psychiatry was. Even in France the first chair specifically devoted to neurology was not created until 1882. M. Gonzalez Echeverría gave a course of lectures on the nervous system at University Medical College in New York in 1861. Harvard created a professorship of "Physiology and Pathology of the Nervous System" for Charles Edouard Brown-

Séquard in 1864. But when Hammond sought to establish a practice in New York that same year, no permanent positions existed there for neurological instruction.[3] The College of Physicians and Surgeons created a post for him as lecturer on diseases of the mind and nervous system during the winter term 1866–67, after his return from Europe. The combination of mental and nervous diseases into one pedagogical unit was an innovation tailored to Hammond's conception of the new field he was attempting to create. At the same time the new "Outdoor Department" of Bellevue Hospital began a clinic for "Nerves" with Hammond (together with W. R. Gillette) in charge.[4] The positions probably brought little direct remuneration, but they allowed the aspiring neurologist to examine a substantial number and variety of cases in his area of interest at a time when he still had few private patients. They also "advertised" the direction of his new practice.

Bellevue Hospital's new Medical College, opened in 1861, already ranked close to the College of Physicians and Surgeons and University Medical College among the leading schools in the city. Bellevue faculty members took pride in their special courses preliminary to the regular winter sessions, in the "union of clinical and didactic teaching" that its students (in theory, at least) received, and in the "Analytical Medical Chemistry Laboratory" outfitted for the use of fifty or sixty students.[5] A new professorship of diseases of the mind and nervous system was created there for Hammond in the fall of 1867 and promoted enthusiastically by his colleagues. Again, the broad scope of the position reflected Hammond's program for neurology. His introductory address "On the Proper Use of the Mind" was widely reported in medical journals across the country.

Hammond's lectures were, according to the Bellevue catalog, "both didactic and clinical." His course began with "the theoretical knowledge of the various diseases to which the brain, the spinal cord, and the nerves are liable." Later, cases were "brought before the class for opinions relative to diagnosis and treatment." Hammond featured the therapeutic use of electricity. He recommended to the students the works of Henry Maudsley, Robert Bentley Todd, and Handfield Jones, but when the course began there was no comprehensive English-language textbook on neurology. Hammond himself published the first one in 1871, his *Treatise on the Diseases of the Nervous System.* The reading list was kept current with the addition of G. Fielding Blandford's *Insanity and Its Treatment* (Am. ed. 1871), Weir Mitchell's *Injuries of Nerves and Their Consequences* (1872), and Hammond's translation of Moritz Meyer, *Electricity in Its Relation to Practical Medicine* (Am. ed. 1869).[6] On paper, this is a rather impressive picture of neurological education. But Charles L. Dana commented acidly in 1900 that a quarter of a century earlier "teaching neurology to medical students . . . [had] consisted measurably [sic] in telling that of which we knew little to those who could not possibly know anything. Neurology was unripe," he continued, "but the medical student was still more so."[7]

Patients, however, were plentiful, and Hammond sharpened and demonstrated his technical skills on them in a variety of settings. In 1869 he began a new Saturday afternoon clinic for the outpatient treatment of insanity. It was modeled on the Berlin facility of Wilhelm Griesinger and was widely (though perhaps inaccurately) noted as the second of its kind in the world.[8] Two years later he opened the New York State Hospital for Diseases of the Nervous System, located at the corner of Second Avenue and St. Marks Place in lower Manhattan. This avowedly charitable institution received initial funding of $2,000 from the state of New York, along with private donations. It had the frank objective of "afford-[ing] an opportunity to physicians and medical students for clinical observation and instruction in the . . . diseases of the brain and nervous system." It even contained a "museum of the normal and pathological anatomy of the nervous system, with Dr. John J. Mason as curator."[9] The institution may well have been modeled on the British "National Hospital for the Paralyzed and Epileptic," established in 1859 and already, under John Hughlings Jackson and William R. Gowers, a major center for neurological research. In fact, George M. Beard had announced in 1869 that "just such an institution is needed in New York."[10]

The in-patient facilities of the New York hospital were never solidly established, primarily because additional funds were not obtained. But the clinics were well attended. T. M. B. Cross, resident physician, reported that 194 patients had made a total of 2,340 visits during the first eight months, and had received over 1,200 prescriptions. Thus the clinic was seeing an average of about one new patient per day, and a total of sixty-seven patients per week. The typical patient made twelve visits to the clinic, with at least six different prescriptions for each case. Active therapeutic intervention was still common practice. Allen McLane Hamilton, physician-in-charge during the second year, reported a 30 percent increase in attendance (372 patients who made 4,592 visits in a twelve-month period) and declared the new dispensary, opened in 1871, a success. Even with this increase, however, the facility only served an average of eighty-eight patients per week. The institution closed during its third year, but it served for a time as a focal point for the emerging specialty of neurology in New York. Hammond's assistants at Bellevue Medical College (Reuben A. Vance, T. M. B. Cross, and C. T. Whybrew) were all among the attending physicians at the hospital, along with four other members of the New York Neurological Society. This group, organized by Hammond in the spring of 1872 as the first specifically neurological association in the United States, held its meetings at the hospital.[11]

Like many aspiring specialists, Hammond taught gratis for several years in the summer sessions of the University of Vermont. He also offered short courses at Bellevue Medical College in the optional sessions preceding each winter term. Here he presented his recent work on whatever interested him at the moment: paralysis, sleep, medical electricity. The latest therapeutic innovations were also shared and debated. These courses were a step toward postgraduate medical education, an innovation that would soon draw much of his attention.

Hammond's colleagues on the Bellevue faculty indicated their confidence in his general clinical ability by appointing him professor of materia medica and therapeutics when the post came open in 1872. But his instruction in this area differed from that of his predecessor, B. F. McCready. According to the *Annual Circular,* he would teach "not only didactically, but, as far as possible, by experiments on living animals, and by clinical observation of the effects of medicinal agents." Despite his new clinical preoccupation, Hammond was clearly still very committed to experimental physiology. Students were reassured that "Materia Medica will not be neglected," but the new professor would emphasize "the physiological and therapeutical properties of the remedies."[12] Here was an attempt to raise the scientific level of medical education, not by institutional reform but by individual initiative. But the innovation did not last. When Hammond resigned from the faculty in August 1873, his successor, the neurologist Edward Janeway, omitted the promise (perhaps never fulfilled) of animal experiments. At the same time, important changes were made in the teaching of Hammond's specialty. The chair of "Diseases of the Mind and Nervous System" was dropped, and John P. Gray of the State Lunatic Asylum at Utica was invited to lecture on "Psychological Medicine and Medical Jurisprudence." Gray was given a chair with this designation in 1875, while Janeway was appointed to a chair of "Diseases of the Nervous System" (not to overlap Gray's course) a year later.[13] The separation of the two fields, psychological medicine and neurology, proved that Hammond had not yet succeeded in establishing his specialty as an intellectually coherent discipline.

POSTGRADUATE MEDICAL EDUCATION

In the fall of 1874 Hammond became professor of diseases of the mind and nervous system at his alma mater, University Medical College. There he and other distinguished specialists were to serve as clinical lecturers, providing instruction in their specialties more advanced than that in the traditional undergraduate course. "Under his urgings," remembered Daniel B. St. John Roosa, "the faculty established what they called a post-graduate faculty."[14] This was Hammond's second sustained attempt to organize a system of medical education aimed at graduate physicians, after his unrealized plan for an "Army Medical School." The arrangement at U.M.C. fared little better, and soon the "Post-Graduate Professors" became dissatisfied with their position. They organized themselves into a separate faculty body with its own president and secretary, and communicated their grievances to the regular faculty. Receiving no satisfaction, the Post-Graduate faculty resigned en masse in 1881 and opened their own school the following year.[15]

Hammond and the others contended that the regular faculty had been unwilling to incur the financial risk entailed in a serious attempt to upgrade undergraduate education. This goal was widely discussed and endorsed (at least in theory) both by the profession and the public.[16] But the secessionists, who were not members of the governing board of U.M.C., also had a personal stake in the matter. As a contemporary noted, they "lent the prestige of their reputation and labor to an institution, and contributed to its prosperity," and were therefore "ill-content to be barred from sharing in its councils."[17] Evidently the specialists were by this time sufficiently well established that their affiliation with a school could be seen as lending prestige to the institution, rather than vice versa.

But despite Hammond's long-standing interest in specifically postgraduate education, his associates first attempted to start a new undergraduate school on the plan already attempted by Harvard and of which the Johns Hopkins was soon to become a model. They gave up on the project because endowment funds failed to materialize and negotiations with Cornell did not produce a workable plan for real university ties.[18]

The Post-Graduate faculty secured premises and began organizing a proprietary school of a new type, the New York Post-Graduate Medical School. Hammond was "the soul of the organization," reported D. B. St. John Roosa twenty years later. "He was really the President, although I had the name. He was thoroughly devoted to the interests of the school, so that the smallest detail of management was not considered by him beneath his notice."[19] This had been his leadership style as surgeon general as well. The neurologist himself told the faculty and students of the Post-Graduate in 1893 that "I am one of the founders of this school. I shall always regard that fact as the most honorable of all the events of my professional life – the one in which I take the most pride."[20] Even allowing for polite hyperbole, it is clear that Hammond had a great deal invested in the enterprise. As an institution, the Post-Graduate was closely identified with the interests of medical specialism. It became a focus for professional controversies over issues such as the upgrading of medical education and the "dispensary abuse" question that sharply divided physicians in New York and elsewhere. The Post-Graduate experience is integral to an understanding of Hammond's neurological practice and research in the 1880s.[21]

The new school intended, according to Hammond, "not to increase the number of Doctors but to add to the qualifications of those already graduated." Only holders of the medical degree would be admitted, and no degrees would be conferred.[22] Its faculty thus avoided the common charges that the "medical clique" which controlled the undergraduate schools enriched itself by "manufacturing doctors" at the expense of the ordinary general practitioner who already faced stiff competition for paying patients. "We have had enough of the high-tone and dignity sham, and now let us have the facts," declared a "Successful Practitioner" in 1875; "colleges and hospitals are run for the fame and pecuniary profit of a few medical men who are to a large degree regardless of the rights of our profession."[23] Rather than attacking American doctors for ignorance and incompetence, the Post-Graduate sympathized with the difficulties they confronted in trying to better themselves. Even a three-year medical course allowed insufficient time for a student to learn to practice "intelligently and safely for his patients."

Wealthy and ambitious students might complete their studies in Europe or in a hospital position, but most did not have these advantages. Besides, even well-prepared physicians would realize that "medical science . . . is progressive, and it is difficult for a practitioner to keep pace." They would scarcely want to sit through undergraduate lectures again, and even if one did so "he would not get what he wants there." The Post-Graduate offered practitioners conscious of their deficiencies an opportunity to remedy them.[24] This appeal to upgrade the medical profession encouraged average, underqualified American physicians to participate, rather than blaming them for an admittedly bad state of affairs. Physicians moving to New York were encouraged to use the school as a mailing address. Visitors were "invited to make the reading room of the Post-Graduate School their headquarters. This room is always open," the faculty urged, "and the medical journals from all parts of the country, together with some from Europe, are kept on file."[25]

The details of the clinical instruction at the Post-Graduate were arranged for the convenience of the experienced physician, perhaps from out of town. It was assumed that students would like to extend their knowledge as much as possible in the little time they could spare from busy practices. Matriculants could attend all the courses of the professors and associate professors in all branches. Or they could specialize in one or two areas, taking extra work with the instructors and members of the dispensary staff. Here was a route to specialty practice open to any paying customer with a medical degree. For example, in 1886–87, those with a particular interest in neurology could use the hour from four to five to observe Professor William A. Hammond on Wednesday and Friday, Professor Charles L. Dana on Tuesday and Friday, and Associate Professor Graeme M. Hammond on Saturday. Ambrose Ranney, professor of the anatomy and physiology of the nervous system, offered clinics from noon to one on Monday and Thursday, while Dr. Brown taught "Electrotherapeutics" Tuesday evenings and "Diseases of the Mind and Nervous System" on Monday afternoons.[26]

Many were skeptical about the financial feasibility of the Post-Graduate, but it proved almost immediately to be a success. Significant numbers of practitioners were apparently convinced both of the importance of advanced medical knowledge and of the qualifications of the specialists. Neither immediate economic advantage nor formal professional recognition followed directly from attendance at the school. Nonetheless, 100 students registered during the winter and summer sessions of 1882–83. About one-third of them came from New York City and neighboring Brooklyn, and the remainder from nineteen states, two foreign countries, and the U.S. Army Medical Corps. By 1890 nearly 850 students were attending the Post-Graduate and its rival, the New York Polyclinic, and a dozen similar institutions had been organized across the United States.[27]

The success of postgraduate education on this model depended heavily on the availability of working-class patients, referred to as "clinical material," attracted by the free or very inexpensive clinics and dispensaries. This brought with it the inevitable charge that the Post-Graduate faculty was contributing to the "abuse of medical charity," seen by many New York practitioners as a threat to their own modest incomes.[28] In the academic year 1883–84, for example, the fourteen professors of the Post-Graduate held a total of at least eighteen positions in hospitals, dispensaries, and other medical charities. The six associate professors held at least four such positions, the seven lecturers held six, and the twenty-seven clinical assistants held eight positions. In contrast, nearly two out of every three regular physicians in New York held no appointments at all, while about 70 percent of all positions were filled by 3 percent of the doctors.[29] Clinics held at the school itself added, although perhaps marginally, to the city's medical facilities for the poor.

Complaints from the lower echelons of the profession were

frequent and bitter. One correspondent to an 1883 issue of the *Medical Record,* who signed himself "Itis," protested against "any institution whereby our means of gaining a livelihood are materially, and even seriously compromised." This irritated physician argued that polyclinics were unnecessary, as facilities for clinical instruction were already more than ample. "The Polyclinic and Post-Graduate School," he complained, "inculcate upon the mind of the rustic physician from the wilds of Bushwick the principles of the various specialties, for a decided quid pro quo, by means of patients expropriated from us." He had recently lost three of his own cases to professors at clinics, and urged other physicians to do everything possible, "consistent with business courtesy and gentlemanly courtesy," to thwart the culprits.[30]

The problem of competition was real, although misconstrued by contemporaries: most dispensary patients could not, in fact, afford private care. Competition in the medical market was aggravated not by deadbeats seeking to avoid payment but by a surplus of practitioners relative to the number of patients who both desired their services and were able to pay for them. Between 1877 and 1886 New York medical schools graduated 6,373 physicians (88 percent of them from "regular" institutions), an average of over 700 new doctors per year. In Chicago, new medical certificates were issued to 924 doctors between 1880 and 1884, of whom only 510 were still listed as practicing physicians in 1885. The attrition rate approached 50 percent after four years.[31]

Charges of "abuse" were not new, of course, and the postgraduate schools may have been in a better position than other institutions to rebut them. In contrast to unaffiliated dispensaries, their patients were not "wasted" solely in the interest of a few publicity-seeking specialists. And unlike the undergraduate medical colleges, they did not increase the number of competitors in a crowded field. Rather, they offered all physicians the chance to acquire knowledge which might give them an edge over their peers. The consistently high enrollments in postgraduate schools suggest that a significant fraction of the New York profession actually took advantage of this opportunity during the 1880s. In the words of Abraham Flexner, the postgraduate schools functioned as a much-needed "undergraduate repair shop."[32] They probably also played an important role in bridging the gap between the elite physician, often a man with a European perspective and scientific aspirations, and the unsophisticated but ambitious graduate of the average American medical college.

The attempt of the Post-Graduate to upgrade the American medical profession institutionalized a vision of medical science that guided much of Hammond's own research as a neurologist. It was not a model that endured. When Flexner conducted his famous survey of medical education in 1910, he found much to criticize even in the best of the postgraduate schools. He declared the teaching "too immediately practical to be scientifically stimulating: it has the air of handicraft, rather than science." Flexner also objected to the emphasis on surgery and the specialties, rather than internal medicine.[33]

Even as Flexner wrote, these schools were already beginning to implement many of the reforms he was suggesting for them. But it is misleading to regard them simply as inferior approximations to the type of medical education that later came to dominate the American scene. Rather, they represented a very different perspective on educational reform. The faculty of the Post-Graduate stated this explicitly in the *Announcement* of 1915–16. They identified "two distinct ideas in the line of medical progress." The first of these was the Flexner program: the upgrading of entrance requirements, the standardization of the curriculum, and the establishment of a hospital year. The second, "of slower growth but of equal importance," was the extension of post-graduate instruction.[34]

Flexner politely rebuked the postgraduate schools for their inattention to science, and it is true that the Post-Graduate stressed clinical rather than laboratory work. "To give instruction in Medicine without the Laboratory as the chief aid in diagnosis is an impossibility in the present scientific age," the faculty admitted in 1905, "and it is a question whether, in the future, those wishing to take some course in Medicine will not be required also to take a ticket for the Laboratory." A new laboratory had, in fact, just been built for work in pathology, bacteriology, and clinical microscopy.[35] But no such requirement was actually instituted.

Further, the next year's *Announcement* included a virtual manifesto of the clinician. The faculty conceded that medicine had recently made great advances as an exact science "in large measure" because of laboratory investigations. But they were sure this had caused "too much reliance to be placed on the laboratory and too little on the clinical aspects of the cases." They did not want to reduce the number of researchers, but "to make our matriculates better diagnosticians and more scientific clinicians. Nothing of moment can be done at the present day without laboratories," they added, "but they are not the only means of diagnostication. We realize fully," they concluded, "that nothing can take the place of painstaking observations and scientific analysis at the bedside."[36] Despite renovation and expansion of laboratory facilities in the next few years, the Post-Graduate did not change this approach. For its faculty, perhaps, "science" and "handicraft" were not mutually exclusive.

The founders of the Post-Graduate intended it as a center for the study and development of medical science. The semimonthly meetings of its Clinical Society provided a forum for faculty, students, and alumni to discuss the latest findings in a variety of burgeoning specialties. Hammond often chaired these meetings. The papers he read, on topics such as hydrophobia and epilepsy, were vigorously debated.[37] The work of the Society was recorded in its journal, the *Quarterly Bulletin* (later titled simply *The Post-Graduate*). But it was a vision of medical science that centered on increasingly exact study of the patient at the bedside rather than in the laboratory. "The day of the haphazard association of clinical facts is passed," declared the *Announcement* for 1915–16. "Modern medical teaching must be scientific and the old fallacious idea of scientific versus practical work is a thing of the past." The up-to-date physician was "essentially practical because scientific knowledge is based upon practical work." And central to the work were "instruments of precision – thermometer, auroscope, cystoscope, etc." and the utilization of "the fundamental methods of observation, palpation, percussion, auscultation and mensuration."[38] The physician trained at the Post-Graduate was not supposed to be simply a skilled craftsman, but a scientist whose data came from his "practical" work with patients. In the Post-Graduate Medical School, Hammond had helped to create an institution that fostered specialism in medicine as a vehicle for medical science as he understood it. This concept of scientific clinical medicine dovetailed neatly with Hammond's own work. It was one to which he became more firmly committed in later years, even as it lost ground among an influential section of the American medical elite.[39]

ORGANIZING MEDICAL SCIENCE IN NEW YORK

Hammond had a strong sense that organization was needed to develop a professional framework for the science he wished to pursue. He had helped to set up the Philadelphia Biological Society in 1858 for this purpose. Ten years later, with the monumental experience of reorganizing the Army Medical Department behind him, his institution-building in New York began in 1868 with an improbable attempt to reconstruct not only New York medicine, but virtually the entire public intellectual life of the nation. As his practice grew and his professional commitment to neurology deepened in the following years, he turned instead to the less grandiose and far more successful concept of the specialty society. His journalistic endeavors during the same years also focused more and more sharply on his specialist concerns.

Hammond shared with Charles W. Elliott and other progressive New York physicians the conviction that American medical scientists were catching up rapidly with their European counterparts, and might soon surpass them. "The time has come," said Elliott, "when it is prophesied that students from abroad may find it as much to their advantage to come here and complete their education, as has before been the necessity for American students to go abroad." But this development could not be left to chance, since most physicians were "hard working busy men, who scarcely have the time and leisure to cultivate those more delightful scientific facts which are identified with all the hopes of progress in medicine." Medical scientists "must have leisure, . . . an atmosphere, they must be stimulated by a band of fellow-workers." Most of all they needed "an audience before whom they can bring their partially developed thoughts so that in the collission [*sic*] of mind with mind, these may be shaped and brightened, and assume the proportions they are destined to assume." The "National Institute of Letters, Arts and Sciences" that Hammond, Elliott, and others worked to establish was intended to serve these purposes.[40]

The organization was designed on a grand scale. "It may be that we are laying the foundation of an institution like the Royal Society of England," an enthusiastic promoter told the well-attended introductory meeting of June 12, 1868, "or it may be an institution like the National Academy of France." Clearly this group did not believe that the National Academy of Sciences fulfilled this role in the United States. The illustrious roster of supporters lent some credence to their hopes. And as several speakers pointed out, New York City was a fitting place for such a project. "The great commercial metropolis of this Western world, the financial centre of the Continent – soon perhaps to be of the world – [ought] also to be the great home of science," as one put it. Civic and national pride not only motivated the formation of the institute, but were reflected in the organizational plan carefully drawn up by Hammond and the members of his committee. In accordance with the "American idea," Hammond said, the new society would be larger and more inclusive than its French model. The United States also differed from Europe in that the indispensable financial support for such an institute could not be expected from the state or national governments. It would come, if at all, from "the vast wealth of the city," from "the men of money, the princes of our country."[41]

An "Academy of Medical Sciences" was actually organized as a division of the fledgling National Institute. The eminent Austin Flint, Sr., agreed to serve as president and Hammond assumed, as he often did, the post of vice-president.[42] But the merchant princes were evidently not convinced by the fervent rhetoric of that "hearty and harmonious" first meeting and subsequent months, for the elaborately designed National Institute never materialized. New York's intellectuals were left "to be a company of Nomads or Bedouins, each one of whom is to go his own way."[43]

Hammond's "own way" was neurology. There was not a well-mapped route, scarcely even a foot trail, and his path meandered through the thickets of the mind and nervous system. His new *Quarterly Journal of Psychological Medicine and Medical Jurisprudence*, founded in 1867, recorded some of the highlights of the trip. It contained a potpourri of original articles, excerpts (primarily from foreign sources), and critical reviews of recent works. Perhaps only the editor himself could have perceived a logical coherence to the contents. The first volume, for example, was largely filled with Hammond's own essays on the nature and seat of instinct, organic infantile paralysis (polio), the famous Johnston will case, and "Merlin and His Influence on the English Character and Literature." Other papers concerned "The Negro as Soldier," medical electricity, insanity, nightmares, and sexual aberrations. The second volume (1868) contained much material on Hammond's new interest, aphasia and language development. There was also an extended discussion of "the law of rape," side by side with neurological articles by Edward C. Seguin, Austin Flint, and others. Hammond's contributions included papers on "The Influence of the Maternal Mind Over the Offspring During Pregnancy and Lactation," two new medical instruments (the dynamometer and dynamograph of Mathieu), "epilepsy due to cerebral anemia," chlorosis, polio again, and the state of the mind during sleep. Nearly all of these topics were of continuing interest to Hammond and fell well within the boundaries of what he considered "neurology."

As neurological teaching and practice came to occupy more and more of Hammond's time, the contents of his journal were gradually limited to clinical issues in neurology and psychiatry. Recognizing this tendency, he changed the title in January 1870 to the *Journal of Psychological Medicine: A Quarterly Review of Diseases of the Nervous System, Medical Jurisprudence, and Anthropology*. In addition to detailed reports of Hammond's clinical lectures at the Bellevue Hospital Medical College, it now contained a great deal of material on insanity. For example, the main articles in the July 1872 issue were "The Composition of Mind," by John Fiske; "Some Medical Questions of the Lawler Will Case," by Roberts Bartholow; "Suggestions Relative to the Sequestration of Alleged Lunatics," by R. W. Parsons; "Theomania," by Allan McLane Hamilton; and a translation of M. Onimus's "On the Phenomena and Movements of Rotation Consecutive upon Removal of the Brain," made by the editor's precocious thirteen-year-old daughter Clara. The "Contemporary Literature" section of the same issue reviewed four works on spiritualism (including Hammond's), *Neuralgia* by F. E. Anstie, *Psychology* by W. D. Wilson, and a collection of essays (in German) by Edward Reich. The "Chronicle" was in two parts: a letter on psychological medicine by George Fielding Blandford of London, and a synopsis of "Physiology and Pathology of the Brain and Nervous System" prepared by H. D. Nichol.

The juxtaposition of what might now be called neuropathology and psychiatry in Hammond's *Journal of Psychological Medicine* can best be appreciated in the context of the highly problematic relations between the two fields in the second half of the nineteenth century. Psychiatry in England was dominated by the Enlightenment view of the restoration of reason to the insane through a combination of moral suasion and social control. Alienists, preoccupied with "humane" treatment, devoted much attention to problems of asylum management. Britain had a strong psychological tradition stretching from the work of Hobbes and Locke to the associationism of David Hartley, and through both the Benthamites and the Scottish philosophers. This academic tradition had so entrenched an idealist perspective that even neurophysiologists like Charles Bell and Hughlings Jackson often could present their work as unrelated to problems of mind. The mutually agreed-upon division of labor between neurology and psychiatry thus minimized friction between the two specialties. Henry Maudsley was probably the most significant exception to this admittedly overschematized view. But his work was received with more enthusiasm in Germany (and, in the United States, by Hammond) than it was in his own Great Britain.[44]

The Continental situation was quite different. In Germany, there was little to speak of in the way of formal psychology or psychiatry before the nineteenth century. By mid-century, "Romanticism" had generally been routed by an upsurge of interest in somatically oriented laboratory research. The field of neurology was consequently defined largely in terms of the experimental psychology of such men as Helmholtz and Wilhelm Wundt, and by the experimental physiology of the nervous system exemplified by Moritz Heinrich Romberg. Wilhelm Griesinger, whose clinics for the insane served as a model for those of Hammond, declared around 1867 that "psychiatry and neuropathology are not merely two closely-related fields; they are but one field in which only one language is spoken and the same laws rule."[45]

In France, too, materialist views prevailed although in notably different forms.[46] Neurophysiology flourished through the work of François Magendie and Claude Bernard, to name two outstanding examples. The movement for reform in the care and treatment of the insane in France, usually associated with Philippe Pinel, differed from the parallel movement in Britain in its thorough domination by physicians and by its corresponding locus in the large Parisian hospitals. A French psychiatric tradition thus developed that (unlike the English one) stressed the neurological study of mental phenomena and functional nervous disorders and that (unlike the German one) was primarily clinical in its orientation. In Hammond's time, Jean Martin Charcot represented this tradition. Hammond was apparently on cordial terms with Charcot, and based his *Treatise on the Diseases of the Nervous System* largely on his lectures. By way of comparison, Sigmund Freud's teacher Pierre Janet was another follower of Charcot. Hammond never referred in print to Freud, a much younger man, but Freud cited Hammond in his early work on cocaine.[47]

By mid-century the United States already had a psychiatric tradition that, if not exactly flourishing, was at least solidly entrenched. Superintendents of institutions for the care and treatment of the insane, whose views on asylum construction and management owed much to British psychiatry, had formed the Association of Medical Superintendents of American Institutions for the Insane in 1844.[48] When Continental neurology, including within its province diseases of the "mind," was imported by men like Hammond after the Civil War, conflict was virtually inevitable. A theoretical debate was already public in 1871, and open strife came several years later.[49]

Hammond explained in a review of John P. Gray's important pamphlet *The Dependence of Insanity on Physical Disease* (1871) that "modern science of psychology . . . is neither more nor less than *the science of mind considered as a physical function*." He found this a "legitimate working hypothesis," in contrast to Gray's "metaphysical" suggestion that mind might be a spiritual entity using the brain as its instrument. "The true road to a medical knowledge of insanity is through pathology," Hammond insisted. At the same time it seemed to him unscientific "to leave mental phenomena out of psychological medicine altogether." He opposed reductionism, arguing that "the aims and methods of physical sciences . . . are essential to psychology, and not its preference for physical facts merely."[50] His *Journal of Psychological Medicine* promoted this conception of one discipline embracing the spectrum of problems ranging from normal psychology through insanity to functional and finally organic nervous disorders.

The *Journal* lapsed again in the fall of 1872. Hammond resurrected it for the last time in July 1874, as *The Psychological and Medico-Legal Journal*. It was to contain more material than formerly on medicolegal affairs, a reflection of the editor's increasing involvement in the New York Medico-Legal Society. The periodical would feature reports of the proceedings of this group and of the New York Neurological Society, as well as original communications. There would be no editorials and no "chronicle" section, as the publication was intended to "increase and diffuse knowledge upon matters pertaining to . . . science."[51]

The Neurological Society was another of Hammond's pet projects. It had been organized informally in March 1872 around the New York State Hospital for Diseases of the Nervous System, but lapsed after a short time. Under the stimulus of competition from the newly reorganized New York Society for Neurology and Electrology, Hammond revived it in 1874 with a distinguished roster of members. The purpose, he declared in his inaugural address as president, was to study "the science of medicine in all its relations to the nervous system." He did not know of "any higher scientific labor than this for a physician to perform." The importance of neurology, he said, "augments daily with the advance of civilization and refinement" that increased the incidence of nervous diseases, "before which all others are of secondary rank."[52] Hammond was boosting his own specialty, but he had chosen this particular specialty precisely because it seemed to him to offer the greatest opportunities for important scientific achievement. Attendance at meetings of the society rarely exceeded a dozen or so members. But its lively discussions justified Hammond's enthusiasm. Topics included hydrophobia, the effects of alcohol and the "insanity of inebriety," "nervous affections of the throat," and reports of interesting neurological cases. The group later became a major force in the movement for insane-asylum reform and a belligerent in the much-publicized quarrels that arose between neurologists and asylum superintendents.[53]

Hammond was sufficiently encouraged by the end of 1874 to take steps to launch a new national organization, the American Neurological Association. Shortly after its first annual meeting in June 1875, Hammond severed his connection with the *Psychological and Medico-Legal Journal.* Thereafter he devoted much attention to the scientific and organizational work of the association. For nearly a decade he contributed at least one, often several, papers to each annual meeting and participated actively in its wide-ranging discussions.[54] When its organ, the *Journal of Nervous and Mental Diseases,* moved from Chicago to New York in 1876, Hammond became an associate editor. Less than ten years after the collapse of the broadly conceived National Institute of Letters, Arts and Sciences, Hammond's organizational activities in the scientific world had come to focus more and more sharply on a field of work that, largely as a result of his own efforts, was beginning to achieve recognition as a distinct medical specialty.

One last venture into editorial work should be noted briefly. The first annual issue of *Neurological Contributions* appeared in 1879, the last in 1881. It was edited by Hammond and his assistant, W. J. Morton, and written almost entirely by the editors. By this time Hammond's busy and lucrative practice, as well as his public quest for vindication from the United States government, had diverted his attention almost entirely from theoretical questions. The contents of the new journal were limited to clinical lectures on diseases of the mind and nervous system and to reports on the asylum reform campaign which was then well under way. By 1882 the asylum controversy had waned and Hammond's attention was occupied with the Post-Graduate Medical School and with medicolegal affairs.

The neurologist was elected a trustee of the New York Medico-Legal Society in January 1882, at a meeting that chose the lawyer Clark Bell as president in a "sharp contest" with disputed results. Hammond's paper on President Garfield's assassin, Charles Guiteau, sparked a lively debate at the March meeting, raising expectations that the society might "improve from its present state of mediocrity," as a medical observer put it. But the May meeting belied the promise. The medical editor E. S. Gaillard, reporting on the proceedings, noted that "the practical value of all this, if evident to the authors of it, is certainly not apparent to anyone else. In the scientific scale," he concluded, "it stands at zero."

Society members returned in September to a "very lively meeting," if not a very scientific one. They waited impatiently for young Graeme Hammond to finish his report on death by hanging, with perhaps a little interest in the experiment he had made on himself, until they could get on with the "real business." This was an "edifying wrangle" over the refusal of the treasurer, E. C. Harwood, to pay a $250 printing bill, on the basis of incorrect minutes prepared by the former secretary. "For four hours the bust of the venerable Mott looked down upon a choppy sea of waving hands and vehement expostulations," reported an observer who hoped the society might "settle down to scientific labors alone."

But the large attendance in December was due to yet another hotly contested presidential election, in which William A. Hammond was defeated by the incumbent, 62–51. Some disgruntled members immediately began to organize a new group, the New York Society of Medical Jurisprudence. Hammond remained in the original organization, continued to served as a trustee, and made another run for the presidency in December 1883. Although Bell was reluctant to serve again and recommended that a physician be found for the post, he stayed in the race to defeat Hammond, who was as unpopular among the lawyers as Bell was among the physicians. The Medico-Legal Society "might make itself useful," commented a physician, "but for 2–3 years factional fighting has completely tied it up." It had been "seriously, if not irretrievably, injured by the fatuous ambition of a lawyer who seems to have no other aim in life than to be its president and manager," complained another medical writer. Some hopes were raised by the election of Professor R. Ogden Doremus at the end of 1884, but apparently not those of Hammond, who resigned as trustee a few months later.[55]

*   *   *   *   *

Hammond might have been the model of "a New York medical man," according to an 1881 parody of Gilbert and Sullivan's *Patience,* "a very much advertised man/A pills-in-variety, talk-in-Society/Each-for-himself young man."[56] He "did not long keep up his connection with medical journals, medical schools, and hospitals," commented medical editor Frank Foster in 1900, "and after a time he was no longer a frequent contributor to medical literature."[57] Medical societies fared somewhat better: he maintained his interest in the neurological and medicolegal associations for periods as long as eight to ten years.

Hammond had a keen sense of what was timely, and was quick to find a link to neurology in almost any issue of public concern. He was an indefatigable organizer who saw clearly that scientific work was a collaborative affair and attempted consciously to build the institutions that could foster it. What he could not see, and should not be faulted for overlooking, was that the base for "big science" did not yet exist in the American society of his day.

VINDICATION

Hammond's medical reputation and his fortune were securely established by 1877, but his clouded military record still troubled him. Probably at his request, and supported by a petition of the

Medical Faculty of New York, New York Congressman Benjamin
A. Willis and Senator Roscoe Conkling introduced bills H.R. 2108
and S. 560 to initiate proceedings to overturn the decision of 1864.
To avoid the imputation of crass motives, the wealthy neurologist
insisted that no financial relief be included. President Rutherford
B. Hayes initiated a review of the case in the spring of 1878, but the
confused proceedings dragged out for most of the year. The military board he appointed confined itself to a reading of the pon-
derous trial transcript and refused to hear additional testimony on
Hammond's intent that had been excluded from the original hearing. In March of 1879 the board endorsed the original findings.[58]

Another flurry of activity ensued, and Secretary of War G. W.
McCrary finally authorized the submission of new evidence,
which Hammond delivered in the form of testimonials and affida-
vits on August 14, 1879. "I think I have a right to regard with
pride my course since I was discharged from the Army," wrote the
neurologist. "I have worked hard against great odds to acchieve
[*sic*] success; but all my efforts would have been in vain but for the
support, the confidence and the substantial aid of those friends
who in the very depth of my troubles came forward with their
assistance."[59] On personal review of this material, McCrary exonerated Hammond and recommended that the original sentence be
annulled. Hayes concurred, and within two weeks it was done.
Hammond had been vindicated just in time for the opening of the
season in New York society.

7

"A laborious and skilful observer"

The common thread running through two decades of Hammond's neurological work was his extensive clinical practice. From the late 1860s through the mid-1880s a steadily increasing stream of patients presented themselves uptown at Hammond's fashionable private office, downtown at the short-lived New York State Hospital for the Diseases of the Nervous System, and at his medical school clinics. Their complaints had to be diagnosed, a prognosis hazarded, and a plan of treatment initiated. Hammond's published works suggest that he kept careful and often detailed case books, but no such records are extant. Any reconstruction of his practice must thus remain somewhat speculative.

A good idea of the range of clients Hammond encountered can be inferred from his published clinical lectures and from the case descriptions that often constituted a large part of his formal papers. More systematic although perhaps less candid was his influential *Treatise on the Diseases of the Nervous System*. The publication of the first edition of this path-breaking English-language neurology textbook in 1871 was a landmark in Hammond's career, and eight later American editions updated his presentation of his specialty to the profession at large.[1]

NEUROLOGICAL PATIENTS AND THEIR COMPLAINTS

The outpatients at the New York State Hospital for Diseases of the Nervous System were probably typical of the clinic patients seen by Hammond over the years. A statistical profile of this group is available from the annual reports of the institution. About three-fifths of the 566 patients were male, two-fifths female. About half were between twenty and forty years of age. More than a quarter

116   *Preserve your love for science*

were over forty, a figure not surprising in view of the degenerative nature of many diseases of the nervous system. This patient profile was quite different from that of the typical general-practice dispensary, which usually attracted larger proportions of women and children. About 40 percent of the patients were native-born Americans, while most of the remainder were Irish. It is safe to assume that most of the clinic patients were from the working class and the unemployed poor of the city, as the hospital was designed for the indigent.

Lists detailing the types of diseases seen at the hospital are available but their utility is limited by our necessary dependence on, and understanding of, the diagnostic skills and concepts of neurologists over a century ago. Probably about one-third of the patients presented with diseases definitely characterized by organic lesions: various forms of paralysis (including polio), sclerosis, and the like. At least that number had clearly functional disorders, diagnosed as cerebral or spinal anemia or congestion, "nervous asthenia," hysteria, or hypochondria. The remainder included sixty-eight cases of "neuralgia," sixty-four of "epilepsy," and sixteen of "lead-poisoning." Cases of insanity, idiocy, and delirium tremens were sent elsewhere. Unfortunately there is no record of the patient population at Hammond's clinic for "insanity."[2]

Some clinic patients apparently consulted Hammond later privately, a practice that lent credence to charges that specialists unethically lured patients aware from their family practitioners. However, the two groups – private and clinic patients – must have differed markedly both in the nature of their complaints and in terms of their social origins. Hammond had no family practice. All of his private neurological patients were referred to him by other physicians or sought his advice on their own for a specific complaint. His well-known practice of charging $10 or more for an office visit would have deterred all but the affluent. Published case notes frequently refer to patients as gentlemen or ladies, as merchants, businessmen, professionals, and elected officials. "Many of our most eminent men, both in public and private life, have to thank him for preservation of mental and physical health," wrote Spencer F. Baird in 1879.[3] The patients resided in all parts of the country. Some made the journey to New York specially to consult the renowned expert, and others took advantage of his services while in the metropolis on business or en route to Europe.

The facial expression is well seen in the accompanying
woodcut (Fig. 32), made from a very accurate sketch of one

FIG. 32.

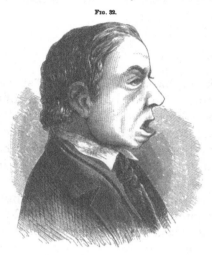

of my patients suffering from the disease in question, and
who entered my consulting-room with his handkerchief to
his mouth to absorb the streams of saliva which were flowing.

Patient with "glosso-labio-laryngeal paralysis," ca. 1873. Hammond's text
calls attention to the patient's facial expression, but his attire also suggests the class of patient typical of the neurologist's private practice.
(William A. Hammond, *Treatise on the Diseases of the Nervous System*, 4th
ed. [New York: Appleton, 1873], p. 680. Courtesy of Middleton Library of the Health Sciences, University of Wisconsin, Madison.)

Some sought little more than a cure for seasickness from the neurologist, an intimation that neurology was in fashion.[4] Probably a
much larger proportion of the private patients suffered from functional disorders, which will be discussed in more detail in the next
chapter.

For those with organic disease, Hammond could often do little
beyond providing an authoritative, though usually not reassuring,
diagnosis and prognosis. This was frequently a difficult task. For
example, a patient brought before the students at University Medical College seemed at first to be a case of spinal irritation (a
functional disorder) but proved on examination and on the basis of
the history to have incipient Pott's disease, an incurable form of

tuberculosis. In another case Hammond expected to find locomotor ataxia or posterior spinal sclerosis. But a simple test of the
patellar tendon reflex (the "knee-jerk") forced him to change the
diagnosis to anterolateral sclerosis.[5]

TOOLS OF THE TRADE

Hammond's textbook emphasized the need for "special means of
investigation and treatment" in the study of diseases of the nervous
system, as in other specialties. Neurology had advanced in the last
decade, "and undoubtedly a great deal of the advancement is due
to the instruments and apparatus by which scientific research in
this direction has become practicable." A thirty-page introduction
to the *Treatise* described the tools of Hammond's new trade.[6]

First among the instruments was the ophthalmoscope, pro-
totype of specialist technics.[7] "If physicians would understand
what they are dealing with," Hammond commented in 1866,
"they must be able either themselves to use these instruments
or . . . ask the help of some professional brother, who, perchance,
may bear the somewhat questionable but not unworthy distinction
of being a specialist."[8] Proper skill was not easily come by. "The
real value of ophthalmoscopy in diseases of the nervous system,"
he warned, "is in danger of being disregarded through the sciolism
of pert pretenders, who read papers and write memoirs without
ever having seen the optic disk to recognize it."[9] Hammond had
learned of the use of the ophthalmoscope in the diagnosis of diseases of the nervous system from French works on the subject
rather than from American ophthalmologists, and most likely had
begun using it in 1866.

Hammond introduced other new medical instruments to the
American profession. Among these were Duchenne's trocar for
muscle biopsy and Henri Becquerel's disks for the precise determination of slight cutaneous temperature differentials. Hammond
modified E. H. Sieveking's recently invented esthesiometer for his
own use. The dynamometer, a device for measuring muscular
strength, could be connected to a sphygmograph to make a dynamograph. Hammond claimed priority in the description of this
compound apparatus.[10] His textbook also mentioned the
cephalohemometer, which he and S. Weir Mitchell had separately

contrived for use in physiological experiments on cerebral circulation in laboratory animals. Fully half of Hammond's introductory discussion concerned electrical apparatus, used mainly in treatment. This will be considered later.

The ophthalmoscope, like many other instruments that helped to define specialist knowledge, enabled the physician to visualize the interior of the body. Most of the devices that Hammond described had a different use. In measuring sensibility with the esthesiometer, strength with the dynamometer, and circulation with the cephalohemometer, Hammond was assessing functions. In this sense, the emphasis was physiological rather than anatomical.

It is unlikely that Hammond relied heavily on technological aids, with the possible exception of the ophthalmoscope, in making difficult diagnoses. Rather, he sharpened his observational skills in neurological illnesses by concentrating on a relatively large number of cases within a limited range of disorders. His study of polio, discussed in the next chapter, will show how his publicly avowed specialist interests led him to extend scientific knowledge of such diseases while simultaneously attracting to his office the case material from which this knowledge could be constructed. Two examples of Hammond's diagnostics, cerebral hemorrhage and athetosis, will illustrate these points here.

Cerebral hemorrhage, said Hammond, was ordinarily not difficult to diagnose. However, the circumstances of a case might create doubt. "Supposing an individual to be found in a state of profound insensibility," he explained, "the condition may be due to compression from injury of the skull, to concussion from a fall or blow, to congestion, to asphyxia, to syncope, to a recent epileptic fit, to uraemic intoxication, to hysteria, to narcotism, or to drunkenness." A mistaken diagnosis of cerebral hemorrhage would be "embarrassing to the physician, and, perhaps, injurious to the patient." A mistaken diagnosis of drunkenness in a stroke patient would be even more embarrassing, but such errors could be avoided by a careful case history. More difficult was the differential diagnosis from embolism, thrombosis, tumor, or abscess. Here, too, the history and course of the illness would help.[11] Nowhere in his discussion of the diagnosis of cerebral hemorrhage did Hammond mention the use of any instrument. The only laboratory test he could recommend was urinalysis in "very doubtful

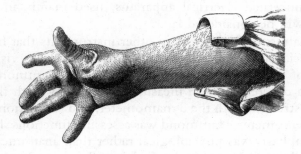

Hand of patient with "athetosis," ca. 1869. J.P.R., a thirty-three-year-old
bookbinder from Holland, originally consulted Dr. Hammond in April
1869 through the Bellevue Hospital Medical College clinic. He later
became one of the first patients in Hammond's New York State Hospital
for Diseases of the Nervous System. This "first-class workman" had a
history of seizures, numbness and pain in his right limbs, and delirium
tremens, and boasted of drinking up to sixty glasses of gin in a day. His
immediate problem – the inability to keep his fingers and toes in a fixed
position – was named by Hammond "athetosis," also known as "Hammond's disease." (William A. Hammond, *Treatise on the Diseases of the
Nervous System,* 4th ed. [New York: Appleton, 1873], p. 657. Courtesy
of Middleton Library of the Health Sciences, University of Wisconsin,
Madison.)

cases" to rule out uremia. In other situations, such as a suspected
case of "cerebral softening," instruments were recommended but
the clinical verdict still rested largely on the case history.

Hammond's description of the disorder he named athetosis is
virtually the only one of his scientific contributions cited (as
"Hammond's disease") by twentieth-century historians of neurology.[12] He characterized it mainly as "an inability to retain the
fingers and toes in any position in which they may be placed, and
by their continual motion." Although he classified it among the
"cerebro-spinal" diseases by analogy with chorea and cerebrospinal sclerosis, he frankly admitted that "relative to the character of the lesion . . . and its exact seat, I am not yet prepared to
speak with any degree of certainty." Since the disease was not fatal,

he had had no opportunity to make a postmortem examination.[13] The nine-page discussion in the *Treatise* consisted mainly of two detailed case histories. One was of a patient he had first seen in 1869 at the New York State Hospital for Diseases of the Nervous System, and the other of a patient described in a report sent to him by Dr. J. C. Hubbard of Ashtabula, Ohio. In later editions he added notes on cases more recently brought to his attention. The symptoms of the disease were "clearly indicated" in the histories, and no diagnostic apparatus was necessary. Hammond reported on the treatment he had given the patients, but candidly admitted doubt as to its efficacy and offered no recommendations.

Once Hammond published the first two cases, others were quickly brought forward. Samuel D. Gross and Fordyce Barker, for example, both claimed to have seen such patients earlier. But it was the aspiring neurologist who had an interest in describing and naming the condition and in claiming the syndrome as a newly discovered disease. Such demonstrations of expertise were the stuff of which a specialist reputation could be built. Beyond this, Hammond's neurologic orientation alerted him to diagnostic subtleties that were unavailable to the nonneurologist. It is ironic that a man who prided himself on the broad scope of his scientific work should figure in the standard history of neurology largely as an eponym for a disease of which he understood neither the etiology, the pathology, nor the therapeutics. Even in 1873 he could do little more than adduce further cases – by this time he knew "positively" of six, excluding those claimed by Gross and Barker – and distinguish athetosis from no fewer than seven other conditions.[14]

NEUROLOGICAL THERAPEUTICS

With a few important exceptions, Hammond was rarely able to give his patients a favorable prognosis. Diseases such as spinal, meningeal, or severe cerebral hemorrhage, cerebral softening, acute or tubercular cerebral meningitis, nonsyphilitic spinal or brain tumors, and acute myelitis would almost certainly result in death. Other conditions were nonfatal but usually incurable: thrombosis, paralysis agitans, atrophy of motor nerve cells, spinal softening, and, more commonly, locomotor ataxia. Still others – such as spinal meningitis, anterolateral spinal sclerosis, and pro-

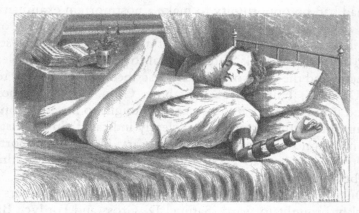

Patient with "spinal meningitis," ca. 1873. The contractions of this patient's limbs had persisted for three years when Hammond first saw him, accompanied by a variety of other symptoms attributed by the neurologist to "chronic spinal meningitis of syphilitic origin." Although the medical symptoms were reported cured by large doses of "iodide of potassium and corrosive chloride of mercury," neither Hammond nor the orthopedist Lewis A. Sayre (called in consultation) was able to reverse the contractions. (William A. Hammond, *Treatise on the Diseases of the Nervous System,* 4th ed. [New York: Appleton, 1873], p. 453. Courtesy of Middleton Library of the Health Sciences, University of Wisconsin, Madison.)

gressive muscular atrophy – could only rarely be cured. Almost no patient suffering from any disease of the nervous system was likely to recover spontaneously.

As Hammond saw it, however, there remained ample scope for active and perhaps even heroic treatment. Even though the prospect of a full cure was virtually nil, the disease might be arrested or the symptoms ameliorated. From the perspective of a century, the attribution of even such limited success to medical intervention might well be questioned. But Hammond was practicing within the framework of nineteenth-century medical assumptions, despite his progressive outlook and technical innovations. For him and for his patients, the notion of remission was less plausible than the obvious (if incorrect) inference that any improvement following treatment must be credited to the physician.[15]

Hammond could on occasion be conservative in his therapeutics and blunt in his condemnation of heroics, as he had been in the calomel controversy. Discussing a stroke victim, for instance, he commented that there was little to do for the patient except to keep him quiet and perhaps give him stimulants. Potassium bromide and other common medicines were "worse than useless," and blistering should be avoided. Under such limited treatment, Hammond said, the patient might possibly recover.[16] He remarked that an early patient suffering from convulsive tremor had previously been subjected to heroic therapy but "notwithstanding the treatment, he continued to survive."[17] He said of glosso-labio-laryngeal paralysis that "regarding the treatment of the condition I have nothing whatsoever to offer and nobody else has any treatment to offer."[18]

His skepticism was more the result of prior unsuccessful therapeutic experimentation of heroic proportions than of a theoretical commitment to the healing power of nature. Hammond's treatments generally combined the use of internal medication with the application of electricity in some form. He also attempted mechanical and surgical procedures, the latter particularly after the advent of aseptic technique. His attempts to cure the stubborn and rather common disease locomotor ataxia included all of these modes of therapy, and will serve as an example.

"A great many medicines have been employed in the treatment of sclerosis of the posterior columns of the spinal cord," Hammond reported in 1871, identifying the disease by its underlying pathology in accordance with the plan of his *Treatise,* "but few have been productive of any material benefit." He recommended "ergot in large doses" and "the bromide of potassium . . . in doses of from thirty grains to a drachm three times a day" in the early stages of the disease. This was to diminish the circulation of the blood. He added cod-liver oil as a tonic, and featured the application of the primary galvanic current.

Additional remedies for locomotor ataxia were directed toward the relief of specific symptoms: bismuth, electricity, or pepsin for "gastric derangements," and codeine for back pains. In more advanced cases, nitrate of silver replaced the ergot. Hammond was understandably not satisfied with the results of this therapy, however, and had experimented with phosphoric acid, phosphorus, and chloride of barium, to his mind with some success. Since he typically resorted to polypharmacy he could not state with certainty what produced his good results, except that the iodide of potassium cured cases with a "syphilitic taint." He could state with the confidence of experience that hydrotherapeutics, counterirritation, the ether spray, faradization, and plasters were ineffective. Crutches were useful, allowing the patients to rest the affected muscles and thus to conserve their nervous force. For all this therapeutic effort, by 1871 Hammond could only report two cures out of the ninety-one cases he had treated. Some of the others were relieved, but in most the disease continued unchecked.[19] The search for new modes of treatment continued.

Hammond's surgical methods were as experimental as his medications, and no more effective. In 1881 he promoted a plan of "elongating" the sciatic nerve by exerting traction from a point under the biceps.[20] Most other members of the American Neurological Association were dubious, if not actually hostile. Eight years later Hammond himself referred to the method as a vogue that had passed. He had meanwhile learned through the newspapers about a new method of treatment that Charcot was teaching in Paris. It was based on the suspension apparatus used by orthopedic surgeons in fitting patients with corrective plaster-of-Paris jackets. Originally patients were suspended with their feet off the ground, supported by chin and arm straps. Hammond and Dr. E. L. Tompkins, his assistant at the new Washington sanatorium, modified the procedure to dispense with the arm straps. Patients were now suspended by the chin and occiput alone, with a spring balance added to measure the traction precisely.

Within a few months Hammond had used this uncomfortable device in five cases of locomotor ataxia. He found "marked benefit" in terms of relief of pain, improved balance, and even restoration of sexual power. He went on to test it in a case of anterolateral sclerosis and in several cases of functional impotence.[21] This was typical: if Hammond found a remedy beneficial in one condition, he was apt to try it on other types of patients as well. His desperate clients presumably were not only willing to submit to these experiments, but to pay for the privilege as well.

Hammond recognized the dangers of the suspension treatment: he was "quite confident that we shall someday hear that a neck has been dislocated and sudden death produced by the unskillful use of the method." Just a week later his fears were confirmed by a report in the *New York Medical Journal* of the death of a medical man who was attempting to treat himself by suspension. Hammond's own apparatus was perfectly safe, readers were reassured. By the end of the year, neurologists had become skeptical. Landon Carter Gray, for example, referred to the method as "the latest neurological fad," although not rejecting it outright. He regretted that it had been introduced to the United States by "the sensationalism of the New York 'Herald.'" A few months later, physicians were told that the fad had passed. Suspension (like nerve-stretching) had been shown to have only transitory benefits and some evil results. It had, however, encouraged the use of safer mechanical means such as massage and simple exercises.[22] By then Hammond was absorbed with his newest enthusiasm, the "animal extracts" of Brown-Séquard, and dropped the matter of suspension.[23]

While Hammond's therapeutics seems in retrospect to be less impressive than his diagnostic skills, they were nonetheless crucial to his success as a clinician, a teacher, and an author. "The professional success attained by Dr. Hammond . . . has been all but phenomenal," noted a reviewer of the eighth edition of the *Treatise* in 1886. His textbook was admired for its "admirable style," "the copious therapeutic recommendations of the work," and its "practical directness . . . that has met the temper of the profession." The reviewer explained that "modern authors have been conservative in naming lists of remedies for diseases of the nervous system." But most of the physicians who rely on textbooks "are like the vast mass of members in the church: they . . . want no uncertainty of sound in talking of prescriptions for particular diseases. Above all writers in this respect," he concluded, "Dr. Hammond has been their man."[24]

Many of Hammond's innovations were widely circulated through the medical journals: new uses for ergot, sulfate of manganese, arsenic, chloral hydrate, and nitroglycerine, to name a few. The neurologist himself emphasized this aspect of his work on appropriate occasions. He recognized that "the science of therapeutics is that in which the busy practitioner finds more enjoyment than in any other branch of medical science, for it is the one of all others that he can make more immediately useful to himself and his patients." Doubtless, he told readers of the *St. Louis Clinical Record*, "if morbid anatomy and pathology were completed sciences they would constitute the basis for therapeutics." But "as they are very far from being even tolerably developed," physicians generally had to rely on "pure empiricism" for progress toward "the end and aim of medicine – the knowledge of how to cure the sick."[25] One may suspect the New York expert of pandering to his audience of western practitioners, but his experiences with contemporary therapeutics were probably at least as frustrating as theirs.

It is sometimes difficult to reconstruct controversial aspects of Hammond's practice, and to assess the responses of his contemporaries. For example, he developed a procedure for the cure of hypochondria by the "aspiration of pus from the liver" using hypodermic needles. Unkind and probably untrue tales circulated about his methods. "The story went," recollected the neurologist Charles L. Dana, "that he once filled his hypodermic syringe with cream, plunged his needle into a patient's liver, showed him the withdrawn 'pus' and cured him of an abscess. The story was not true," Dana added, "but its recital was popular and gave comfort to the malevolent." Was this an example of an attempt to cure by suggestion? The procedure was respectable enough for the noted medical editor E. S. Gaillard to submit to it at the hands of J. Marion Sims, with Hammond assisting, and for Sims to present the case before the Virginia Medical Society. In 1880 Hammond described nine other patients who had undergone the treatment. One was an Ohio state senator, and the others had come to him from Maine, Pennsylvania, Michigan, North Carolina, Virginia, and Alabama. Hammond's theoretical defense of the procedure was controverted, but the operation had a great deal of publicity, and some credibility as well.[26]

By the 1880s such practice was coming under serious attack. Dana, who had been Hammond's student, declared in 1886 that "the incompetence of a medical or surgical specialty is indicated, in a measure, by the variety and novelty of its therapeutic armamentarium. Judged by this test," he continued bluntly, "I fear neurology would have to suffer in scientific estimation."[27] Even the first edition of Hammond's text had been charged in 1871 with such faults as "unwonted signs of individuality of thought stamped on almost every page" and even "*overpositiveness, amounting to recklessness*."[28]

But active treatments with conspicuous results were generally considered the proper work of a physician, by medical and lay persons alike. Even a sophisticated clinician like Hammond could not adhere to an extreme therapeutic nihilism, although general hygienic treatment and regimen, and in many conditions the avoidance of bloodletting and counterirritation, figure conspicuously in his text. The variety and novelty of his therapeutics may even have seemed to many evidence that the neurologist was thoroughly up-to-date, a complimentary adjective almost synonymous with "scientific." Hammond's use of instruments was clearly more central in treatment than in diagnosis, and could well have reinforced such impressions. In this respect, as in so many others, Hammond stood with one foot in the medical world of his student years and the other in the very changed world of the last decades of the century.

George Rosen's classic work on the specialization of medicine emphasized two key developments: the conception of a localized solidistic pathology that made the special study of particular organs plausible, and the invention of instruments with which the interior of the body could be visually apprehended. At least in the case of the ophthalmologist, Rosen showed, knowledge of such instruments and their subsequent therapeutic application constituted the characteristic expertise of the specialist.[29] In the case of neurology, the process of specialization was rather more complex.

The next chapters will show how conventional lesion-oriented pathology coexisted in Hammond's work with a new and rather vague functionalism rooted in his physiological experience. The latter may have been implied by his focus on the nervous *system* rather than on any one particular organ. In fact a nonlocalized pathology was almost prerequisite to the plausible practice of neurology, since lesions of the nervous system were, even a century ago, recognized as generally irreversible. The neurologist could consistently hold out hope for recovery only if the disorder were functional rather than the result of organic damage. Hammond's theories of "cerebral hyperaemia" and "spinal irritation" make sense as attempts to reconcile the apparent contradiction between the imperatives of contemporary medical science and those of the consulting room.

NEUROLOGY AND ELECTROTHERAPEUTICS

While instruments and apparatus did play a prominent part in Hammond's practice, they were at least as useful in conveying a sense of the neurologist's presumed authority as they were in actually arriving at a diagnosis or producing a cure. If any one technic – diagnostic or therapeutic – can be said to have characterized early American neurology, it was the medical use of electricity. No other was either as closely connected to the field or as omnipresent in its practice. It thus deserves more careful examination as an element of Hammond's work.

Medical electricity had already been studied for some time when European neurologists began its systematic development in the mid-nineteenth century. Duchenne used the induced ("faradic") current in 1849, and his treatise *De l'électrisation localisée* first appeared six years later. Robert Remak introduced the use of the primary ("galvanic") current in 1856, publishing his *Galvanotherapie der Nerven- und Muskelkrankheiten* two years later.[30] Experiments with medical electricity in the United States can be traced back to Benjamin Franklin and were the subject of much interest. But electricity remained a novelty among respectable American physicians until after the Civil War.

Hammond was one of the persons most responsible for the New York debut of the works of Duchenne and Remak. The eminent Fordyce Barker, addressing the New York Obstetrical Society in February 1865, acknowledged "his indebtedness to Dr. W. A. Hammond, not only for calling his attention to the subject [of faradization], but for much valuable information and instruction as to the modes of applying this agent."[31] Hammond claimed to have used galvanism in the treatment of bedsores while surgeon to the Baltimore Infirmary in the winter of 1860–61. In March of 1861 he described its use in a clinical lecture on a case of chronic myelitis. After the war, the October 1867 issue of Hammond's *Quarterly Journal of Psychological Medicine* carried a translation of Henri Becquerel's long paper on "the application of electricity to therapeutics," which had appeared in Paris in May and which the editor considered the best available work on the subject.[32]

But Hammond was soon suspicious of "a subject which is almost becoming threadbare from the number of unscientific attempts which are being made to enlighten the medical profession in regard to its mysteries." Commenting on George Beard and A. D. Rockwell's new book on medical electricity early in 1868, he stopped short of accusing the authors of being unscientific but doubted "if they are warranted . . . in claiming the power they do for the very important therapeutical agent of which they treat."[33]

These rather harsh comments may have been inspired, at least in part, by the imminent publication of Charles F. Morgan's posthumous book *Electrophysiology and Therapeutics,* the proofs of which Hammond had corrected. "There is nothing in the English language," boasted the editor, "which at all approaches it as regards the scientific treatment of the whole subject of electricity." The book received favorable notices from less partial critics as well.[34]

Hammond had another work in press by November: his annotated translation of Moritz Meyer's *Electricity in Its Relations to Practical Medicine.* This book was already in its third German edition and the author was, according to George Beard, "the best known of the electro-therapeutists in Berlin." The American edition was an immediate hit. It was "admirably adapted to the requirements of the medical profession," declared one reviewer. "On the intricate subject of Electrotherapeutics no higher authority exists than Dr. Moritz Meyer," gushed another, "nor could a better exponent of his researches and views be found than Dr. Hammond, whose own investigations in this field have developed many practical results."[35]

Many ill-educated physicians were probably content to leave increasingly complex and expensive electrical machinery to an expert. To some extent, then, the technique of medical electricity would have fostered nascent neurological specialism. But the reverse was also true: the prestige and scientific background of the neurologist lent credibility to methods previously associated with the quack. "After a long struggle with prejudice and indifference," editorialized the *New York Medical Journal* early in 1870, "electricity has deservedly won a position in legitimate therapeutics." Physicians' distrust had been justifiable "so long as electricity as a remedial agent was in the hands of crafty, ignorant, and money-getting men – quacks." But the value of the remedy had been tested and proved "by men whose motives are beyond mistrust, who are as thorough clinicians as they are accomplished scientists." That neurologists were also "money-getting men" apparently was not seen as relevant. Later that year the *Medical Gazette* reported that "a wave of enthusiasm on the subject of electrotherapeutics is rolling over the world," adding that nowhere else was interest "so widely diffused as in the United States."[36]

Electrotherapy was applied in a variety of cases, but it was so

closely associated with diseases of the nervous system that an en-
thusiast could speak in 1874 of neurology and "electrology" as
"the Siamese twins of science." But twins, even if linked, are
distinct individuals. If medical electricity characterized any one
specialty, it was "electrology" or "electrotherapeutics" and not
neurology. An Electrotherapeutical Society of New York had been
organized in 1871 with the endorsement and participation of many
distinguished physicians. By that time, too, positions were to be
had as "electrologist," "electrotherapeutist," or even "electrician"
in a number of important medical institutions.[37] Two years later
the society expanded its scope to include the study of the nervous
system. It was formally reorganized as the New York Society of
Neurology and Electrology in January 1874, with the new journal
Archives of Neurology and Electrology appearing soon after.

Hammond remained aloof from these efforts, most likely because of his ongoing feud with George Beard, although nearly
everyone else interested in neurology and psychiatry joined. Instead, Hammond reactivated the moribund New York Neurological Society that he had founded in 1872. Ostensibly Hammond's group was to concern itself with practical problems and
cases, while the other was more interested in theoretical questions.
It is doubtful, however, whether such a distinction ever really
existed. The two groups had a largely overlapping membership
and were frequently confused by the profession. Hammond's ri-
valry with Beard became a durable standing joke. "Sweet Peace,"
heralded the *Medical Record* in 1882. "Two New York neurologists
were recently seen to shake hands with each other in a cordial
manner. It is thought now," the editorial wit continued, "that it
will not be necessary to organize a third neurological society." The
item was reprinted in the *Cincinnati Lancet and Clinic* with the
addendum, "We are so glad. Utterly two-two." This, in turn,
reappeared in the *New England Medical Monthly.* There can be little
doubt that the butts of the joke were Hammond and Beard.[38]

Electrology did not long survive as a recognized specialty. At a
time when specialism was by no means generally accepted, it was
unable to defend successfully its existence to other members of the
profession. This failure cannot be attributed entirely to the inefficiency of its therapeutics, because the same could be said about
neurology. Nor was there any insurmountable obstacle, theoretical or practical, to the emergence of a specialty organized

around a technique. Surgical specialties even in the 1870s, radiology several decades later, and endoscopy more recently did so with success. The particular difficulties that beset electrology are suggested in an 1875 review of the second edition of the Beard-Rockwell treatise.

The reviewer reported himself "fatigued but not convinced." The authors apparently wanted "to show that electrotherapeutics is a science which had made great progress since Remak's time, and that long and patient study is required before its details are mastered." He disagreed, arguing that "electrotherapeutics is not a science" and that "no great progress has been made." Furthermore, "any sensible doctor of medicine can fit himself in a month's time, at most, to make all of the applications as well as the so-called masters." The claim of electrology to scientific specialty status must have been further undermined by Rockwell's insistence that electrotherapeutics need not be based on electrophysiology.[39] Electrology quickly took second place to its "twin" in meetings of the New York Society of Neurology and Electrology, and when this group merged with Hammond's a few years later electrology seems to have met its formal end as a would-be specialty.

Even among neurologists electricity was gradually falling into disfavor. By 1879 electrotherapeutics was a matter of so much dissension that had neurologists depended on it for their credibility their cause would long since have been lost. A debate at the fourth annual meeting of the American Neurological Association in that year disclosed to the medical world that the alleged experts could not agree among themselves on which direction to apply the electric current to the patient, nor even whether that mattered. One Dr. J. D. S. Smith of Bridgeport, Connecticut, complained emphatically that the textbooks "*muddle* more than they enlighten the general practitioner." The A.N.A. discussion showed "that the muddle is not confined *alone* to those who *learn,* for those who *have* and *do teach* seem to make muddle doubly muddling."[40]

* * * * *

The rhetoric of Hammond and his contemporaries leaves a clear impression that technological accessories played an important role, and perhaps even a crucial one, in the establishment of recognized neurological expertise. They did so both by giving skilled specialists a margin of actual technical superiority over general practitioners, and by providing their patients with visible evidence that the specialty was thoroughly scientific and up-to-date. But in neurology it was not the case that "the tool made the specialist no less than the specialist made the tool." Nor was neurology in the United States "dependent upon the invention of instruments which are indispensable to physical diagnosis of disease and of the organs which they involve."[41] In their dealings with patients presenting with organic diseases of the nervous system, neurologists' special expertise rested far more on focused clinical experience and judgment than it did on esoteric technics.

There is an irony in the fact that Hammond, whose first interests were in basic medical science and whose first researches were performed in comparative isolation, should ultimately have achieved prominence in neurology as a clinician and as an organizer. He brought to the new specialty, said Joseph Collins, "an uncommon literary capacity, a rare power of narrative, and more important than all, an intuitive clinical insight, coupled with a capacity for detail." These were "all united with colossal physical strength and tireless mental activity." A neurologist reviewing the sixth edition of Hammond's *Treatise* in 1876 suggested that its "fullness and practical excellence in . . . therapeutics, is one of the chief reasons for the favor with which the work has been received by the profession." He found Dr. Hammond "a laborious and skilful observer, bold and inventive, but too often hasty in reaching conclusions" and "in a measure, deficient in analytical and generalizing powers." Despite this, "no single member of the profession in the United States," the reviewer declared, "has done more to develop neurological medicine, or . . . to attract the favorable attention of the profession abroad."[42]

Ten years later, J. Leonard Corning considered Hammond's neurology to have a special national character. "Contrast," he suggested, "this direct, this lucid, this American method of treatment with the nebular manner of handling things neurological so characteristic of the metaphysical dogmatism of certain cerebral anatomists." Hammond, he concluded, "has risen to fame, borne by the momentum of his own gifted understanding." And yet the very years during which Hammond seemed to be "tracing indelibly upon the tablet of clinical neurology a record of his existence" soon came to be regarded as part of the prehistory of the specialty. Louis J. Casamajor wrote in 1943 that in 1883 "neurology was still learned mostly from the rear section of textbooks on general medicine, for neurology was still a province of medicine and hence respectable." Charles L. Dana reminisced in 1924 that "neurology became almost respected in New England and New York in 1890."[43] Hammond's overly ambitious vision of neurology, based on fairly mechanical extrapolation from limited data, faltered in much the same way as had his program for biology a quarter of a century earlier.

8

"So great her science"

"The man of medicine stands midway between the lawyer on the one hand and the devotee of abstract science on the other," editorialized the *Therapeutic Gazette* in 1886. "The fashionable practitioner, the great specialist, who annually receives his many thousands of dollars, is the man of the present. Often, however, his present success is founded upon his past labors for science."[1] A more skeptical observer rhyming in a humorous vein about "The Specialist" put it differently: "For here Neurology had ta'en her part/So great her science, and so small her art!"[2] Either writer might have had Hammond in mind. When the former surgeon general moved to New York in 1864 he established himself in private practice, the only way he could use his medical skills to support himself and his family. But scientific investigation remained central to his view of medicine. And in the absence of efficacious therapeutics for most neurological disorders, the scientific reputation of the neurologist might be one of his greatest assets.

The scientific problems to which Hammond turned after the Civil War were among those of current interest and controversy in European medical circles. But from the clinical vantage point virtually mandated by his circumstances, he saw these issues differently and produced results significantly dissimilar from those of his laboratory-based counterparts. Hammond's researches on organic infantile paralysis (polio), on aphasia (loss of speech), and on sleep all illustrate this point. While not definitive, his conclusions were often consistent with some of the best work of his contemporaries. Taken as a whole, these scientific labors were plausible enough to sustain the scientific reputation he had built up before the Civil War with his experiments in physiological chemistry.

Hammond first applied clinical tools and methods to current problems of medical science in the study of infantile paralysis.[3] It was an appropriate choice for an aspiring specialist. The illness had been described as early as 1789 by Michael Underwood, a London obstetrician who paid special attention to diseases of children. The orthopedist Jacob von Heine published a clinical description in 1840 that was thereafter regarded as definitive. The illness was especially dreaded since it typically attacked otherwise healthy children, crippling them suddenly and usually for life. There is some evidence that by mid-century its incidence was increasing in the United States.[4]

Heine neither made pathological observations nor proposed a specific lesion to characterize the putative disease. "Infantile paralysis" therefore had dubious ontological status in terms of contemporary medical science. Heine did claim that a specific lesion existed, and urged the publication of more autopsies through which it could be identified. G.-B.-A. Duchenne argued for a spinal lesion, reasoning by analogy with cases of known lesion to the cord, but could not demonstrate this hypothesis experimentally. There was a major difficulty in solving the problem by orthodox methods: infantile paralysis rarely killed its young victims. Thus few physicians ever had an opportunity to conduct an autopsy, at least until decades after the illness, when the results might well have been regarded as inconclusive. In the face of this obstacle to research, the pediatricians Frederic Rilliet and A.-C.-E. Barthez and others broke from the Paris tradition. They recognized the disease but postulated that no lesion existed, promulgating the term *paralysie essentielle*.[5] Like the parallel term *fièvre essentielle*, this purely clinical description did little to elucidate the pathological issue.

Infantile paralysis attracted little interest in the United States before the Civil War. By 1858, the only American medical contributions on the subject were case reports by J. M. Paul (1829) and G. Colman (1843).[6] By the time Hammond began to publish on the subject in 1867, however, six more articles had appeared, and they were not simply case reports. The spurt in medical journalism was related to the rise of specialism. As Charles F. Taylor wrote in 1867, medical knowledge of infantile paralysis could be gleaned from scattered cases "only when some enthusiastic 'specialist' calls them from their hiding-places."[7] But which specialist? Infantile paralysis could plausibly be claimed by the pediatrician, the neurologist, or the orthopedist. Abraham Jacobi discussed it in a review of "recent works relating to infantile pathology and therapeutics" in 1858. The young author had recently begun to lecture on pediatrics at the College of Physicians and Surgeons of New York and would soon take the first American chair in that field.[8] Taylor had recently returned to New York from Sweden, and was busily promoting the "movement cure." He would play an important role in the development of orthopedics as a specialty.

Taylor considered infantile paralysis to be a distinct disease. Unlike other paralyses, "there is no evidence whatever . . . of any organic lesion in the brain or spinal cord." He, too, noted that "such cases seldom die, and the opportunities for post-mortem examinations are very few indeed." From his perspective, the unanswered physiological questions could be ignored and the pathology summarized as a deficiency of "nerve force" leading to malnutrition and atrophy of the muscles. More important to his practice, deformities could be prevented by proper management.[9] In contrast to Taylor, the neurologist M. Gonzalez Echeverría said that the condition was the last phase of "reflex paralysis" and not a distinct disease. He did agree with Taylor that no lesion of the central nervous system could be assumed.[10] The different professional interests of these specialists resulted in the development of pathological speculations along different, even contradictory lines, although all worked within a general framework of shared assumptions.

Hammond's initial emphasis was practical. "I shall not at present dwell upon the many points connected with the pathology of the affection in question," he wrote in December 1865. He had "no very definite ideas upon the subject." Previously published opinions were "in the main based on conjectures," and his own had no "more solid foundation." His purpose was to present a therapeutic breakthrough: the use of "the continuous galvanic current of great intensity in exciting muscular irritability when it has been apparently altogether lost."[11] By May 1867 Hammond had seen at least twenty-two cases of the disease for himself. He accepted an invitation to present his views on its pathology before the New York Medical Journal Association. Following Duchenne, the Paris clinician who had already won recognition for his contributions to French neurology, Hammond used purely clinical methods. He first distinguished "true" infantile paralysis from another condition described in a case report by a Dr. Kennedy by contrasting the easy cure of the latter with tonics (iron and strychnia) with the obstinacy of the true disease. Hammond also reported that he had devised a sensitive instrument to measure the slight temperature differentials between the healthy and diseased limbs of patients with true infantile paralysis.

With the clinical evidence in front of him, Hammond was more willing to discuss pathology. He endorsed Duchenne's views, arguing that the substance of the spinal cord became diseased, impairing the contractile power of the muscles and leading to their atrophy. Nerve function itself was not affected. Instead, malnutrition of the muscles occurred because "the proper stimulus has not been sent through the nerves . . . for so long" that the muscles had "lost the power of being excited by their natural motor influences" and were "incapable of recovering their tone and healthy condition." Hammond differed from Duchenne in claiming that fatty degeneration of the muscles was not always present. He thus preferred the designation "organic infantile paralysis" to Duchenne's *paralysie atrophique graisseuse de l'enfance*.[12]

Hammond's hypothesis had the advantage of being demonstrable without resort to the autopsy that was so difficult to obtain. Duchenne had invented an instrument, introduced in America by Hammond as "Duchenne's trocar," with which microscopical sections of muscle tissue could be obtained from the patient at various stages of the disease. Hammond's drawings of specimens thus obtained demonstrated to his satisfaction the degenerative course of the illness. Beyond this, it was clear to him that the characteristic lower back pain "marks the seat of the disease of the spinal cord." He did not venture to guess as to its exact character. He had had only one opportunity to examine the cord postmortem, and knew of no examinations by others. Omitting microscopical analysis, he had discerned a gross lesion only. But possible spinal lesions played a secondary role in the pathology he had outlined. This question could, in his terms, reasonably be left unsolved.

Muscular damage and therefore paralysis could be explained physiologically even if the acute phase of the disease left no permanent
scar. Duchenne, said Hammond, had "very abundantly settled"
the pathology of organic infantile paralysis "by examination of
tissue taken from the living subject."[13] The scientific clinician
seemed to have resolved a question at the bedside that had previously been studied, without signal success, in the pathological
laboratory.

In this case Hammond's methods were more significant than the
results. The neurologist himself quickly revised his opinion as new
microscopical findings came to hand. The account of infantile
paralysis published in his *Treatise* four years later acknowledged
the "remarkable series of observations on the minute anatomy of
the spinal cord, made by Dr. Lockhart Clarke," as well as the
"recent observations" of Charcot and Joffroy. Hammond no longer considered the "essential feature" of infantile paralysis to be
muscular degeneration. He wrote that "the lesion . . . consists
essentially of atrophy and disappearance of nerve cells."[14] In accordance with this new view, the disease was classified in the text as
one of "nerve cells," although Hammond's muscle biopsies were
still included. The clinical portions of this chapter did not differ
significantly from the corresponding remarks on symptoms, diagnosis, prognosis, and treatment in the paper of 1867. Here Hammond could speak with even greater authority. In the five years
between 1865 and 1870 he had seen at least ninety-eight cases of
the disease. His scientific papers on polio had certainly contributed
to his reputation as an expert, and hence to the influx of cases. In
the long run, however, his expertise was based far more on his
clinical experience than on his attempts to elucidate pathology.

APHASIA, LATERALIZATION, AND THE
EVOLUTION OF LANGUAGE

Aphasia, unlike polio, never contributed significantly to Hammond's caseload. But when he began his study of this intricate
problem in 1864, a heated debate was raging in Parisian scientific
circles. Aphasia was seen as an important test of the doctrine of
cerebral localization. This anatomical controversy had, in turn,
philosophical overtones and, less overtly, political implications.
And it was an issue that anatomy itself had failed to resolve. In the

1860s, dissectors from opposing camps could not always agree even on their observations of brain structure, let alone on interpretations of these data.[15]

But pathology also presented relevant evidence. French physicians, using the fundamental Paris technique of correlating clinical symptoms with autopsy results, searched for specific brain lesions in cases of linguistic derangement. Jean-Baptiste Bouillaud, in 1825, correlated aphasia with injury of the anterior lobes of the brain. Paul Broca announced to the Parisian Société d'Anthropologie in 1861 his conversion to the doctrine of localization. He believed he had more precisely located the "speech center" in the third frontal convolution. Broca was generally defended by younger men, Liberals and Republicans, while the older and more conservative faction, led by A. Trousseau, upheld the position that the brain acts as a whole.[16] Hammond noted that the pathological evidence was also ambiguous. Most of the aphasic cases that had been described supported Broca's position, but there were many troubling exceptions.[17] Aphasia was thus an important scientific problem for which the traditional research methods of European medicine were unable to provide a solution. Hammond's application of clinical analysis again suggested a way out of the dilemma.

Aphasia was the topic of a special meeting of the New York County Medical Society convened at the College of Physicians and Surgeons in December 1870. Hammond's "lengthy but interesting paper," in the words of a medical reporter, set the tone for the subsequent discussion.[18] He began by distinguishing between the intellectual aspect of speech (memory of words) and its physiological aspect (articulation, phonation, sign language, mimicry). This was the only point on which the members of the French Académie de Médecine had agreed in an argument over aphasia in 1864–65. Hammond called derangement of the physiological aspect of speech "ataxic" aphasia. He noted that this form was found when hemiplegia (generally left hemiplegia) was present. In other cases, the aphasia was of the "amnesic" form. Here the patient lost the idea of language and the memory of words. "This is a point," he said, "which had not hitherto been noted. The phenomena indicate . . . very clearly, the seat of the lesion, and the physiology of the parts involved."[19] When the lesion affected the gray matter of the brain, he concluded, the idea of language was damaged but motor function was not impaired. Since hemiplegia indicated a lesion of the corpus striatum, ataxic aphasia must be caused by the extension of the lesion into the immediately neighboring parts. These, in turn, must be regarded as the seat or center of the physiological aspect of language function. This was substantially the conclusion reached by John Hughlings Jackson, on whose work Henry Head based his classic analysis of aphasia.[20]

Hammond's paper on aphasia had not actually tried to locate the speech "center" or "faculty" in the brain. Instead he specified the putative site of a lesion that could derange speech. This was a subtle and crucial point to Hughlings Jackson, who articulated it as the dictum that "to locate the damage which destroys speech and to localize speech are two different things."[21] Hammond and Jackson avoided the knotty problem of the nature of language, on which the Académie had foundered.[22] They treated speech as a function or behavior that could be observed clinically. This "*comparative method* of clinical analysis" proved very productive in Jackson's hands. Jackson "was, first and foremost, a clinician by deliberate intent. The clinic, the bedside, and the autopsy room were his only laboratories."[23] Hammond's work was contemporaneous with Jackson's but largely independent. While original in some respects, it by no means invites comparison in regard to importance. However, Hammond's work on aphasia does deserve attention as an attempt to carry out scientific work in neurology at the bedside at a time when few facilities were available in America for medical research. Hammond, no longer a laboratory physiologist, was attacking current problems of medical science with the tools and methods of the clinical specialist.

Hammond's New York colleagues expressed interest in his discussion of aphasia but were not convinced. John C. Dalton, for example, upheld the conservative view. "If we were to depend alone on the anatomy of the fibres of the brain," he said, "I do not think we could form any *a priori* notion of the possibility of locating any faculty in any one part." He thought it "possible that the brain may act always as a whole." Dr. W. B. Neftel responded with the position that would become dominant in the following decade. He argued that the existence of a "center of speech" could be inferred from the demonstrated existence of other centers. "But the centre of speech is certainly the most interesting of all," he conceded, "being at the threshold between the motor and the intellectual functions."[24]

For reasons that have yet to be explored adequately, most neurological work on aphasia after about 1869 came to depend on "diagram-making." Henry Head reported that by 1886 most British neurologists "believed that every sign and symptom could be deduced from a local lesion in some cortical centre or injury to the paths between them." German work, following Carl Wernicke, took a similar course. By 1926, Head wrote, neurology had "become frozen stiffly in the grip of pseudo-metaphorical classifications which neither explain the conditions nor correspond to the clinical facts." Head's own landmark work on aphasia grew out of his increasing dissatisfaction with this "diagram-making" and his rediscovery of Jackson's work.[25] In Head's time, functional approaches to the body and disease were a critical part of "bedside medicine" as it was counterpoised to laboratory research. In this context it is significant that the eighth edition of Hammond's *Treatise* (1886) did not turn away from the line he and Jackson had originally taken.

Hammond differed from Jackson in that he was more strongly drawn to the psychological, social, and medicolegal implications of aphasia, while the Englishman did not stray far from the narrower neurological path. Hammond assumed that even the most abstract findings of medical science would have immediate practical consequences. In this respect, too, he was a transitional figure. While his specific scientific insights were consistent with the most advanced work of his time, his overall perspective on science was more characteristic of an earlier period. This facet of Hammond's neurology is evident in two aspects of his work on language: analysis of unilateral brain phenomena and the application of language studies to evolutionary theory.

Hammond noted in 1870 that "the left hemisphere [of the brain] is more intimately connected with the faculty of speech than the right." This point – which Hammond seems to have stressed more in the oral than in the printed version of the paper – particularly impressed the otherwise critical Dalton. "A point new to me, and of the greatest interest," the eminent physiologist commented, "is the ingenious explanation given of the habitual occurrence of aphasia as a result of lesion of the left hemisphere, taken in connection with its occasional occurrence of the right." Hammond's explanation was that "this is analogous to right- and left-handedness, and not due to original difference in function of the two hemispheres, but to their independent action, and to the earlier or stronger development of the left."[26] Jackson also adopted this hypothesis. His efforts to understand aphasia in the context of other unilateral phenomena (including handedness) played an important part in his notable successes in epilepsy and localization during the 1870s and 1880s.[27]

Hammond followed up on the insight in a different way. He dropped the matter for close to fifteen years, then returned to it in a widely publicized paper on "unilateral hallucinations" read before the New York Neurological Society on December 1, 1885. He defended A. L. Wigan's theory "that there are in fact two brains, the two hemispheres having independent though similar functions, ordinarily acting together, though capable of isolated and even different action." It was not a popular position, and the neuroanatomist E. C. Spitzka led a chorus of opposition.[28] Undaunted, Hammond told the lay readers of *Forum* in 1887 that the theory that the mind was dual "is supported by many facts in the anatomy, physiology, and pathology of the brain." When one hemisphere is injured, he explained, the two halves of the brain can act independently. He thought this explained some cases of missing persons. These individuals "suddenly disappear from their homes and as suddenly find that they have been unconscious of their acts."[29]

The social complexities that could result from such a neurological state had been vividly portrayed in an 1881 novel by Hammond's twenty-two-year-old daughter Clara Lanza. This work was dedicated to her father and prefaced with the assurance that "the state of 'double consciousness' . . . [is] a phenomenon well known to neurological physicians." The novel and Dr. Hammond's connection to it were widely noted in New York medical journals. Hammond stated confidently that unfortunates like the heroine could be cured with remedies for epilepsy. "The dual existence would cease and the impulse to run away be abolished."[30] Thus even his rather esoteric scientific work on aphasia served to advertise Hammond's practice. But it also illustrated the continuity he saw between narrowly technical neurological issues and broader social ones. Hammond seems eventually to have lost interest in the idea of double consciousness, for when he wrote a four-act play twenty years later about a man who leads a double life, the neurological theme was absent. Rather, the hero is an impecunious gentleman supporting his daughter on the proceeds of an impeccably reputable gambling house while perfecting a new chemical explosive that will make his fortune. He maintains a dual persona so that the gambling parlor does not dishonor the family.[31]

As an expert on aphasia, Hammond was also able to contribute to the discussion of Darwin's theory of human descent. The occasion was the publication in 1877 of Frederick Bateman's *Darwinism Tested by Language*. The author contended that articulate speech was a universal characteristic of humanity that distinguished it from other species. The faculty of speech could not be explained in terms of material phenomena, he said, citing as evidence Broca's failure to locate it in the brain. Bateman concluded that humans were not only quantitatively but qualitatively different from the animals and could not have evolved from them. Hammond had been an evolutionist for some time, and here was a chance to jump into the argument.

The neurologist countered Bateman's argument in a lengthy book review for the *Journal of Nervous and Mental Diseases*. He argued first that at least some animal language, such as the song of the nightingale, was sufficiently complex to be regarded as articulate speech. He thought that apes were physiologically capable of learning human speech, although so far no one had attempted to teach it to them. But Hammond's main point was that Bateman had attacked a straw man. Even Broca no longer held to the particular version of speech localization that Bateman criticized. Hammond drew on his previously published work on aphasia for a lengthy history of language localization studies. He reiterated that the lesion that caused speech to become deranged could be localized to the region of the middle cerebral artery, an area recently labeled by Adolf Kussmaul as the "speech tract." Bateman's antievolutionary argument thus collapsed. Hammond was no more sophisticated than his opponent in conceptualizing the relations between quantitative and qualitative differences, maintaining that the differences between people and animals were purely quantitative. They were not distinguished primarily by "the mental faculties, or the intellectual characteristics." Rather, there were structural differences in the bodies and "the degree of development of the several organs by which both mental and physical acts are performed." He reminded his neurological audience that one "can only regard [mind] as the product of nervous action."[32]

Hammond pursued this theme in a perhaps unfortunate talk at the first annual commencement of the reorganized but still "irregular" New York College of Veterinary Surgeons in March 1878. His topic was "Equine Psychology," caricatured by one reporter as "horse sense." The neurologist reminded the new homeopathic veterinarians that the horse was noted for its docility and intelligence. Its brain was remarkable for the depth and number of its convolutions, as well as for its large weight relative to the body. He related anecdotes to illustrate the point that "the intelligence of the animal differed only in degree (not in kind) from that of man, passing to the interesting question of language." He mentioned the nightingale again to buttress his contention that "there was no rational doubt that animals were able to convey very specific ideas to each other by means of sounds."[33] Hammond's scientific views were perhaps no less unorthodox than his willingness to associate with a homeopathic institution.

SLEEP AND INSOMNIA

Hammond first studied the theory of sleep as a young army surgeon in Kansas. A unique patient consulted him in 1854 with a large cranial fissure resulting from a railway accident. Hammond noticed that while his patient was comatose the scalp over the fissure was elevated, that during normal sleep it was depressed, and that when the man was awake the scalp was on a level with the cranium. He later made analogous observations of infants (possibly his own Graeme and Clara) with unclosed fontanelles.[34] These findings contradicted the view of most contemporary physiologists that vascular congestion of the brain caused sleep. Earlier authors had suggested that congestion caused sleep mechanically, by compression of the brain or a part of it. But by mid-century most physicians accepted the "Monro-Kellie doctrine" that since the skull is rigid and the brain substance relatively incompressible, the total quantity of blood in the brain must be constant. Then both "congestion" and "anemia" of the brain would be impossible. Perhaps venous congestion coinciding with diminished arterial circulation caused sleep through a deficiency of oxygenated blood.

Johann Blumenbach had advanced the theory that diminished flow of oxygenated blood caused sleep as early as 1779, but he did not tie this to venous congestion. He based it instead on observations of the exposed brain of a patient with massive cranial trauma. His *Principles of Physiology* provided the starting point for Hammond, Arthur E. Durham, and other physiologists seeking an approach to sleep that would be neither metaphysical nor superficially mechanistic. Hammond may have read Blumenbach as early as the 1850s, when his efforts to assist his Philadelphia colleagues' research on racial craniology could easily have led him to the German master of race theory.

Another thread leading to Hammond's theory of sleep was his chemical study of metabolic wastes. He assumed that the brain tissue is consumed in the process of thought in amounts proportional to the intensity of mental exertion. He liked to explain this with the analogy of a steam engine, which consumed coal, generated electricity, and left ashes as a by-product. Likewise, the brain metabolized its own tissue, generated mind, and left the waste products of metabolism as measurable traces in the blood. Then the brain would need to repair or rebuild itself, and this process might plausibly take place during sleep. Hammond claimed that his experimental results were consistent with this hypothesis.

Still another link was Hammond's collaboration with Weir Mitchell on the effects of poisons, and by extension narcotic drugs. A key source cited by Hammond in reference to sleep was an article by an Irish practitioner, Alexander Fleming, who reported compressing the carotid arteries to produce deep sleep. Hammond said that this work, and the experiences of the Virginia physician Bedford Brown with ether and chloroform, illustrated the "important fact" that the quantity of blood in the brain decreased during sleep. His own experiments included observations of the effects of ether, chloroform, and opium, which he believed to produce stupor rather than true sleep.[35]

More broadly, Hammond's interest in sleep developed from a physiological approach to psychology. Here again he chose a research topic close to the heart of a contemporary scientific debate. As Lorraine Daston has shown, a central intellectual issue within

British (and consequently much American) psychology in the last third of the century was a "perceived tension between the moral necessity of free will and a law-governed mental science." This problem troubled even the most enthusiastic supporters of psychophysiology, who concentrated much of their effort on trying to solve it.[36] But if any one fact seemed clear about sleep, it was that the faculty of volition was suspended. Thus sleep might prove more readily amenable to a purely physiological explanation than other psychological states. "It is only by studying the behavior of the mind during the coming and going of sleep," wrote the geologist Nathaniel Shaler in the *International Review*, "that we can hope to understand the peculiar relations of the will to the rest of the mental capacities."[37] Moreover, sleep was conspicuously resistant to analysis by introspection, the central method of philosophical psychology. While sleep remained a mystery to traditional psychological writers, it was a fertile field for physiologists (including Hammond) interested in elaborating a materialist psychology.

A British researcher, Arthur E. Durham, took the lead in sleep physiology with a paper presented at the June 1860 meeting of the British Association for the Advancement of Science in Oxford, and published that fall in *Guy's Hospital Reports*. Hammond began his own experiments on sleep in the summer of 1860. He insisted that they had been conceived and performed independently of Durham's. This is certainly possible, but there is also a possible link through John William Draper, an eminent physiologist who had supplied Durham with some of his unpublished results and who was at the Oxford meeting.[38] Draper had been Hammond's teacher fifteen years earlier, and could easily have brought word of Durham's seminal paper across the Atlantic. When Hammond found time five years later to publish his results, he generously and truthfully acknowledged that Durham's investigations had been more detailed and probing than his own. Most contemporaries seemed satisfied to couple the two men as coauthors of a position that, despite differing emphases, they shared.

Durham defined sleep in physiological terms as "that period of cerebral inactivity during which nutrition of the brain substance takes place." He designed a series of experiments, based on the ideas of Blumenbach, in which holes were drilled in the crania of dogs and other animals and fitted with watch glasses to form airtight windows on the brain. Hammond did the same on dogs and rabbits, omitting the glass and attributing the technique to the Dutch ophthalmologist Franz Cornelius Donders.[39] He observed the color of the brain and its position in relation to the skull. Durham supplemented the observations of the unaided eye with those of the microscope. Both researchers concluded that sleep was a comparatively bloodless condition of the brain. For the second part of his argument, Durham cited direct experimental evidence that mental exertion affected the waste products of the nerves, and declared himself convinced that "oxidation of the brain-substance is concomitant with, and directly proportionate to, the development of cerebral activity" – that is, to thought. Hammond cited his own Kansas experiments which, though less direct and conclusive, made the same point.

Hammond devoted nearly a quarter of his 1865 article "On Sleep and Insomnia" to a summary of Durham's conclusions. Their outline of the sleep cycle was as follows. Increased stimulation of the brain might cause (or permit to come into play) greater chemical affinity of the brain tissue for oxygen. This increased rate of oxidation of brain tissue would draw oxygenated arterial blood more rapidly into the brain, mechanically distending the cerebral capillaries and permitting an increased quantity and velocity of blood to circulate in the brain. This condition, "circulation of function," favored the endosmosis of waste products from brain tissues into the blood, and worked against the exosmosis of nutrients into the tissues. Then when the brain stimulation decreased or the "tendency to oxidation . . . diminished," less blood would be drawn into the brain, the capillaries would contract due to their normal elasticity, and "circulation of nutrition" would supervene with more nutrients flowing into the tissues of the brain. Thus whatever increases cerebral circulation can induce wakefulness and whatever decreases it (consistent with health) can induce sleep. Such causes could act directly through the vascular system or (as with sense impressions and exciting ideas) through the nervous system.[40]

Like Durham, Hammond thought that sleep allowed "the nutrition of the nervous tissue to go on at a greater rate than its destructive metamorphosis," that the quantity of blood in the brain decreased during sleep, and that sleep could be induced by arresting the flow of blood to the brain. Unlike Durham, he was not especially interested in the possibility of chemical regulation of the sleep cycle. His more modest goal was to establish only "that sleep is directly caused by the circulation of a less quantity of blood through the cerebral tissues than traverses them whilst we are awake." He called this the "immediate" cause of sleep, and the "necessity for repair" was the "exciting" cause.[41] For Durham, in contrast, the "proximate cause" of sleep was (probably) the buildup of metabolic wastes, or anything else that interfered with the mutual affinity of brain tissue and oxygen. Hammond's formulation was more narrowly mechanical, representing a less sophisticated concept of causality in physiology.

The Hammond–Durham theory of sleep was widely discussed in lay magazines as well as in the medical press. Many physicians were favorably impressed by Hammond's work, which was endorsed by the influential British physician J. Milner Fothergill. J. Leonard Corning, a neurologist who had at one time worked with Hammond, declared in 1882 that "of the various writers who have contributed to our knowledge on this subject, there is not one who has done more for our physiological enlightenment respecting the nature of sleep and its accompanying phenomena than Dr. William A. Hammond."[42]

As late as 1894, Henry Wurtz cited Hammond favorably in *Popular Science Monthly*. He explained that "normal sleep and sleepiness . . . are due to a small increase over the average of the carbonic acid in solution in the blood, arising through its overproduction from the greater amount of muscular and other tissue that undergoes oxidation during the waking hours." Unlike Hammond, he did not single out brain tissue.[43] Other popularizers were more cautious in endorsing the idea that sleep depended on reduced circulation of blood in the brain. "Only within the last ten years or so," wrote the young neurologist Henry Charleton Bastian in *Appleton's Journal* in 1869, have "physiologists . . . begun to entertain this view."[44]

Other writers remained skeptical of the physiological approach. Shaler stated in the *International Review* in 1879 that science had learned something of the evolutionary history of sleep and of "the methods of its action upon the machinery of the body," but still knew nothing about its relation to the "machinery of the mind," since introspection was not available as a tool of investigation.[45] The sharpest critic of Hammond's physiology of sleep was the

South Carolina physician Samuel Henry Dickson, an elder states-
man of American medical literature. Resting his case on the
Monro-Kellie doctrine, which his generation so took for granted
that he found it unnecessary to cite references, Dickson claimed
that Hammond's experiments had proved (if anything) only
Blumenbach's view that sleep could be produced by a decrease in
oxygenated blood flowing to the brain. His general approach reflected the same medical conservatism. For example, he assumed
as "received and reasonable" the idea that the necessity for repair
of brain tissue was the "sole use and final cause of sleep." Neither
Hammond nor Durham spoke of "final causes" and Durham had
shunned the Aristotelian terminology altogether. Volition, Dickson asserted, was not caused by the decomposition of brain tissue.
Rather, it caused actions that could cause decomposition. The
mental was for him both prior to and primary over the physical.[46]

Others were more cautious in their appraisals. Hammond's colleague Edward C. Seguin questioned his reasoning. He had personally "verified the exactness of Dr. Hammond's and Mr. Durham's observations," but thought it "most hasty and in conflict
with general physiological laws to have concluded *post hoc* that this
anemia is a *cause* of sleep." He called for more "experimental and
logical study."[47] Benjamin Ward Richardson, F.R.S., declared in
the first volume of *Popular Science Monthly* his dissatisfaction with
all existing accounts of sleep, including that of Durham and Hammond. But unlike Dickson and other conservative thinkers, and in
common with Hammond and Durham, Seguin and Richardson
expected physiological science to come forth eventually with a full
explanation of sleep and other mental phenomena.

Neither Hammond nor Durham conducted serious laboratory
work on sleep after 1860, and the physiological problem proved to
be quite difficult to unravel.[48] When Hammond began publishing
on the issue in 1865, his focus had already begun to shift to the
clinical: treatment of insomniac patients. A somewhat conservative
reviewer for the *New York Medical Journal* noted that "the physiological views respecting the *immediate* cause of sleep, maintained
by Dr. Hammond, are . . . at variance with those of most physiologists." However, he continued, "whatever difference of opinion may exist regarding Dr. Hammond's physiology, there can be
none respecting his therapeutics."[49] Clearly this physician did not
accept the idea of Hammond and others that the efficacy of the

therapeutics counted as evidence in favor of the physiological theory from which they were ostensibly derived.[50]

By the 1880s the increasingly significant interface between laboratory and clinic had begun to elicit self-conscious debate among leading American physicians on the question, at once methodological and ideological, of how science ought to enter medical work. The functionalism of German clinicians such as Friedrich von Frerichs and Adolf Kussmaul, for whom scientific medicine was a "bedside" affair, competed in subsequent decades with the "bench" orientation of disciplines such as bacteriology and laboratory physiology. When Hammond articulated his views on polio, aphasia, and sleep between 1864 and 1871, laboratory science was as yet neither an option nor a threat to American physicians, as his own experiences indicated. The results of clinical investigations he and others carried out during this short period were not incorporated into twentieth-century medical science in any important way. Correspondingly, they have been omitted from most standard histories of medicine, and America has been stigmatized as "indifferent to basic science" at least until the last decades of the nineteenth century.

Hammond was in many respects exceptional among American physicians in the postbellum period, as he was in the 1850s. His story does suggest, however, that the American scientific landscape was far less barren than has often been supposed. It supports recent reinterpretations that invite us to consider the nature of the ideology of scientific medicine as problematical, and to take more seriously the clinically oriented researches of mid-nineteenth-century physicians in Europe and the United States. Clinical specialism, as Hammond was to develop his neurology, entailed not only a different way to organize practice but new ways of viewing the human body as well.[51]

9

"Systems of cures and wonderful remedies"

Hammond based his influential *Treatise on the Diseases of the Nervous System* (1871) on the assumption that illnesses could be distinguished and classified on the basis of the morbid changes found in specific tissues of specific organs. His detailed discussions under the head "morbid anatomy" in nearly every chapter testify to his competence in dissection and microscopical inspection as well as to his familiarity with British and Continental medical literature. In many instances, pathology and morbid anatomy are discussed together. In others, the pathological explanation is a restatement of the tenets of the Paris Clinical School.[1] "Doubtless, if we had the opportunity of more thorough study of the symptoms of diffused cerebral sclerosis," he wrote, "and comparing them with the condition of the brain as found by post-mortem examination, we should find that they varied considerably in character, according to the part affected." He expected that "the nervous cells which had disappeared – motor, sensitive, or trophic – were in exact pathological relation with the symptoms observed."[2]

But the text itself also reveals the inconsistency of Hammond's position on the appropriate form of pathological explanation. For example, in the section on "cerebro-spinal diseases" he discusses at some length the prevalent view that there were "two kinds of chorea – one which is entirely functional, belonging to the so-called neuroses, the other the result of organic disease of the brain or spinal cord, or both." While he felt that the pathology of chorea could not yet be defined accurately, he had "strong evidence to support the view that it is not a neurosis or functional affection – *if, indeed, there are any such* – and that it is the result of changes taking place in the cerebro-spinal system."[3] But the section on "diseases of nerve cells" in the same volume contains a chapter on "functional derangements of motor nerve-cells." Here Hammond expresses the opinion that paralysis agitans "is due to an irregular and diminished evolution of nerve-force from the motor nerve-cells in relation with the nerves supplying the muscles in which the agitation exists." He adds that "the pathology of tremor, *not the result of structural lesions,* is . . . not yet clearly understood."[4]

The problem here is not merely inconsistency. Rather, Hammond's struggle to systematize neurology on a scientific basis reflects the tension between two conflicting pathological concepts. One was the tradition of pathological anatomy that had come to symbolize scientific medicine in the first half of the nineteenth century. The other was a less conventional physiological approach, consistent with Hammond's earlier laboratory research. The first was necessary for Hammond to convince his contemporaries (and most likely himself) that his work was truly scientific. The second, however, offered far more immediate opportunities to explain the cases of the patients he was seeing daily.

Ironically, the success of the *Treatise* rested primarily on its practical suggestions and its general scientific tone. A contemporary critic declared in 1881 with much justice that Hammond had "extensive knowledge, though it is more varied than profound." The author's strengths were that "his practical experience is large, his convictions are positive, and he can set them forth clearly and attractively." On the other hand, "with all his acuteness and wide observation, [he] is not . . . an accomplished physiologist or a thorough pathologist, and he is, therefore, often a superficial reasoner upon points involving these sciences."[5] "Science" was central to the neurologist's self-perception, and he often referred to himself as a physiologist. But his neurological work was most vulnerable precisely on the grounds of incorrect or even incompetent basic science, and this vulnerability increased over the years.

There is a further irony. The vast bulk of Hammond's *Treatise* was devoted to diseases for which discrete lesions of the nervous system could be found or, at least, were presumed to exist. Despite the most vigorous therapeutic efforts, such cases were unlikely to improve much. However, patients with such progressive illnesses could not have constituted more than one-third of those who consulted Hammond privately, even excluding "insane" patients. Far more of his clients suffered from illnesses he diagnosed as cerebral or spinal congestion or anemia, from "that protean disease" hysteria, or from epilepsy.[6] These were also virtually the only conditions for which he gave a favorable prognosis. Hammond never doubted (at least publicly) that these illnesses, like insanity, had a physical basis in some disorder of the nervous system. His problem was to elaborate convincing diagnostic categories that could make medical sense out of collections of vague and seemingly trivial symptoms which nonetheless were real enough to the patient. Hammond's pathological explanations of these diagnoses were uncompromisingly materialistic, though unsatisfactory to the scientifically minded physician steeped in mainstream European methods, and disconcertingly obscure to the less educated doctor. "Cerebral hyperaemia," in particular, furnished the rationale for a huge portion of the neurologist's practice. In this respect it was very similar to "neurasthenia."[7] Correspondingly, active medical intervention was an important element in producing cures, since it afforded tangible evidence that the physician was taking the illness as seriously as the patient did.

One early patient in New York was a sixteen-year-old girl brought to the neurologist by her mother in December 1864 "to be treated for spinal irritation." Her health had been failing, supposedly from excess study. "She had become very irritable, had lost her appetite, felt an indisposition to exertion of any kind, and was troubled with severe dyspepsia." To Hammond, her appearance seemed "chlorotic." He examined her spine, asked about her menstrual history, auscultated her heart and examined her blood miscroscopically. He then prescribed iron and quinine (to be taken as tonics) and recommended a full and nutritious diet. At first the patient improved, but later her condition worsened. A second examination showed edema, swollen feet, a bellows murmur of the heart, and a recent history of "epileptiform seizures." Under a new therapeutic regimen including strychnia, "potassae arsenicalis," and ale, she was reportedly restored to health in less than a month.[8]

Ten years later, this young lady would almost certainly have been diagnosed as neurasthenic, if not by her family physician then by a neurological consultant. But Hammond never accepted the diagnosis of neurasthenia. He objected strongly to "the proposal of obscure theories of lithaemia, or nervous prostration, or brain exhaustion, or neurasthenia, or any similar hypothesis which consists of mere words."[9] Hammond saw thousands of patients

who complained of insomnia and headache, dizzy spells or noises
in their ears, of lapses of memory or judgment, of transitory
illusions or delusions, of heaviness in the limbs or pain in the back,
of stomachache and general malaise. In "cerebral hyperaemia" he
thought he had the key to understanding the physical disease from
which these unfortunates suffered. As a medical scientist, he expected no less.

CEREBRAL HYPERAEMIA AND ITS TREATMENT

Hammond saw insomnia as the crucial symptom, the one universally present and increasing rapidly in frequency. "The state of
excitement in which people of the present day live, the demands of
business, the struggle for wealth and position," he wrote, "produce just that state of the brain which, if continued not only
through the day but far into the night, makes sound and healthy
sleep an impossibility."[10] One of his earliest New York patients,
for example, was a busy stockbroker "in whose case the only
deviation from health which could be observed was an utter inability to sleep."[11] Insomnia was common, but by no means trivial, and Hammond pressed the idea that professional treatment
was urgent. In his novel *Robert Severne* (1867), he has the scientific
physician Dr. Lawrence describe how "a well-known literary gentleman consulted me . . . 'For God's sake, put me to sleep,' he
said, 'I have not closed my eyes for two weeks!'" Lawrence remarks sadly that "he was too late; yesterday he was taken to
Bloomingdale." In case readers were not sufficiently alarmed by
the prospect of an insane asylum, Hammond reminded them of
"the danger attending long-continued concentration of the mind
upon one line of thought; how the brain, feeding as it were upon
the products of its own decay, wears itself away little by little, but
with awful certainty." In the end "either nothing but the shadow
of its pristine greatness remains, or else the reason . . . finally
becomes extinguished."[12]

To Hammond, a recognized expert on the physiology of sleep,
the insomnia universally present in these cases had an obvious
cause. Sleeplessness resulted, he said, from an excess of blood
circulating in the brain, or "cerebral hyperaemia." On this foundation an entire pathology could be built to explicate the links between social stress, mental disturbance, and physical symptoms.

Hammond's views on sleep physiology were published in the *New York Medical Journal* in 1865. The monograph based on these articles was not on sleep, however, but *On Wakefulness; with an Introductory Chapter on the Physiology of Sleep* (1866). The neurologist was rapidly orienting himself to the institution of private practice, and the clinical aspects of his subject became primary. His remedies for insomnia were appreciated by the profession, but from the perspective of medical science insomnia was a symptom rather than a disease.[13] In *Sleep and Its Derangements* (1869), an enlarged edition of the same book, "primary insomnia" was identified as a "functional disorder of the brain, arising from inordinate mental activity."[14] But in the more systematic *Treatise on the Diseases of the Nervous System* (1871), insomnia became the characteristic symptom of the first stage of a specific disease, "cerebral congestion of the active form." This stage was called "cerebral hyperaemia."

As Hammond had pointed out in his novel, the prognosis for primary cerebral congestion was not good. Before long, further physical and mental symptoms would appear: confused memory, weakened judgment and will, transitory illusions, hallucinations and delusions, headache, vertigo, noises in the ear, heaviness in the limbs, slurred speech. Hammond believed that in the first stage of the disease, patients might continue to lead a normal life, but they would not recover spontaneously. They would deteriorate to a second stage, where the disease took on an apoplectic, epileptic, maniacal, soporific, or aphasic form. Without proper medical attention, the third stage would supervene with a variety of secondary lesions, including tumors or softening of the brain, resulting in death.

Hammond was careful to cite earlier discussions of cerebral congestion, especially those by French authors. His own main contribution was the ascription of a psychological etiology to the disease. This was developed in detail in his book *Cerebral Hyperaemia the Result of Mental Strain or Emotional Disturbance* (1878). In particular, Hammond claimed originality in describing the "prodromatic stage" of cerebral congestion, in which wakefulness "may be for a time the only evidence of disorder which attracts the attention of the patient."[15] In other words, cerebral hyperaemia was precisely equivalent to insomnia.

Hammond recorded 622 cases of cerebral hyperaemia in a six-year period, an average of two new patients per week. Of these, 507 were of the "active" form, and 478 were reported cured by appropriate treatment (none spontaneously) before going beyond the first stage. This group of patients, who consulted Hammond for insomnia with a variety of other nondisabling physical and mental symptoms, may have accounted for 20 percent or more of his private practice, excluding cases of insanity, and for a far higher percentage of his recorded cures.[16] During the 1880s other physicians also took advantage of this convenient and respectably scientific diagnosis, although it never achieved the popularity of neurasthenia.[17]

Hammond developed the disease concept in a way that highlighted the expertise of the neurological specialist. He stressed the diagnostic use of sophisticated instruments: the esthesiometer, the ophthalmoscope, the aural speculum, and "Lombard's thermoelectric differential calorimeter" to identify the characteristic heat of the head. Yet a careful reading of both the *Treatise* and *Cerebral Hyperaemia* shows that neither recognition of characteristic symptoms (except cerebral heat) nor differential diagnosis of the disease depended crucially on this impressive arsenal. The longest chapter in the little book is a listing of symptoms that might or might not accompany insomnia in a particular case. How the physician was actually to distinguish cerebral hyperaemia from a host of other conditions – "*nervousness, dyspepsia, chlorosis, malarial disease, and . . . cerebral anemia*" – was left rather vague. Hammond also claimed that many cases of so-called menstrual neuroses, cerebral excitement, and "neuropathie cérébrocardiaque" were really cerebral hyperaemia. It is not clear from his discussion whether he regarded these terms as legitimate diagnoses to be distinguished from his own, or whether he meant his terminology to supplant them altogether. When he remarked with studied casualness that "there are few diseases so distinctly marked by their symptoms and clinical history," he was implicitly claiming privileged status for his pathological theory rather than providing, as the chapter head had promised, a differential diagnosis.[18]

Cerebral Hyperaemia gave Hammond a chance to explore the links between the mental and the physical in the context of scientific medicine. He drew upon the experience of over a decade in neurological practice to explain how his patients literally worried themselves sick. "The condition in which the brain is left after very intense or protracted mental application, or as a consequence of powerful emotional disturbances, is one of very great importance," he began. His self-experiments of the 1850s showed that brain tissue is "decomposed" as a result of mental exertion, as coal is in a furnace. Changing metaphors for his affluent clientele, he explained that had the experiments continued, "I would have been living . . . on my brain capital instead of the income, and brain bankruptcy would have been only a question of time."[19]

Hammond also emphasized a direct connection between thought and cerebral circulation. Circulation increased, he said, during mental activity and could result in permanent overdistension of the cerebral blood vessels, eventually producing "profound interstitial changes . . . in the brain substance." He did not explore Arthur E. Durham's detailed explanation of this process, nor the psychology of sleep, possibly considering these topics too abstract or technical for the general audience of the book. Instead he moved quickly to the conclusion that persons who overstrained their brains, such as inventors, female students, and Wall Street speculators, would fall victim to the disease.[20] This conclusion was consistent with prevailing views on neurasthenia and the "rest cure," as well as with contemporary class and gender prejudices.

It was obvious that insomnia could result from overly intense study or strong emotions. Hammond's problem was to show that increased cerebral circulation could be so caused, and that this accounted for the insomnia and other symptoms. Additionally, he was still nagged by the thought that an essentially functional pathology was insufficient. "The morbid anatomy and pathology" of cerebral hyperaemia "must remain to some extent a subject for speculation until *post-mortem* examinations enlighten us as to its real nature."[21]

The only direct evidence Hammond had to defend the pathology he suggested for cerebral hyperaemia was "the redness of the face, and throbbing of the cephalic arteries" and "the sensation of fulness of the head." Hammond also cited the "persistent insomnia always present" as evidence that cerebral circulation was disturbed, but here the argument was dangerously close to circularity. His strongest claim for the term *cerebral hyperaemia* was an *a posteriori* conclusion based on therapeutics. "Agents which we know increase the amount of blood in the brain . . . aggravated the symptoms of the disease," and those with the opposite effect on cerebral circulation relieved them.[22] Even this did not convince many of Hammond's colleagues, who commended his therapeutics while rejecting his scientific speculations.

Hammond's treatment of cerebral hyperaemia began with "external agents" like gentle friction and soothing sounds, but he favored agents that reduced cerebral circulation. A late supper, for example, might divert blood from the brain to the stomach. "The sensible physician will hardly resort to drugs," remarked Hammond, a well-known gourmet, "if such pleasant medicine as a good supper can be given with equally good effect." Often it did not, and then the physician might prescribe warm baths, mustard plasters, alcohol, strong coffee, or a variety of other drugs. Hammond's remedies of choice were the bromides of potassium and sodium, in doses as high as thirty grains, in spite of their unpleasant side effects. His treatments were energetic and often heroic, as a case history will demonstrate below. But he claimed to find bloodletting undesirable, despite its plausibility as a straightforward way to reduce circulation. There is some evidence that he did use it on occasion, but bleeding was associated with an earlier, uncomfortable, and apparently less scientific era.

A "hygienic regimen" was also imposed and mental exertion proscribed, although (unlike the "rest cure") amusement was encouraged. A month of such treatment, and probably a dozen visits to Hammond's elaborately decorated office, would usually suffice to cure the cerebral hyperaemia. In convalescents, however, "there is usually a state of physical debility present," requiring further treatment.[23] The bromides would have guaranteed the debility, and possibly the psychotic symptoms that Hammond said might attend the later stages of the disease.[24] But unlike the patients who came to Hammond with demonstrable organic disease of the nervous system, those with cerebral hyperaemia were encouragingly curable.

Hammond's treatment of a young man from Georgia was probably typical, except that the patient's outraged cousin, Dr. J. G. Hopkins, took the case to the medical press. Hopkins had brought his cousin to Hammond for depression and a "morbid fear" of being away from the doctor. Physical symptoms included headache, dizziness, a sense of constriction around the cranium, and gastrointestinal problems. Hammond examined him with the ophthalmoscope and Lombard's calorimeter, and analyzed the blood microscopically for traces of uric acid. He diagnosed the illness as "passive cerebral congestion," and embarked on an active course of treatment. In his own words, he "cauterized the nape of the neck, applied statical electricity to the same part and the cervical and dorsal regions generally, advised the use of ice to the nucha, and gave internally a mixture of bromide of sodium, pepsin, powdered charcoal and water."[25] This was Hammond's trademark medication, recalled by Charles L. Dana in 1900 as "the famous black mixture, whose inky trail has followed in the wake of neurological therapeutics in New York ever since." The pepsin and charcoal were for the stomach.[26]

Dr. Hopkins was so outraged by Hammond's proceedings that he wrote "a spicy letter" to the *Atlanta Medical and Surgical Journal* denouncing the neurologist as a fraud. The Georgia physician called the diagnostic procedure "too ridiculous for comment," the New York specialist a "clown," and the treatment a "circus." He complained particularly that Hammond had told the patient in the course of the treatment that "'Tis all damn nonsense, and I shall write your father to send you to the asylum. Do you suppose God is going to help you and you sit down on your tail and not help yourself?'" To this charge Hammond replied that "I did on one occasion speak harshly to him because on the day before he had not sufficiently exerted himself to do without the society of the Doctor, but this was my duty." Thus "moral treatment," or what might now be termed "behavioral therapy," also played a large part in the management of this case. The patient's own view of the proceedings is not recorded.[27]

NEUROLOGY AND PSYCHOTHERAPEUTICS

Hammond did not often discuss publicly his use of psychotherapeutics, and it is difficult to reconstruct his private attitude. The image of neurology that he projected emphasized that mental disorders had an underlying physical pathology in the nervous system and that they required tangible cures. Yet published case reports indicate that a psychological approach frequently complemented the physical treatment. One example is the case of a young woman who claimed to have an irresistible compulsion to swallow pins and needles that later emerged (she said) through her skin. Hammond diagnosed "hysterical deception" and noted that such patients indeed suffered from a real illness, although not from the ones they thought they had. "I wished to subject her to medical treatment for a few days before accusing her of deception and thus losing her confidence," he explained. It was "a deception for which . . . she was not altogether responsible."[28] Clearly the neurologist held his patient partly "responsible," and meant eventually to confront her. But was the "medical treatment" intended merely to gain her confidence by appearing to take her complaint seriously? More likely the neurologist honestly believed in the efficacy of his medications and external applications, although he was far too perceptive as a clinician to neglect psychological means when they seemed appropriate.

This interpretation is supported by Hammond's famous conflict with George M. Beard, another New York neurologist whose views and interests paralleled Hammond's in many respects. At the second annual meeting of the American Neurological Association in 1876, Beard read a paper intended "to call attention to a special means of using the mind in the treatment of disease – namely, producing definite expectation." Beard emphasized that this "was not to supplant other methods," but Hammond still objected bitterly. "If the doctrine advanced by Dr. Beard was to be accepted," he reportedly complained, "he should feel like throwing his diploma away and joining the theologians." Physicians could not use such nebulous mental therapeutics to cure real organic disease. "If the ideas of Dr. Beard were adopted," he warned the meeting, "we should be descending to the level of all sorts of humbuggery," and he hoped that "the paper would not go to the public with the endorsement of the Society."[29]

The vehemence of this response invites closer analysis. Beard's remarks on mental influences in causing as well as curing disease were consistent with conventional medical wisdom. Moreover, Hammond's own M.D. thesis (now lost) was entitled "The Etiological and Therapeutical Influence of the Imagination." His physiological studies had included analysis of the physical effects of mental exertion. As recently as 1868 he had published an article on "The Influence of the Maternal Mind over the Offspring during Pregnancy and Lactation." In it he had argued that "the blood can undergo change through the influence of the mind, and can serve as a means for the transmission of mental impressions." An 1870 paper "On Some of the Effects of Excessive Intellectual Exertion" maintained that mental effort could cause physical disease. His book *Cerebral Hyperaemia,* published early in 1878, was largely concerned with the mental causation of what he took to be an organic disorder.

Only a few years later, Hammond would also concede that mental influences could be therapeutic as well as pathological. "The history of medicine abounds with relations of famous systems of cures and wonderful remedies," he wrote in 1881, "whose whole power depends upon suggestion and expectant attention." He said he favored the use of "all honorable means," including placebos and other psychological cures, in medical practice.[30] Nine years later he marveled that "there seems to be . . . no limit to the power of the principle of suggestion with some persons." He told readers of the *North American Review* that cases of false hydrophobia, induced by fear of the real disease, could prove fatal to the highly suggestible patient.[31]

Why, then, did Hammond lock horns with Beard over psychotherapeutics? Perhaps it seemed to him that Beard had not made it sufficiently clear that the efficacy of mental influences rested on their essentially physical nature. He thus undercut neurological somaticism at a time when philosophical considerations were still crucially important to the new and still controversial specialty. Beard's remarks seemed both to encourage self-appointed spiritual healers and to have blurred the distinctions between such quacks and the scientific neurologist. While discussion of mental therapeutics might have been tolerable within neurological circles, it would be dangerous for the public to associate mental therapeutics with neurology. Once neurologists were more securely established, open discussion might be safer.

*   *   *   *   *

By 1890 both "cerebral hyperaemia" and the theory of sleep on which it rested had been seriously undermined.[32] Hammond had not altered his views, but the medical world was changing rapidly. He thought of himself still as a physiologist, but the American Physiological Association had formed without him, and its interests had little to do with his.[33] Landon Carter Gray challenged Hammond's expertise directly in his inaugural address as president of the New York Neurological Society in May 1890. "Can we diagnosticate hyperaemia or anaemia of the brain and cord?" he

asked, and answered the question with a resounding "no." Even
Hammond had trouble distinguishing two presumably opposite
conditions, Gray noted, and the symptoms he attributed to cerebral hyperaemia were found in many diseases.

Other members of the Neurological Society, all (like Gray) a
generation younger than Hammond, joined the chorus of disapproval. M. Allan Starr, for example, said that to pretend to diagnosticate between cerebral anemia and hyperaemia "was merely an
evidence of incompetency on the part of the physician."[34] At this
meeting of a society that Hammond himself had founded when
Starr was a Princeton schoolboy, not one voice was recorded as
speaking in the older man's defense.

The onslaught prompted Hammond to take precious time away
from his busy Washington sanatorium to defend his favorite
medical theory at the October meeting of the society. The self-
identified physiologist rehearsed experimental evidence (none of it
new) that he thought supported his views. But he relied more
heavily on his clinical experience. "When I have a patient suffering
from insomnia, pain in the head, vertigo, hallucinations, suffusion
of the face, cephalic heat, and other striking symptoms," he insisted in a tone mixing pathos and bluster, "and when I find that these
symptoms disappear under the influence of remedies such as the
bromides, ergot, ice, and douches of cold water to the nape of the
neck, cups in the same locality, nasal bloodletting, or spontaneous
hemorrhage, position, and other means calculated to diminish the
amount of intracranial blood," he continued, "I do not see how an
escape is possible from the conclusion that the patient suffers from
cerebral hyperaemia."[35]

The *post hoc* argument from therapeutics (including bloodletting) was still Hammond's most compelling one. He reminded his
colleagues of his long years in practice, treating thousands of patients and teaching thousands of medical students and doctors, and
of his "more than a score of books and monographs, which have
been translated into nearly every language of the civilized world."
These entitled him, he pleaded, "to something more than dogmatic denial, and certainly should shield me from the charge of
incompetence, or a too fertile imagination." He protested that "it
is not true science to dispute these results on mere theoretical
grounds, or to bring forward in explanation theories which have
nothing whatever to support them." Cerebral hyperaemia was

well-grounded and thus "not to be dismissed by . . . the proposal of obscure theories of lithaemia, or nervous prostration, or brain exhaustion, or neurasthenia, or any similar hypothesis which consists of mere words."[36]

The difference between Hammond and his neurological critics was not only one of information, but of ideology or outlook as well. He saw dogma where his juniors saw scientific skepticism, and science where they saw dogmatism. While "neurasthenia" was for most of the younger men an unproblematic diagnosis, Hammond saw it as unscientific speculation. Gray saw neurology as becoming at once a more precise and a more complex science, but at the same time he was far less sanguine than Hammond about the possibility of comprehending such "an exquisitely and almost inconceivably complex organ" as the brain. The ebullience and optimism of the older man constituted a central element in his vision of the scientific enterprise, while Gray's skepticism similarly loomed large in his newer – and in a sense more professional – orientation.

Hammond's work – theoretical, clinical, and organizational – provided the basis for the establishment of neurology in the United States. But the process he helped to set in motion soon turned the specialty into a field of work quite different from – and in some respects even opposed to – his original conceptions.

10

"A positive mental science"

"I used to say in my lectures to medical students," Hammond reminisced in 1895, "that if I should ever be disposed to make for myself a god, I would select a piece of gray nerve-tissue as the object of my adoration." It was, he continued, "the most wonderful substance, so far as we know, in the whole universe, surpassing in its grandeur sun and moon and stars and everything else of which we have any knowledge."[1] The wonder was that, in Hammond's view, gray nerve tissue gave rise to the human mind. Neurology was thus the foundation of psychology, and psychology the key to society. His research on sleep and insomnia had been one effort to approach psychology on a scientific clinical basis. The study of insanity seemed even more promising.

PHYSIOLOGICAL PSYCHOLOGY AND PSYCHOLOGICAL MEDICINE

Advances in neuroanatomy and neurophysiology in the mid-nineteenth century, as well as the evolutionary thought of Spencer and Darwin, suggested to Hammond new possibilities for the scientific study of mind.[2] In this he may be compared to Alexander Bain, John Stuart Mill, and others. But while Bain's influential work is noted for its attempt to unite traditional psychology with the newer physiology, Hammond found the two approaches to be directly opposed. "The one necessitates no knowledge of the structure of the brain or of the functions of its several parts," he wrote, "the other requires no acquaintance with metaphysical subtleties or the principles of thought; the one regards the mind as an abstract property common to all mankind, and pays no heed to the numberless varieties due to inherent differences of organization," he continued, "the other takes it up as the resultant of certain functions the organs of which are tangible facts." Further, "the one has been followed by the greatest thinkers and philosophers the world has produced, the other has been trod by but few enquirers." Consequently "the one has resulted in the foundation of a science which has apparently reached its utmost stage of development, the other has as yet scarcely approached the confines of true scientific inquiry."[3] Hammond's polarization of the two approaches emphasized his main point: the metaphysical approach to psychology was played out. Who, after all, could do better with Plato's method than Plato?

Hammond expected progress in psychology to come only from physiology, or psychological medicine. He took Henry Maudsley's new book on *The Physiology and Pathology of the Mind* as a model for such research. He found Maudsley's concept of mind to be far more subtle than the incorrect view of Pierre Jean Georges Cabanis that the brain secreted mind as the liver supposedly secreted bile. Perhaps mind "results from the action of the brain," or perhaps the brain is "the organ – the tool by which mind does its work." There are crucial differences between these two possibilities, but for Hammond the important point was that "whether in health or disease, the mind is to be studied from a purely material standpoint, and not as a mysterious principle to be looked upon with awe as something entirely beyond our reach." These comments were addressed to the broad audience of *Nation* magazine, but Hammond directed similar comments to his medical readers. "Above all things," he wrote, "it is now necessary that the unholy barrier set up between psychical and physical nature be broken down." He called for the formation of "a first conception of mind . . . founded on a faithful recognition of all those phenomena of nature which had by imperceptible gradations [led] up to this its highest evolution." The "biology" that had been on the positivist agenda of Hammond's Philadelphia group ten years earlier had taken a somewhat different form than the youthful physicians had anticipated. But it had succeeded in laying the basis for the next step, a "positive mental science." Physiology could not (yet) fully explain human thought and action, but it could "overthrow the data of a false psychology."[4]

Hammond's psychological theory was not simply an abstract issue, nor was it the subject of purely academic debate. A trans-atlantic furor over George M. Beard's demonstrations of hypnosis in 1881 brought the philosophical controversy into the public view. Beard had brought a "trained subject" to London, where fifty of the leading physicians of the city gathered to watch their hypnotic performance. The audience was not entranced. Beard claimed that its obvious hostility had made the subject nervous and had ruined the experiment, but the eminent medical psychologist Crichton Browne pronounced him a fake and demanded that Beard repudiate him. This the New York neurologist refused to do, partly on principle and partly, it seems, because his poor hearing kept him from fully understanding the situation. Hammond leaped, uninvited, into the ensuing intercontinental fray. "But, think of Hammond fighting for Beard," chortled an American editor, "it's too good!"[5]

Beard's critics contended that mental processes were purely subjective. The only proof that a person had been hypnotized could be his or her own assertion that it was so. But Beard's subject admitted that he was traveling under an assumed name and that he had previously participated in mesmeric and spiritualistic experiments. Browne, John C. Bucknill, and others argued that he must therefore be considered personally unreliable, and his testimony discounted. "Phenomena connected with or attributable to abnormal states of consciousness," insisted Bucknill, "cannot be appreciated with any satisfactory degree of exactness without some knowledge of the moral character of the hypnotized subject." He stressed that there could be no physiological test of consciousness. Browne made the same point: the subject "was exhibited to illustrate a condition recognizable by subjective symptoms alone, and which might be physiological, pathological, or criminal." Hence "his style and designation become facts of extreme significance."[6]

Such statements constituted a frontal assault on the basic premises of psychological medicine as Hammond understood it. In his view, neurologists employing a "physiological" approach to psychology were almost by definition more knowledgeable than even the best of the physicians adhering to a "metaphysical" approach. Beard had refused to respond to Browne's challenge on the grounds that he would not discuss scientific subjects in public with nonexperts. Hammond agreed, but probably realized that few physicians or members of the public would accept the designation of Browne and Bucknill as amateurs in psychological medicine. He therefore attempted to rebut their arguments.[7]

Hammond contended that the moral character of hypnotic subjects was irrelevant because hypnotic trance was, like other psychological states, a physiological condition that could be detected by objective tests. For example, the hand of a hypnotized person could be burned with a red-hot iron without response, and the indifference could scarcely be feigned when the sore might remain open and painful a month afterward. "It is no wonder," he added, "that these people shrink from such experiments." According to Hammond, neurologists like Beard and J. M. Charcot, not medical psychologists like Bucknill and Browne or general practitioners, were qualified to judge hypnotic demonstrations.[8]

Beard's opponents were also offended by the showmanship with which he – like Hammond – staged his demonstrations. Beard had behaved, said Dr. H. Donkin, "after the manner of a platform exhibitor rather than of a clinical demonstrator."[9] There was much justice to this charge. Hammond's own rather spectacular demonstrations at the University Medical College in January 1881 and before the Medico-Legal Society several months later drew large crowds and extensive newspaper coverage. "How Patients Might Be Led to Commit Crimes by Unscrupulous Persons," trumpeted the *New York Times,* headlining its graphic account of proceedings which at times resembled a three-ring circus.[10] Even Hammond's closest associates were wary: the publication committee of the Medico-Legal Society withheld a report of Hammond's performance that was already in type, and it only appeared six years later.[11] Hammond clearly relished the theatrical, and probably justified it as a way to bring important scientific truths before the public. Hypnotism was, he said, "one of the most important powers of nature." In Beard's words it was, "next to evolution . . . the supreme scientific question of this century."[12] Few medical issues could have captured popular interest and imagination as effectively as hypnotism.

For the most part, Hammond developed his psychological theory in the context of his neurological practice. Patients suffering from "cerebral hyperaemia" and "spinal irritation" had recognizably physical symptoms, and while Hammond was sensitive to their psychological dimension he had no trouble accounting for

168	*Preserve your love for science*

them physiologically. Insane patients posed a greater challenge, for their symptoms were in the first instance mental or behavioral. Hammond worked hard over the next two decades to develop an appropriate theory of insanity.

CLASSIFICATIONS OF THE INSANITIES

Insanity, he declared in 1866, was "a general or particular derangement of one or more faculties of the mind, which whilst not abolishing consciousness, prevents freedom of mind or of action." This definition made no reference at all to a material basis for such "faculties." Four years later he remedied this deficiency. "I regard insanity," he then wrote, "as a manifestation of disease of the brain characterized by a general or partial derangement of one or more faculties of the mind, and in which, while consciousness is not abolished, mental freedom is perverted, weakened, or destroyed."[13] He left this statement essentially unchanged through the first edition of the *Treatise on the Diseases of the Nervous System* (1871), the greatly revised sixth edition (1876), and the *Treatise on Insanity* (1883). In the latter he also accepted the simpler definition, "a psychic manifestation of brain disease unattended by loss of consciousness."[14] Even these definitions did little more than invoke the assumption that the behavior disorders that he classified in terms of mental functions had a physical basis in the brain.

Hammond took seriously the idea that mind was material in nature. An early essay on the cerebellum used an electrical metaphor to argue that the organ functioned as "an additional generator of nervous power."[15] In the *Treatise* he admitted the generation of "nervous force" in all gray matter, including the spinal cord and ganglia. But he denied that noncranial gray matter bore on questions of insanity. Over the next few years he apparently changed his opinion, for he argued in May 1875, in his inaugural address as president of the New York Neurological Society, that the brain "is not the sole organ of the mind." Here he claimed that all gray matter was identical, generating the same force.[16] The 1876 edition of the *Treatise* promoted this new opinion and described perception in particular as partially a function of the spinal cord. At the same time the author increased his emphasis on perception and "perceptional insanities" in his discussion of abnormal psychology.[17]

Perception played a steadily growing role in Hammond's psychology. He described "thalamic epilepsy" for the American Neurological Association in 1880 as characterized by "hallucinations and loss of consciousness." He located its "morbid anatomical basis" in the optic thalamus, which he believed to be a "center for perception."[18] In earlier writings, Hammond had considered the "primary manifestation of mind" to be the will, suggesting that his research on sleep was strongly motivated by an interest in psychology. Later he gave intellect the first place in this hierarchical scheme, but in 1884 he awarded the title to perception.[19] Hammond's changing views on the physical function of the spinal cord corresponded with his changing psychological notions in spite of his continued inability to formulate, much less demonstrate, a thoroughly physiological psychology.

Hammond realized, at least by 1880, that his somaticism logically called for a classification of the forms of insanity based on their morbid anatomy and physiology. This was the plan, however imperfectly realized, underlying his discussion of other diseases of the nervous system. In the case of insanity it was clear to him that this was not practicable, even on a tentative basis. "It is to be regretted," he apologized to his readers, "that the present state of cerebral anatomy and physiology is such as to prevent our making any precise localizations of the several forces and faculties which go to make up the mind." Of the six ways he could imagine attempting a classification of insanity, the anatomical was that "preferred to all others, but, unfortunately, our knowledge is not yet sufficient to enable us to adopt it to any considerable extent." He considered a physiological model to be second-best, but also not feasible. An etiological classification he found neither theoretically satisfactory nor practical.

Hammond thought a psychological classification of mental illness was somewhat more plausible, with specific illnesses arranged in accordance with the several mental faculties. This had "some advantages . . . but there are disadvantages which more than overbalance them." Physicians had tried this method since the late eighteenth century, including Wilhelm Griesinger and Hammond himself in the earlier editions of his textbook of nervous diseases. "Mature reflection has, however, convinced me," he confessed, "that it cannot be exclusively followed." It was only satisfactory "in the present state of our knowledge of brain anatomy, physiology, and pathology." While the neurologist was known for holding tenaciously to unpopular views, he was not dogmatic, for these views were subject to change in the light of practical experience.

He was fascinated with recent attempts to classify the insanities on a pathological basis "according to the morbid conditions of the brain, which are supposed to be in immediate relation with them as causes and effects." The attempts of A. Voisin and J. Luys were "ingenious," but Hammond could not regard them as either final or practical. Like most of his contemporaries, he resorted in the end to a "clinical, or symptomatological" plan. He admitted that his categories were ambiguous and even overlapping. But some system was more useful to practitioners than none at all, and might suggest deeper insights. Hammond tried to compensate for the lack of scientific clarity on insanity by incorporating long sections of previous works on the nature of mind and sleep, about which he probably felt more confident.

Hammond's nosology relied on a rather traditional psychology of mental functions. Derangement primarily of one mental faculty constituted a simple form of insanity. It would be classed as perceptional (illusions and hallucinations), intellectual (including intellectual monomania or morbid impulse, and reasoning mania), emotional (such as melancholia, hypochondria, and hysterical mania), or volitional (so-called aboulomania). Conditions involving two or more faculties were considered "compound." These included acute mania, catatonia, dementia, periodical and circular insanities, and hebephrenia. But there was a separate category of "constitutional" insanities, comprising epileptic, puerperal, and choreic forms. Finally there was "arrest of mental development," which Hammond included among the insanities although considering it to require a different sort of special expertise.[20]

There was a commonsensical logic to this scheme, but it was a far cry from the physiologically or anatomically based plans that would have been consistent with the theoretical structure of Hammond's psychological argument. An explicit material basis for illness was conspicuously absent. Further, his descriptions of some conditions lacked reference even to his analysis of mental functions. For example, mysophobia was "morbid, overpowering fear of defilement" and hebephrenia was "mental derangement of puberty." These clinical entities were described in purely behavioral terms.[21]

If such inconsistency troubled Hammond, it was far more objectionable to outsiders. One physician testified in court that although Dr. Hammond was a recognized authority on diseases of the nervous system, his work on insanity was less satisfactory than the rest of his neurology. While reviewers of the *Treatise on Insanity* were generally respectful of the author, they were also critical of the book itself. Perhaps because the recommendations for case management were not seen as helpful, it never approached the popularity of Hammond's *Treatise on the Diseases of the Nervous System.*[22]

NEUROLOGISTS AND ASYLUM SUPERINTENDENTS IN CONFLICT

The most pressing practical matter in the care of the insane was where and by whom they would be treated. The Association of Medical Superintendents of American Institutions for the Insane (AMSAII), founded in 1844, had virtually monopolized psychiatry in the United States for thirty years. Their thoughtful, considered, and tested opinions on hospital construction and management defined medical expertise on the subject of insanity.[23] But when John P. Gray, the forceful and articulate superintendent of the Utica (New York) Asylum, became president of AMSAII in 1875 he took on the task of leading the group through a period of increasing crisis. It was under attack by such leading medical psychologists as John C. Bucknill of England for its failure not only to make good its extravagant claims of the curability of insanity in the asylum, but also to apply consistently its own theoretical principles. Its exclusion of all but superintendents of insane asylums left an increasing proportion of American alienists (including assistant superintendents and directors of institutions for the "feebleminded") outside the fold, and fostered a limited and conservative outlook among the members of the association.[24] The formation and consolidation of neurological societies between 1872 and 1876 represented a new challenge and a potential threat. Gray had commented approvingly in 1871 on the establishment of a chair in medical psychology for Hammond at University Medical College.[25] But within the next few years Hammond's increasing visibility, combined with his aggressively materialist views, must have begun to distress the outspokenly conservative superintendent.

In March 1878 Hammond and his neurologist friends launched the first offensive of a five-year war against the superintendents.[26] Edward C. Spitzka presented a paper to the New York Neurological Society on "The Study of Insanity Considered as a Branch of Neurology, and the Relations of the General Medical Body to this Branch." This call for far-reaching psychiatric reform was referred on Hammond's motion to a committee including himself. Under his leadership it recommended to the neurologists at their next monthly meeting a full-scale legislative and public-relations campaign for "asylum reform." By June a ten-member committee had been formed to compose a "statement of facts and presumptions regarding insane asylums." This committee must have included, at least on paper, most of the active core of the Neurological Society, and it was authorized to co-opt additional physicians who were not neurologists. The neurological specialists clearly hoped that general practitioners would ally with them against the asylum superintendents.[27]

Perhaps Hammond was impatient with the ins and outs of committee work, or perhaps he simply wished to provoke his colleagues to sharper action. In any case, he took it on himself to write an editorial that appeared anonymously in the New York *Herald*. In it he pointed out alleged abuses at the Utica Asylum, which, under Gray's superintendence, was generally regarded as a model institution. He also called for a state senate investigation. The authorship of the editorial was an open secret. Three weeks later Eugene Grissom, superintendent of the North Carolina State Asylum, delivered a vituperative attack on Hammond to a large audience at the annual AMSAII meeting in Washington, D.C. This fusillade was summarized the next day in the D.C. *National Standard* and, together with Hammond's equally colorful response, received immense publicity.[28] The rhetoric on both sides was itself abusive, but real issues underlay this "indulgence in personalities."

In an argument he would elaborate elsewhere, Hammond castigated the asylum system as inhumane in principle. He found it wrong and degrading to deprive insane persons of their liberty and dignity when they were not dangerous. Grissom, in turn, found

Hammond unsympathetic to the insane because of his narrow construction of legal insanity and his insistence on the punishability of insane criminals. He charged the neurologist with inconsistency in his expert testimony and cupidity in his acceptance of large fees for it. Grissom lambasted Hammond as a "moral monster whose baleful eyes gleamed with a delusive light," and an atheist as well. Hammond did not deny the charge of infidelity, but cited it as evidence that his opponent was ignorant and unscientific, if not actually insane. He defended with alacrity the rewards he received for his valuable services. Hammond did not press libel charges against Grissom, claiming it was not worth his while to travel to North Carolina to do so. Instead he sued his main opponent, John P. Gray, who had published Grissom's speech in the *American Journal of Insanity* and who was widely suspected of having coached Grissom.[29]

Grissom had also reminded his Washington audience that Hammond had left that city in disgrace fifteen years earlier, found guilty of misconduct as surgeon general. A lobbying campaign for Hammond's "vindication" had begun some months earlier, and would result a year later in his restoration by congressional action to an honorable position on the "retired" list with his old rank of brigadier general. Still, the Southerner's accusation must have stung.[30]

The anti-asylum crusade resumed in October. The monthly meeting of the Neurological Society was turned into a sort of medical press conference, with reporters invited to hear Spitzka represent the New York neurologists. This time he concluded with a twenty-point program for the scientific reform of insane asylums.[31] Hammond and others backed him up, and their Committee on Asylum Abuses presented its formal indictment. The society accepted the report and voted to have copies of it, as well as a petition to the state legislature, printed for distribution.

The campaign proceeded more slowly than Hammond had perhaps anticipated, but in February 1879 he appeared by invitation before the annual meeting of the New York State Medical Society. His remarks on "The Non-Asylum Treatment of the Insane" stressed the competence of all well-educated physicians to treat insanity as well as they could any other disease. "There is nothing surprisingly difficult, obscure, or mysterious about diseases of the brain which can only be learned within the walls of the asylum," he urged. "A general practitioner of good common sense, well-grounded in the principles of medicine, with such a knowledge of the human mind and of cerebral physiology and pathology as can be obtained by study, and familiar with all the clinical factors in his patient's history, is more capable of treating successfully a case of insanity than the average asylum physician." The opposition opinion was promoted mainly by medical officers of asylums, he charged, who had "very diligently inculcated the idea that they alone . . . are qualified."[32]

How many members of the New York State Medical Society were prepared to teach themselves the latest in psychology and neurophysiology? How many, for that matter, would Hammond have considered "well-grounded in the principles of medicine"? At least since his tenure as surgeon general he had shown no great faith in the abilities of most general practitioners. The portrait of the family doctor in his novel *Robert Severne* (1867), for example, was particularly unflattering.[33] But there is reason to believe that Hammond was not simply pandering to his audience to win their support. For one thing, he would soon become interested in postgraduate medical education, helping physicians such as these to remedy the defects in their training and instructing them in his specialty. For another, he had articulated a similar position earlier, before the conflict with the superintendents had surfaced.

As early as 1871 Hammond had suggested placing insane patients in physicians' homes, rather than asylums, for treatment. He treated them himself on an outpatient basis in his study. But he still found asylums necessary for some cases, and compared American institutions favorably with European ones.[34] In 1876 he had written that "many insane persons are sent to lunatic asylums who could with regard to every consideration affecting their comfort and health be better attended to in their own homes under the care of the family physician."[35] These assertions did not rest on charges of asylum abuse or mismanagement, but on the assumption that the patient was suffering from an ordinary physical disease of the brain. And Hammond apparently never rejected the idea that asylums would always be needed to care for less prosperous patients whose families and friends could not afford private care.[36]

In Hammond's own practice, treatment of the well-to-do insane might even be incorporated into his social life. He relished the story of a married couple who "consulted him separately as to the sanity of the other," as he told it to dinner guests, "each inviting him to dinner with a view to the doctor's watching the suspected person for a diagnosis of his or her mental condition." Perhaps he recommended treatment for both, since "on their separate visits to the doctor's study, the one who arrived first had to be let out at a side door to avoid meeting the other sitting in the parlor."[37]

While Hammond encouraged the distrust many New York general practitioners may have had for asylum specialists, he was also careful to point out the many "eminent alienists," including Edward Seguin, E. C. Spitzka, George Beard, Weir Mitchell, and J. S. Jewell, who practiced the "science and art of psychiatry" without asylum affiliation. If the average doctor found a case to be beyond his patience or skill, he would be well-advised to consult with a neurologist before surrendering it to the asylum in despair. Hammond left a clear impression that there was such a thing as expertise ("knowledge of the human mind and of cerebral physiology and pathology"), but that the neurological specialist was both more knowledgeable and more approachable than the manager of an institution.

A few months later, with asylum reform legislation pending in Connecticut, Hammond traveled to Hartford to represent the Neurological Society at the annual meeting of the state medical society there. Formerly, he explained, asylums had been built as prisons and the insane had been treated as criminals. Sadly, current practice was little better. In the future, as Hammond described it, physicians might consider "that asylums are but sorry substitutes for the skill and care which should be exercised towards lunatics in their own homes." Meanwhile, "the absolute and irresponsible power of the superintendents must be taken away, and hospitals for the insane must be organized exactly as are all other hospitals." The tedious discussions of asylum construction that occupied AMSAII meetings were unscientific and irrelevant, he said, since the architecture was not curative anyhow. The legislative priority should not be new construction, as superintendents frequently urged, but reorganization.

Hammond encouraged the Connecticut physicians with reports of recent successes in the reform crusade. The "hundreds of letters" he had received "from eminent physicians in all parts of the country" since the meeting of the New York State Medical Society convinced him that "the seed then planted had taken root." Later he told the Neurological Society that his appeal for a legislative campaign in the neighboring state had been "kindly received." Influential alienists blocked the publication of Hammond's remarks in the *Transactions* of the Connecticut society, but they appeared (at the urging of Connecticut friends) in his short-lived journal *Neurological Contributions*.[38]

The petition circulated by the Committee on Asylum Abuses of the Neurological Society was submitted to the New York state senate in March of 1879, and referred to a two-member committee. By the early summer the senators, one of whom represented the district including Utica, brought back a "piece of special pleading, miscalled a report," as the neurologists' committee described it, that completely exonerated the New York superintendents. Perhaps Hammond was still naive about politics, but he and his friends were outraged. Worse, some signers of their petition had withdrawn their names under pressure. The neurologists were suddenly on the defensive. The situation worsened in the fall, when a board of consulting physicians was appointed to the New York City asylum system, as the neurologists had demanded, but without a single neurologist on it. Hammond came into the October meeting of the Neurological Society with a strongly worded resolution of protest and easily persuaded his colleagues to pass and publicize it.[39]

In the following weeks several members of the small society began to believe that approval of Hammond's resolution had been precipitous. Dr. Seguin moved reconsideration at the November meeting, and after some discussion it was decided to seek more information. A month later, however, the Commissioner of Charities and Corrections had still not responded. Moreover, the *New York Times* had confirmed Hammond's worst apprehensions that neurology was being slighted. A page-three story on November 14 declared that the board did represent "all" the specialties, and promoted the superintendents' position that insanity was not, generally speaking, a disease of the brain at all. "Direct medicament of the brain and nervous system is malpractice in [many] cases," reported the paper, "and yet the system has been to dose with bromides and narcotics." It quoted the board members to the effect that "the cant of psychological medicine and the eloquent talk about the wonderful properties of nerve-cells and their laws of action have held the attention of medical men all too long." They wanted to "dismiss this high-sounding rigmarole from the literature of science," and saw the formation of the board as "a turning-point in the doctrines, literature, and treatment of insanity."[40]

A medical correspondent signing himself "D" (probably one of the neurologists) took the unusual step of debating a scientific issue in the popular press. In a calm and carefully worded letter he explained that the board's view was "as old as the hills" and scarcely more helpful than "the misty regions of metaphysics" in understanding or treating insanity. The *Times* editor responded on a less theoretical plane, cheerfully (and perhaps prematurely) announcing the failure of a campaign he attributed to "a single filibustering expert and his hungry followers." The uncomplimentary reference to Hammond must have been unmistakable.

Landon Carter Gray, a member of the Neurological Society, tried to bring the theoretical controversy over insanity back into the professional arena. In a letter to the *Medical Record* he defended the prominent role neurologists were playing in the broad-based reform movement that would soon consolidate around the National Association for the Protection of the Insane and the Prevention of Insanity.[41] In an editorial response, the *Medical Record* probably spoke for many New York physicians in agreeing with the goals of the Neurological Society without condoning its "newspaper notoriety" and "unhappy mode of getting signers" to its petitions. The editors encouraged what they called "lunacy reform," but clearly did not accept the leadership of the neurologists.[42] While some of the neurologists themselves were having second thoughts about the lunacy reform project, Hammond pressed on with his efforts to keep the campaign moving. With Spitzka and Morton he prepared a report for the January 1880 meeting of the Neurological Society. After some discussion it was accepted for publication and distribution in an edition of 3,000 copies.

The asylum reform crusade was upstaged in the spring of 1880 by the trial of Abraham Gosling. The case itself was newsworthy but not especially momentous: the elderly defendant was charged with smashing the windows of a hotel at which he had been kept waiting by a clerk. It was mainly the expert testimony of neurologists and superintendents that lent excitement to the trial. Hammond testified, in court and in a paper read before the

Medico-Legal Society, that a clearer case of paralytic insanity (that is, tertiary syphilis) could hardly be found. "If Mr. Abraham Gosling does not die of General Paresis within three years," the neurologist proclaimed melodramatically, "I will burn my diploma and retire from the medical profession." Asylum superintendents, however, had given Gosling a far more favorable prognosis, discharging him "cured" from a series of institutions in Great Britain, New York, and Pennsylvania. Several testified in court that he was sane and could be held responsible for his destructive acts. Spitzka, supporting Hammond, insisted that neurologists could read subtle diagnostic signs indicating brain disease and therefore (in their view) insanity. He suggested that the superintendents were either ignorant or dishonest.[43] Hammond's prognosis proved correct: Gosling died soon after the trial. But the neurologists had by no means won over a medical profession skeptical of their claims to expertise.

Stories of alleged asylum abuses from New York to Nevada continued to enliven both neurological society meetings and the popular press. An apparent homicide at Blackwell's Island Asylum in May (the Maria Ottmer case) even spurred the creation of a new state senate investigating committee. Hammond confronted his fellow neurologists at their October meeting with the question of how they would conduct themselves in relation to its forthcoming hearings.

Hammond wanted his colleagues to testify before the committee, and brought pamphlets to the meeting to equip them for this ordeal. Seguin and Gray balked, the former threatening to resign from the Committee on Asylum Abuses if he were summoned by the senate. Spitzka reassured them that their role was to be consultants, not witnesses. But when the hearings opened in December the neurologists (including Seguin) testified after all.

Hammond took the stage on the first afternoon with wide-ranging prepared remarks. His own experiences with insane patients convinced him that most inmates' complaints were not based in fact. But he discoursed at length on the evils of forced feeding, forcible restraint ("except in the most extreme cases") and the withholding of patients' mail. He thought competent superintendents to be the exception and drew appreciative laughter with his remark that "the office of Medical Superintendent should be abolished and a lay superintendent appointed to raise turnips, lobby in the Legislature, and entertain the friends of visitors."

The omissions in Hammond's testimony are also significant. He did not elaborate on his views of the pathology or prevalence of insanity, except to criticize a new law by which persons with a single harmless delusion could be committed. Nor did he advocate the nonasylum treatment of the insane. Perhaps this was because the asylums under investigation housed indigent patients who would not have been able to afford home care. Perhaps his colleagues had convinced him that the cause would be harmed by the deification of gray matter or pronouncements that all men were insane. He challenged the superintendents on their own ground, criticizing their managerial competence and leaving it to Spitzka to charge them with ignorance or indifference to science.[44]

The senate's star witness was not a neurologist but the Reverend William G. French, who had visited the New York City asylums for years as a representative of the Protestant Episcopal City Mission and had kept a diary of his observations. The investigation continued for several years, but the neurologists were not further involved. In the end the results were inconclusive. Charges of abuses seemed to have been magnified out of proportion, but many felt that the inquiry itself had prompted recent reform. Hammond probably recognized that the neurologists had failed to establish themselves as the sole legitimate authority on the care of the insane. He and Spitzka reported to the Neurological Society that the National Association for the Protection of the Insane and the Prevention of Insanity, formed partly on their initiative, was making progress. They implied that the asylum reform issue could safely be left in the hands of others. Nothing further was said about "reform in the scientific study of psychology."[45]

After the senate hearings, Hammond shifted the focus of his work on insanity to the medicolegal arena, which will be discussed in the next chapter. But he was never able to overcome the main difficulty inherent in his theory: it was impossible for him to ground his views of insanity in the anatomy or physiology of the brain. His neurological success depended largely on the presentation of a convincingly materialist – and thus "scientific" – explanation of everyday mental phenomena, and his claim to expertise in the area of insanity was similarly founded. Yet, as he was very much aware, he and his colleagues could not even ask, much less answer, many of the questions in which they were most interested without resort to the language and concepts of the traditional psychology which they were attempting to overthrow.

11

"All men are insane"

"What are the morbid conditions of mind fairly attributable to corporeal disorder?" Hammond asked in 1867. "Here is a question leading to truths, as yet but partially ascertained, which enter into not only mental pathology and psychology, but jurisprudence, religion, social life, and the domestic relations." He told Samuel Francis that medicine was "the profession of all others which affords the greatest fields for study." He regarded neurology as "the most important department of medical science." In it he saw not only an opportunity for the scientific study of medicine, but also the seductive possibility of a scientific psychology, and hence an understanding of society itself. In the words of a skeptical critic, "the history of the human race could be written under the caption of psychiatry so defined."[1]

The prominent lawyer and editor Whitelaw Reid reminded the assembled alumni of University Medical College in 1876 that Professor Hammond "is best-known to us all for his well-known theory that all men are insane."[2] This was an exaggeration, but not a great one. "Insanity and nervous affections are more common in the United States than in any other country," Hammond had told the readers of *Galaxy* magazine in 1868. This was because "Americans are preeminently an emotional people," he explained, "and we work our brains and nerves as no other nation has worked them since the world began." Thus "emotional diseases – and chief among them dyspepsia – are so widespread that the individual who is not affected with some one of them is looked upon as a marvel in anthropology."[3]

A medical reviewer of Hammond's *Treatise on Insanity* complained that it seemed to be "the intention of the author to widen the sphere of insanity as much as possible."[4] There was much truth to this charge. Hammond introduced the *Treatise* with the note that it started "from the points that all normal mental phenomena are the result of the action of a healthy brain, and that all abnormal manifestations of mind are the result of the functionation of a diseased or deranged brain." If healthy brain function was sanity, he continued, then an unhealthy brain surely signified insanity. "There can be no middle ground, for the brain is either in a healthy or in an unhealthy condition." Thus, "there are very few people who have not at some time or other, perhaps for a moment only, been medically insane."[5] Hammond's sound clinical insight prompted him to count insomnia and dyspepsia as "nervous affections," and his materialist bent in psychology led him to presume these to be evidence of an unhealthy brain. Such minor ailments could develop, if untreated, into outright insanity. From this point of view, his allegation of widespread insanity was plausible.

Hammond's neurological perspective gave psychological medicine an important role in society, one that he would scarcely shirk. Medicolegal controversies provided natural openings, but Hammond also interested himself in the "woman question," in debunking spiritualism, and even in sniping at Christianity. While these efforts logically extended his neurological theory, the result was frequently to undermine still further a specialty already overextended even within the narrower clinical realm.

INSANITY AND THE LAW

Hammond's first publication on insanity (1866) had been inspired by the famous case of James C. Johnston. The North Carolinian died soon after writing a will disinheriting relatives with whom he had previously been on good terms. Hammond was called in as an expert witness for the disappointed kin, who contested the will on the grounds of insanity of the testator. He testified that the deceased had not been "of sound and disposing mind, but was, on the contrary, the subject of such a degree of mental derangement as to destroy his freedom of will and consequently his testamentary capacity." His diagnosis, on the authority of prominent British and French psychologists, was monomania, a type of "affective mania" or moral or emotional insanity.

Hammond was aware of his responsibility to the Johnston family, but his personal interest in the case was to establish the legitimacy of monomania as a clinical entity. Moral insanity, he explained, was usually accompanied by intellectual derangement. The monomaniac might appear normal because he could control "the paroxysms of delirium to which he is subject, or conceal the particular manifestations of his insanity." There were no true "lucid intervals." Hammond considered the prima facie illogic (as he and the relatives saw it) of Johnston's action to be a sign of delusion, and the most direct evidence of his insanity.[6]

Hammond's first published novel, *Robert Severne: His Friends and His Enemies* (1867), brought his neurological contributions on testamentary capacity to the literary public. The hero of the story has veered to the edge of insanity by overattention to his philosophical studies and consequent insomnia. In this state he confesses in writing to the murder of his wife, who had died of poison. Severne's dishonest and vindictive business manager obtains this confession and brings the scholar to trial. Fortunately, however, Severne and his friends are able to show conclusively that the woman had poisoned herself in an attempt to have her husband hanged. The incidents of the novel may well have been inspired by the trial of one Calvin M. Northrup in Westchester, New York, a few years earlier. In any case, Hammond packed into one lively story not only his medicolegal views on the reliability of confession, but also the perils of untreated insomnia and the rapid development of toxicology, which he regarded as a branch of physiology.[7]

Hammond used false confessions to highlight the value of neurological testimony. He told the New York Medico-Legal Society in 1871 that, contrary to the popular view, full and voluntary confession was not convincing evidence of guilt. "There are forces in operation in the human mind," he warned, "which may prompt to the making of a false confession, even when by so doing, life, liberty or property be put in danger." Confessions of persons constrained by their own mental makeup should be regarded as involuntary and hence inadmissible. Much as Hammond would later regard subjective assertions about states of consciousness as inconclusive and unnecessary tests of the hypnotic state, he considered "confession unsupported by collateral evidence" to be "very unreliable testimony."[8]

Another novel by Hammond, *Doctor Grattan* (1885), mixes romance with the legal problems of false confession and contested wills. The doctor has been treating his friend Lamar for an assortment of minor neurological symptoms when Lamar confesses that he had previously been engaged in the Cuban slave trade. He now believes, as does Grattan, that such activity is shockingly immoral as well as illegal. He wishes to atone by willing his estate to the establishment of a college for black Americans. Lamar, though unshaken in his confession, is finally convinced by the doctor's racist arguments that his plan is illogical and impractical. He decides to bequeath the property instead to his medical adviser, and does so before his sudden death. Grattan is later able to prove that Lamar's confession had been the result of an insane delusion and had lacked any basis in fact. His will is thus invalid, but his honor intact.[9] The novel concludes with the marriage of the young doctor to Lamar's daughter and heir, after the discovery that the estate had been reduced to practically nothing through unwise investments in fraudulent companies. Hammond could write with the authority of sad experience. Four years earlier he had lost $3,500 on a purchase of 1,000 shares of Wyandotte Silver Mine stock, and had also lost his lawsuit to regain the sum from a publisher on whose "false representations" he had relied.[10]

The novel was tolerably well received. A literary critic remarked that the psychological message was one of the strong points of the book, "distinctively a creation of Dr. Hammond's knowledge and taste in matters of a physiologico-psychological sort." He added respectfully that "what he finds it worth while to write it must be worth our while to read." On the literary side, the novel lacked a "solid, coherent, and masterful subject" but contained "some wit, a good deal of pleasantry, an underlying scientific vein, and an enveloping psychological atmosphere."[11]

Real life could be only a bit less dramatic. One of Hammond's interesting patients of 1886 was the proprietor of a large manufacturing business whose first symptom of distress was uncertainty about specific actions he had taken. He later developed a general state of uncertainty that made it difficult for him to function at all. While the patient had previously been healthy, there was a family history of assorted "neuroses" including migraine, chorea, and epilepsy. The crucial episode occurred when the patient was called upon to testify in court and was unable to state whether he had signed a document in question.[12]

Hammond considered this a form of insanity that he labeled "aboulomania," characterized by morbid doubts about acts already performed. He compared it to "mysophobia," in which the patient hesitated to act for fear of defilement or contamination.[13] Both conditions stood "on what may be called the doubtful ground between sanity and insanity – though both are in fact in the domain of mental unsoundness." Between either condition and insanity, he wrote, "there is apparently only the difference of degree, but all our knowledge of brain and mental disorders goes to show that some change in the structure of the organ has been initiated." He thought that the accompanying physical symptoms, including insomnia, pointed to congestion as the most likely culprit.[14] Here is a clear statement of Hammond's contention that neurologists were the appropriate authorities to consult for an understanding of a very broad range of behavior.

In a sense Hammond was contributing to the so-called medicalization of society that has attracted much critical attention in the late twentieth century. But for Hammond himself medical considerations did not necessarily determine social policy. This was especially clear in his well-publicized views on the management of insane murderers. He, like many others, realized that if such people were committed to the asylum rather than to the prison or the gallows, they would be in the hands of superintendents who regarded them as eminently curable. Thus the perpetrator of some atrocious crime might well be on the street a few years (or even months) later.

The more bizarre the crime, therefore, the greater the public anxiety that the criminal be declared sane and subjected to the full consequences of the law. Social imperatives, embodied in legal practice as the M'Naghten rule, pressured the physician called as an expert witness to abandon the principles of his own profession. For Hammond and other neurologists with a special interest in broadening the definition of insanity, the dilemma was especially pointed.

Hammond had considered these issues as early as 1870, sketching his views on "Society vs. Insanity" for the readers of *Putnam's Magazine*. The book-length version, *Insanity in Its Relation to Crime* (1873), bore on its title page the slogan "*salus populi suprema lex est.*" The crux of its argument was the distinction between legal and moral guilt, between crime and sin. Intention, and therefore sanity, were factors in judging moral responsibility. But crime was simply any violation of the laws society had established, Hammond said, to protect itself. The object of punishment was self-defense, not abstract justice. He concluded that insane criminals should be punished "even though they be morally irresponsible for their acts." An offender capable of knowing "that an act which he contemplates is contrary to law . . . should be deemed legally responsible and should suffer punishment." One lacking this capacity "ought not to be allowed to go at large," as liberty is denied to "wild and ferocious beasts" and rabid dogs.[15] Hammond predicted that attempts to integrate pathology and law were doomed to failure, since the two endeavors had different standpoints and different aims.

Not all sins, the broad-minded neurologist told readers of the *International Review* in 1881, should be considered crimes. But all criminals should be punished, for the sake of "safety to the lives and property of the majority." He explained once more that "an individual may be medically insane, and yet not a lunatic in the legal sense. His brain is diseased," Hammond continued, "either temporarily or permanently; his mind is not in all respects normal in its action – and yet he is responsible for his acts."[16]

The notorious case of Charles J. Guiteau, assassin of President Garfield, brought these issues into national headlines in 1882.[17] Hammond's well-known views suited neither the defense nor the prosecution, and he did not appear officially in the case. But he jumped into the fray with a paper read before a well-attended meeting of the New York Medico-Legal Society on March 1, 1882. "Probably no other paper," reported the *New England Medical Monthly*, "has been read in a long while in the United States that has been more widely copied by the medical and lay press than this one."[18]

Hammond was very sure that Guiteau was insane, a "reasoning maniac," and therefore a social danger. He suggested that the simple fact of insanity should not be sufficient to acquit. "The only forms of insanity which should absolve from responsibility and therefore from any punishment except sequestration, are such a degree of idiocy, dementia, or mania as prevents the individual understanding the nature and consequences of his act" – the M'Naghten test – "or the existence of a delusion in regard to a matter of fact which if true, would justify the fact." But the neurologist insisted that this narrow and conservative rule defined only legal responsibility, not medical insanity. "Let Guiteau suffer the full legal penalty for his crime," Hammond concluded, "but let him be executed with the distinct understanding that he is a lunatic deserving of punishment."

This accommodationist position might have done more to enhance the status of neurology than a narrower insistence that the specialist was to be the supreme authority in the courtroom. Hammond noted that judges and juries already recognized that "the motives of a person committing a crime are not to be considered in the estimate we may form of his criminality." They interpreted insanity to support their intuitive views on each particular case.[19] Further, the presiding judge in the Guiteau case had refused to allow the neurologist Edward C. Spitzka to testify as to the defendant's legal responsibility. The jurist insisted this was not a medical matter.[20] Physicians who dogmatically insisted on the insanity of notorious criminals without addressing the social concerns at the heart of the issue undermined their credibility with their manifest impracticality.

Hammond's conviction that insane persons were punishable also corresponded with his pessimistic view of human nature. He believed that there was a "natural selfishness existing in the human race in all parts of the world . . . which, being inborn, is a part of its organization." He added that "the propensity to kill exists to a greater or less extent in the mind of every human being without exception." Since these tendencies could easily lead to crime, he found it necessary to control them by punishing individuals who gave in to their natural impulses. Hammond may have had his own practice in mind when he wrote that "some physicians, scarcely ever meeting with a human being of perfectly sound mind in every respect," would label as insane "five-sixths of the human race."[21]

But even the mentally ill could exercise control, or order could not be maintained in insane asylums. They could therefore be held responsible for their actions. It was the duty of a person who felt an irresistible criminal urge to consult a physician and request at least restraint, if not a cure. Thus Hammond proposed his own modification of M'Naghten. The court would still consider whether a perpetrator knew the nature and consequences of his act. But in the case of an "alleged morbid impulse" it would also want to know whether the defendant did "everything in his power to make the yielding to this impulse an impossibility." If not, "he ought to suffer the full penalty of the law."[22] And for Hammond, the "full penalty" might be extreme: if not capital punishment, he suggested, then perhaps castration.[23]

Hammond supplied several vivid examples of patients who had wisely consulted him in such cases, and it must have been obvious to everyone that the neurologist's comfortable study was far preferable to the inconvenience and humiliation of an asylum. When Hammond argued in the much-publicized legal sphere that "all the insane are not the violent and ferocious beings they are popularly supposed to be," he was again promoting his own practice.[24]

Despite its commonsense logic, Hammond's position on the punishability of insane criminals was anathema to many alienists. "To divide lunatics into two classes, one of which shall be amenable to penal discipline, and the other only to medical treatment . . . would be to run counter to all advances hitherto made in the medical jurisprudence of insanity," declared a British writer on "Guiteaumania." "Efforts have heretofore been directed to reconcile the legal definition of insanity with the scientific description of it; and the attempt to force these two asunder can only end in inextricable confusion." An American reporter on clinical and forensic psychiatry wrote that "perhaps none of the articles . . . has excited as much comment as that of Dr. W. A. Hammond," but noted that "few alienists . . . will agree with him."[25]

The parade of neurologists through the witness stands helped to publicize their practice, but their conspicuous lack of consensus undercut the effectiveness of the publicity. A case in point was that of the convicted murderer John Reynolds, who tried to plead mental incompetence in 1870. Hammond appeared for the prosecution while his friend and fellow neurologist M. Gonzalez Echeverría testified for the defense. The editor of the *Medical Gazette* called attention to this disagreement "to indicate the inevitable conclusion that psychological medicine is as yet wanting in the first elements necessary for any branch of scientific investigation, viz., exact methods of observation." He questioned the source of the disagreement. "Of two observers whose positions should entitle their opinions to equal weight, either one has been deceived by assumed symptoms which the other was shrewd enough to detect, or else both combine to show the uncertainty of the very groundwork on which these opinions rest."[26]

Hammond tried to place himself on more secure ground by

using the most up-to-date tools for neurological analysis. One case in which he "took extraordinary means" to determine the state of mind of the defendant was the spectacular one of Daniel McFarland, which would become a *"cause célèbre* in the annals of psychological as well as of criminal literature." McFarland was charged in 1870 with shooting Albert Richardson, who had allegedly seduced Mrs. McFarland. The *New York Times* reported how Hammond, the star witness for the defense, used the ophthalmoscope, the dynamograph, and other apparatus to test McFarland's nervous system. The neurologist concluded that the prisoner suffered from "temporary insanity" brought on by cerebral congestion.[27]

A decade later, with neurological societies, journals, and practices more securely established, conflicts among the neurologists occasioned mirth within the medical profession. The distinguished otologist D. B. St. John Roosa, who had been an officer in both New York neurological societies, told an alumni dinner of the University Medical College in 1882 that "there is no question of insanity that we cannot get on both sides of, and illustrate the resources of medical minds and independence of thought inspired by the chairs of neurology and medical jurisprudence." His good-natured barbs were reported verbatim for the enjoyment of colleagues in New England.[28]

Roosa hinted, and many believed, that alienists' testimony was fundamentally opportunistic. But for Hammond the distinction between insanity and immorality was an important one. In his novel *Robert Severne* he has the hero wonder whether or not his late wife had been insane. "I thought it would be charitable to attribute her conduct to mental aberration," Severne reflects, but "she was so systematic, so calm and logical in her judgments, so cool and collected in her demeanor, that I could not in my conscience give her the benefit of this supposition." Rather, "her conduct was the result of bad principles which had been instilled into her from childhood. . . . She knew her conduct was wrong, she admitted it to be on several occasions; she says so repeatedly in her journal, and yet she willfully persevered in her depraved and reckless course." He concluded that he could not extenuate her "wicked, her very wicked behavior."[29]

In Hammond's nosology, therefore, "dipsomania" was recognized as a disease but distinguished from vicious drunkenness. The kleptomaniac should not be confused with a thief who "stole for a living." Persons with the insane delusion that they belonged to the opposite sex could be treated medically, but homosexuals and transsexuals who were content with their life-styles were, Hammond said, morally degenerate.[30] His main criterion for making such distinctions in practice seems to have been his informal estimate of the patient's social and moral status. Respectable deviants who admitted the error of their ways were ill, the victims of some form of morbid emotional or volitional impulse. Others were simply wicked. Take, for example, the case of Alice Mitchell, convicted of murdering her lesbian lover. Hammond served as an expert witness in the case. On the basis of his deposition and those of Charcot and the family doctor, Mitchell was declared insane on the basis of her general conduct rather than on the fact of her sexual deviance alone. As the neurologist Charles H. Hughes explained it, Mitchell's actions did not in themselves constitute medical symptoms. The burden of proof was on psychiatry to show that they were actually founded in a pathological condition.[31]

HAMMOND AND THE "WOMAN QUESTION"

Hammond tried to promote and defend his views on social issues using his neurological expertise, but without signal success. An outstanding case in point is his active opposition to the women's rights movement in the 1880s. Hammond's well-known views were already a matter of some amusement among medical men in 1876, when the neurologist was chosen to respond to the toast to "Woman" at the fifth annual reunion dinner of the University Medical College. "Why should the handsome gentleman who sits with such dignity . . . speak for women?" asked Whitelaw Reid. "He is accredited with the wild belief that women get too much praise," he continued. "I have even heard him talk about the fewer convolutions in their brains, as if they didn't always have enough to get the rest of mankind into dreadful and perpetual convolutions, anyway."[32] But the eminent neurologist took his assignment seriously, even on so convivial an occasion. His "chivalrous courtesy" did not prevent him from proclaiming what he took to be important truths. "There are some things just as much beyond her reach mentally as there are others to which her physical organization is not adapted," he generalized. A few exceptional women might excel in the learned professions. But such a course hardened them, so that they were "not exactly the sort of women from whom we would select our wives." In Hammond's novels *Lal* (1884) and *A Strong-Minded Woman* (1885), he has a male character express similar sentiments: the "doctress" Theodora would be a perfect wife except that she "had dissected all manner of creatures from worms to man." Single women, Hammond told the medical alumni, should be free to attempt any career they wished. "It is wholly a matter of expediency," he remarked confidently, "and in the long race she is sure to be beaten."[33]

When Hammond attempted to back up these contentions with medical data, he ran into technical difficulties. Women's brains, he pointed out, averaged six ounces lighter than men's, "and if brain means anything, that fact means something."[34] But he had recently concluded from other studies that brain was not the only source of mind: extracranial gray nerve tissue also generated mental power. He had even declared categorically that "there is no definite relation existing between the intelligence of animals and the absolute or relative size of the brain."[35] Thus his neurological analysis of female intellect hinged on differences in quality rather than quantity. Women were "quicker" but lacked intellectual force, he said. They were intuitive, automatic, and emotional. "Sympathy and emotion are the strong points of woman's mental organization, and in the peculiar sphere which she fills so well they stand her in better stead than would a higher degree of intellectual development."[36]

There was little actual neurology in Hammond's toast, but in the comfortably male atmosphere of the medical alumni reunion he could voice his antifeminist opinions without fear of serious contradiction. The case was different when he addressed the wider audience of the *North American Review* on the same subject a few years later. He began his article on "Women in Politics" by vehemently denouncing "energetic and unscrupulous" female-rights activists. A detailed comparison of men's and women's brains then laid the foundation for the author's views on the sphere of women's activity, and brought the article to the attention of the medical press.[37] But to make his point Hammond had to distort his own scientific views.

The "governing power of the world is to be found in the brain of mankind," Hammond declared. Brain tissue was "the matter which by its inherent power of evolving the mind places the beings possessing it in the highest degree of perfection at the head of creation." He thought it important, therefore, to study male–female differences in "the mind-producing organ." On the average, he found a significant difference in absolute brain size, and contended that this (and not size relative to body weight) counted. Hammond did not "insist upon the fact that as man has more brain than woman he must possess more mind," probably because it flatly contradicted his well-known views on the extracranial generation of mind.

Instead he moved quickly to supposed qualitative differences in men's and women's brains: "Difference of structure necessarily involves difference of function." Hammond did not supply anatomical details, but had no doubts himself that the brain of woman "is perfectly adapted to the proper status of woman in the established plan of nature, and for that very reason it is not suited to the work which is required of man's brain. It is a brain," he continued, "from which emotion rather than intellect is evolved." Besides that it was, "like that of the quadrumana, an imitative brain." Nor were females capable of exact thought, said Hammond, and for this reason life insurance companies often declined to issue policies to them.

This is an interesting although scarcely compelling argument. In comparing women to monkeys (as he had once done with black people) Hammond suggests a lower stage of evolutionary development. But his evolutionism was very unsophisticated, and his rhetoric evokes less a sense of Darwin or even Spencer than of the natural theology of the first part of the century. Brains must be examined to determine women's proper place, but it could be assumed in advance that anatomical differences would be found to account for functional differences adapted to different stations in everyday life. By the early 1880s Hammond himself was pleased enough with Gilded Age society to consider it the "established plan of nature."

The neurologist also brought in his clinical experience. He pointed to a "peculiar neurotic condition called the hysterical which is engrafted on the organization of woman." Within limits, this was "a normal feature of her being, . . . met with in a greater or lesser degree in all females of the human species." As a result a woman was "not unlike a package of dynamite." Perhaps this was the counterpart to Hammond's famous theory that all men are

insane. The antifeminist views he articulated as justification for
sex-role stereotyping also reinforced his perennial message of the
ubiquitous importance of his specialty.

Hammond's main lesson was that "grave anatomical and physiological reasons demand not only that the progress of the
[feminist] revolution should be arrested, but that, contrary to the
ordinary course of procedure in other revolutions, this one should
go backward." The self-proclaimed reactionary concluded optimistically that "while women remain in the sphere of life for
which nature intended them we shall continue to see, as the ages
roll on, better women, and, above all, better men to look after the
interests of humanity according to their natural and unchangeable
powers."[38]

Hammond's neurological authority did not entirely shield him
from an angry response. Lillie Devereaux Blake, President of the
New York State Woman Suffrage Association, found his "loose-
ness of argument and incorrectness of statement surprising . . . in
one who so strongly contends for scientific accuracy in others."
Nina Morais accused him, with much justification, of making
"appeals to popular prejudice." Together with Sara A. Underwood and the prominent physician-reformer Clemence Sophia
Lozier, she contradicted Hammond's characterization of the history, status, and goals of the woman suffrage movement.[39]

But Blake was not quite ready to challenge Hammond's scientific analysis openly. "No doubt," she wrote with perhaps a note
of sarcasm, "the eminent anatomist is as exact in the facts and
figures here given, as the most rigid truthfulness would demand;
we would not venture to question the statements of so distinguished a specialist in a department so peculiarly his own." She
argued instead from historical and scientific evidence that his conclusions did not follow from his premises.

Morais briefly criticized the brain-weight argument but concentrated on the ideas that "brain structures are not reliable standards
of qualification for voting" and that the government should represent the governed, whatever their mental capacity. She turned
Hammond's argument around by suggesting that if "woman is so
unlike man in her physical, mental and social nature" then "she
needs preeminently a special representation." But Morais was not
prepared to compromise the principle of female equality for the
sake of the narrower goal of suffrage. "All fair trials of mental

endowments, thus far," she added, "have shown that the mind of the girl is as good as that of the boy." Underwood more forthrightly attacked "the exploded theory of brain weight determining the amount of intelligence in individuals," and she was on firm ground in doing so. Lozier considered his craniology and physiology incorrect, but in any case irrelevant. "Physiology," she insisted, "can never decide moral or political rights."

Nor did these women accept Hammond's expert testimony on hysteria. "The distinguished alienist," said Blake, "is largely influenced by the studies of dementia and hysteria, to which he has devoted a large portion of his life. His acquaintance with normal and healthy women must be limited." Lozier elaborated on this idea. "Dr. Hammond's experience as a specialist in nervous diseases had apparently been painful," she commented. "Perhaps Dr. Hammond's practice among sick, weak, abnormally emotional and artificially stimulated patients, forming a wealthy clientele, account[s] for his views of women." Less vocal than the feminists were officers of life insurance companies, but they too disagreed with Hammond. Their reluctance to insure women was, they said, due to the increased mortality of the childbearing years rather than to mental peculiarities.[40]

Hammond might ignore the feminists: Dr. Lozier was a homeopath and Underwood later became a spiritualist. But his quasiphrenological arguments also embarrassed his neurological associates. When he addressed a large crowd at the Nineteenth Century Club in February 1884 on the subject of "The Brain and Its Functions" he was flatly contradicted by E. C. Spitzka on the weight differences between men's and women's brains.[41] Other neurologists may well have agreed with much of Hammond's social philosophy. But by claiming too much for neurology he was rendering its scientific status suspect among a large portion of the educated public. Declarations that all men were insane and all women hysterical did little to encourage patronage of the neurological specialist.

In the next years, Hammond turned instead to literature as a vehicle for his antifeminism. His novel *A Strong-Minded Woman* (1885) was a sequel to the popular *Lal* (1884), but unlike its predecessor it paid little attention to plot or character development. Instead it promoted Hammond's opposition to women in public life and his support for free trade. The novel's woman in politics is a coarse and ignorant heiress who runs a meatpacking business built up by her late father. Hammond usually favored entrepreneurship, but he found the slaughterhouse to be a distinctly unhealthy and unaesthetic enterprise, a fitting – perhaps even symbolic – occupation for his antiheroine.[42]

The heiress is contrasted with the altogether admirable "doctress" Theodora, who has been called to a professorship at a female medical college on the basis of her scientific studies. Theodora's enlightened husband understandably (in the author's view) finds this prospect distasteful, but liberally allows her to accept the position. He even attends her overwhelmingly successful introductory lecture, delivered before an audience including a thousand New York socialites. His patience is rewarded: she announces on the way home that she will resign the position because she is pregnant. The message is made explicit: a true woman might be able to compete with men, but she would be conscious that her special role is motherhood. It is interesting that Hammond often gave his female heroines feminized male names: Theodora in *Lal* and *A Strong-Minded Woman*, Alana in *On the Susquehanna* (New York, 1887).

Hammond's last major foray into antifeminism was a return to the Nineteenth Century Club in January 1887. His remarks were published in the *Popular Science Monthly* as "Brain-Forcing in Childhood." He again warned against excessive study, especially for women, with a vivid story of a woman patient who had violated his precept with sad results. Some of the neurologist's pedagogical suggestions were consistent with the new ideas of educational reformers such as John Dewey: object lessons rather than book lessons, for example, and the dictum that students should "be taught to think, and not as at present to absorb without understanding." But the burden of his argument was that girls' brains, in particular, ought not to be forced to work like those of boys. Once again he fell back on the claim that men's and women's brains were anatomically and hence physiologically different. This time he argued that men's brains had more gray matter, sidestepping earlier difficulties involving comparisons of total brain weight. He thus returned to a simple quantitative assessment.[43] The changing details of his theory that mind "evolved" from nervous tissue may even have originated in his efforts to deal satisfactorily with the "woman question."

The eminent neurologist's assurance and expertise clearly impressed a large part of his audience. But it was easier to argue in print with the sharp-tongued expert than to confront him directly. The magazine article drew fire from Helen H. Gardener and at least twenty other readers. Gardener was so incensed that she personally undertook a large-scale study of "Sex in Brain." For this she enlisted the aid of no lesser a figure than the neurologist E. C. Spitzka. The resulting paper, read before the International Council of Women in Washington, D.C., propelled the author into a leadership role in the feminist movement.[44]

Hammond responded to the predictable rebuttals somewhat inconsistently. He admitted that female mentality as a whole was equal to that of man, but revived the argument that differences in brain structure implied mental differences and hence different plans of education. But he also insisted that it was possible to generalize sex differences in absolute brain weight, and even added some passing remarks on supposed differences in the specific gravity of the brain substance.[45] He seemed to be floundering. Although he persevered in his attempts to extend neurological authority to a broad social context, he was unequal to the task – or perhaps the task was an impossible one. In exceeding the limits of the plausible he became an embarrassment to more cautious supporters of both causes he embraced, neurology and antifeminism.

NEUROLOGY, SPIRITUALISM, AND ORGANIZED RELIGION

If anything annoyed Hammond more than women's rights, it was the vogue of spiritualism in the 1870s. Not only did spiritualists claim that another world existed beyond the physical one, in flat contradiction of Hammond's aggressive materialism, but they generally refused to subject their claims to experimental scrutiny. Hammond did not deny the existence of mystifying phenomena, but he found it extremely important that a theory should be "based upon facts." For him this meant that it should rely wholly on observable or potentially observable events in the material world. If observations seemed to contradict materialist common sense, he claimed, the results must have been viewed "unequally." That is, uncontrolled variables must not have been taken into account. He gave the example of the German physiologist Joseph N. Czermak, who had demonstrated that the "magnetic passes" with which a friend had "hypnotized" crayfish were superfluous. "His friend had not thoroughly investigated the phenomenon in all its relations," commented Hammond, "and that is just what is done every day by certain people calling themselves 'inquirers', who make imperfect attempts to solve the pseudo-mysteries of mesmerism, spiritualism, etc."[46]

Hammond published a small book on *The Physics and Physiology of Spiritualism* (1871) to unmask such impostors, and an expanded edition appeared five years later. Another small volume on *Fasting Girls* (1879) exposed the fallacies of what he considered to be ridiculous and unscientific claims that certain young women could live indefinitely without food. The girls themselves (many of whom would now be regarded as anorexic) might have believed their claims. He had seen cases of what he called "hysterical deception" in his own practice that might have fooled a gullible public. Other "fasters" might be conscious frauds, such as a Dr. Tanner of Indiana who refused in 1880 to submit his claims to the test of rigid observation. Hammond included among these the unfortunate young Sarah Jacob, who had starved to death in Wales in 1869 rather than admit that her supposed prolonged fasting was a deception.[47] While uncompromising in his attacks on contemporary disreputable miracle-mongers and unpopular revivalist sects, he exploited popular interest in them with his long and graphic accounts of their more picturesque antics.

Hammond was also interested in historical accounts of bizarre behavior, which he regarded as accurate observations viewed "unequally." Supposed victims of demonic possession were, he argued, hysterics or epileptics who could have been cured with prosaic medications such as the bromide of potassium. "Were it not that there is such a condition as hysteria," he remarked, "we should be disposed to take the other alternative of demoniacal possession as an explanation." The famed figure of Merlin, from British traditional literature, was diagnosed retrospectively as a cataleptic.[48]

When Hammond presented his scientific materialism as an alternative to spiritualism or demonic possession, his medical colleagues most likely found this unexceptionable, if perhaps undignified. But many feared that materialism in medical science would tend dangerously toward atheism.[49] In Hammond's case their fears were justified. Despite his conventional religious upbringing and

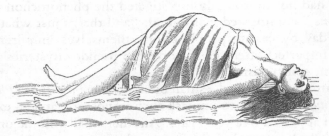

In this case there is a distinct aura starting from the left ovary, and strong pressure exerted upon this organ suffices generally, though not always, to cut short the series of paroxysms.

Patient with "hystero-epilepsy," ca. 1880. Hammond frequently used his neurological expertise as the basis for social or historical comment. Here a woman under his care for daily paroxysms of "hystero-epilepsy" provided an occasion to explain an episode of alleged demonic possession several centuries earlier as an epidemic of neurological disease. (William A. Hammond, *Treatise on the Diseases of the Nervous System,* 7th ed. [New York: Appleton, 1881], p. 788. Courtesy of Middleton Library of the Health Sciences, University of Wisconsin, Madison.)

his habitual affiliation with some fashionable Protestant church, Hammond found much to criticize in Christian traditions. For example, he considered celibacy to be an unnatural and antisocial practice that often led to insanity, suicide, and crime. He found this to be especially true of cloistered women, citing an "epidemic of hysterical chorea with catalepsy" among Ursuline nuns in sixteenth-century Europe and the famous case of the "Devils of Loudon." But such outbreaks were not "restricted to convents or catholic lands," he hurried to explain. "Protestants of the straitest sects have been visited, and our country has afforded many notable examples."[50]

Hammond took a scholarly interest in the history of religion, and his neurological interpretations were sometimes shockingly disrespectful. He claimed that many of the canonized saints of the Catholic Church were, like the "fasting girls," victims of that "remarkable manifestation" of hysteria, the delusion of the ability to live without food. He diagnosed as ecstatics and cataleptics the saints Gertrude, Bridget, Catherine of Siena, Theresa, and Joan of Arc. But he had little sympathy for either side in the bloody religious conflicts that had swept Europe centuries earlier. "While the Catholic ecstatics inveighed against the heretical sects which were springing up on all sides, and consigned them to torture and the flames," he commented, "the Calvinists, Camisards, Pre-adamites, Jumpers, Anabaptists, Bewailers, Sanguinarians, Tremblers, etc. etc., denounced the Pope as Anti-Christ, desecrated churches and exhibited a ferocity which, in its sanguinary character, has rarely been equalled in the history of the world."[51]

Perhaps there were limits to the neurologist's willingness to engage in controversy, for he casually understated what must have been by far his most provocative diagnosis. He said he had personally seen cases of the "hysteroid affection" ecstasy in which there was "a relaxation of all the muscles of the face concerned in expression, and . . . suffusion of the eyes and dilatation of the pupils." Hammond remarked offhandedly that "undoubtedly the instances mentioned in the bible as transfigurations (see Ex. 34:29–35; Matt. 17:1–2; Mk. 9:2–3; Lk. 9:29) were of this character."[52] Jesus himself, he implied, might have benefited from the bromides.

Hammond skirmished incidentally with a Catholic theologian in 1886 when, probably in response to the growing militancy of the eight-hour movement, he attacked workers' use of the boycott and the strike by comparing them to the church's practices of excommunication and interdiction. The bulk of his *Forum* article on "The Evolution of the Boycott" related in an unsympathetic tone incidents from the history of the medieval church. He was taken to task by Henry A. Brann in the pages of *Catholic World* for what Brann took to be damaging inaccuracies in his account.[53] Hammond, more interested in defending capital against labor than in theological disputes, did not respond. By then he was probably working on his new novel *On the Susquehanna* (1887), in which the ironworks of the businesswoman Alana Honeywood are beset by labor troubles instigated by an unscrupulous character.

In later years Hammond became bolder in his challenge to conventional religious sensibilities. His last published novel, *The Son of Perdition,* which appeared just in time for Christmas 1898, retold the story of the betrayal of Christ. Judas is the central character, whose romantic adventures with Sapphira and the converted Mary Magdalene occupy a large portion of the narrative. Some critics admired the work, but others denounced it bitterly. "Novelists choosing to embroider the plain Gospel narrative of the life of Jesus Christ have hitherto been handicapped by conscience or by tradition, or even by conventional respect for names of persons not in themselves impeccably respectable," one wrote acerbically. "Long before beginning this novel, Dr. Hammond must have got rid of sentimental impediments to free interpretation, and reached a point of view which has the possibly doubtful merit of being exclusively his own." Another was even angrier. "We fail of words," he sputtered, "which are strong enough to express our detestation of the daring irreverence which employs the sacred tragedy of the New Testament as the material for vulgar fiction. . . . Putting the American flag on cakes of soap and biscuits is a mild insult compared with this."[54] Hammond, who had at least refrained from including his neurological speculations about Christ, must have been amused.

* * * * *

Despite Hammond's intellectual commitment to the materialism underpinning his clinical neurology, the worship of gray nervous tissue served more to justify than to inspire his rather conventional morality and his less conventional religious views. He could sketch in broad strokes a unified picture of human life and thought from the perspective of neurological science, but its details generally eluded him. His eminence as a physician was based on clinical skill and experience rather than on his broader scientific attainments or philosophy. Whenever he stepped beyond the bounds of neurology, narrowly defined, his authority was challenged and his reputation began to suffer. Younger neurologists with more modest claims for the specialty may have been somewhat relieved at Hammond's announcement in 1883 that he "would rather be a novelist than a doctor." His gradual withdrawal from active participation in the American Neurological Association was rewarded with election to honorary membership in 1887, apparently delayed by the blackball of a young antagonist.[55] A year later he retired from his large and prosperous New York practice and moved to Washington, D.C., to launch still another stage of his variegated career.

12

"I said that I would be back"

"You may recollect," Hammond wrote to his old friend Walter F. Atlee in 1888, "that when I left Washington nearly twenty-five years ago I said that I would be back there within that period as Surgeon General of the Army. I am going back in accordance with that assertion," he continued, "although there are other inducements." His new "large and costly private residence," called Belcourt, was scheduled for completion in May of 1889. He had "always liked Washington," and looked forward to plunging into medical work there.[1]

The Washington correspondent for the *New York Medical Journal* wrote late in 1888 that "medical matters here are not very lively this winter, but with the establishment of Dr. Hammond's new hospital and the war on the Georgetown Medical College dissecting-room, we manage to keep up interest."[2] The eminent neurologist's New York practice had made him a wealthy man, and the Hammond Sanitarium was constructed on a lavish scale. Its large lot at Fourteenth and Sheridan Streets NW, near the National Zoological Garden in Columbia Heights, was valued at almost $30,000. The ornate building cost over $110,000 more, exclusive of gas fixtures and other furnishings. According to the proprietor, the location was both healthful and convenient: the "highest in the immediate vicinity of Washington, the soil is dry, and all the surroundings are free from noxious influences." It was carefully ventilated, and could easily be reached by the Fourteenth Street cable railway.[3]

The hospital could accommodate seventy patients, who paid between $55 and $150 per week apiece. These charges included all expenses except surgical fees. Relations and friends of out-of-town patients could sometimes be accommodated at a cost of $25 per

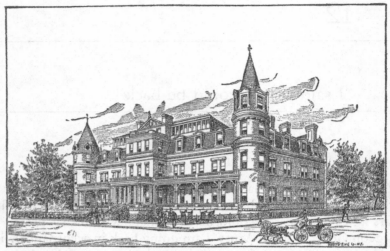

Dr. William A. Hammond's Sanitarium
FOR
DISEASES OF THE NERVOUS SYSTEM,
WASHINGTON, D. C.

For further information Dr. Hammond can be addressed at The Sanitarium, Four-
eenth Street and Sheridan Avenue, Washington, D. C.

> *Advertisement for Hammond Sanitarium, 1889.* Hammond's elegant new
> sanitarium in Washington, D.C., incorporated all the latest conve-
> niences and luxuries. While this notice in a medical journal solicited
> patient referrals from colleagues, the sanitarium – and the "animal ex-
> tract" therapy developed there – were also advertised directly to the
> public. (*Journal of Nervous and Mental Diseases,* n.s., 14, no. 11
> [November 1889]. Courtesy of Middleton Library of the Health Sci-
> ences, University of Wisconsin, Madison.)

week for lodging and board. Both the building and the regimen
were thoroughly modern. There was steam heat, a solarium atop
the main building, and an elevator. "Electricity in all its forms,
baths, douches, massage, inhalations, nursing, etc. are provided . . . in addition to such other medical treatment as may be
deemed advisable." There was even a gymnasium with a variable
treadmill, although Hammond considered such exercise stultify-
ing.[4]

The hospital received its first patients in January 1889 and was almost too successful. After a few years Hammond, always restless, found the work "more onerous and confining than he had thought it would be." He took sole professional charge of the hospital, with the assistance only of one young resident physician. Thus he found "no opportunity, even in the hot months of summer, for . . . needed rest and recreation." He was not away for more than a week at a time during the first five years of the sanitarium's existence. But the financial rewards were great: up to $70,000 annually.[5]

At the sanitarium Hammond expanded the range of his therapeutic experiments. His efforts with the suspension apparatus in the cure of locomotor ataxia and other diseases of the nervous system have already been mentioned. He also took an interest in brain surgery. This new technique stood, he said, with anesthesia, antisepsis, and the germ theory in the front rank of medical progress. Until recently, Hammond told readers of the *North American Review* in 1893, brain surgery had been unthinkable since the brain "was regarded as being the seat not only of the mind but of the soul." It had been blocked by those doctors "of whom there are always many – who stand in the way of progress" and by "still more narrow-minded and unprogressive theologians." But he thought that "the spirit of the age is different now," in spite of eternal "jealousy and ultra-conservatism" among physicians and "mental stagnation and ignorance of science" among the clergy. He was confident that the "skilful, the conscientious and the bold investigator" could "hold his own against all attacks." Most physicians and even many surgeons were ignorant of recent advances and were thus overcautious. That was never Hammond's problem. He predicted that surgery on "this preeminent organ of the body" would add "to the triumphs which scientific medicine and surgery are continually achieving."[6]

New techniques in brain surgery encouraged Hammond to return to the question of cerebral localization. Most of his surgical cases were epileptics whom he treated by trephination. He referred occasionally to "paring the convolutions" at the site of the "suspected lesion." Hammond also trephined a patient suffering from "merycism," described as "the abnormal act or habit of raising the food from the stomach and re-masticating it." He reasoned that there might exist a "regurgitating center" in the human brain.[7]

Hammond told the American Neurological Association in 1891

that in the seven cases he was about to describe, "the seat of a real or supposed injury" was only one "factor in determining where to operate." He worked on the assumption that "the symptoms, their nature and location, were even of more importance" in deciding on the site and extent of the operation.[8] That is, the surgical methods were to be informed by a combination of cerebral anatomy and clinical judgment, rather than by simple empirical observation of superficial injuries. In fact, cerebral localization was one area in which clinical methods could contribute significantly to medical science.

Hammond soon dispensed with elaborate antiseptic techniques, relying instead on scrupulous cleanliness (if not exactly asepsis). Brigadier General Hammond (ret.) reported to the Section on Military and Naval Medicine and Hygiene of the Pan-American Medical Congress in 1893 on thirty cases in which he opened the skull without antiseptic precaution. The results had been at least as good as in the fifteen cases where such measures were used. Displaying his medicoliterary erudition, he compared contemporary antiseptic procedures to the "Power of Sympathy" of Sir Kenelm Digby in the seventeenth century.[9]

Hammond's most extensive therapeutic experiments at the sanitarium involved the use of "animal extracts." In June 1889 Charles Edouard Brown-Séquard had reported to the Société de Biologie on the preliminary results of his administration of a preparation of animal testes injected subcutaneously for the relief of senescent debility. It was a plausible experiment in the context of late nineteenth-century conventional wisdom on the debilitating effects of masturbation, excessive sexual activity, and the like. Beyond this, Brown-Séquard saw in his work a possible proof of his new physiological theory of the "internal secretions." This was the notion that all tissues of the body secreted substances directly into the blood which were necessary for the nutrition of the other tissues. If debility could be cured by supplying the body with a missing nutrient, he reasoned, this would show that an original deficiency had caused the weakness. The seventy-two-year-old physiologist, whose first experimental subject had been himself, called on other elderly physicians (presumably male) to conduct similar self-experiments.[10]

Brown-Séquard's announcement, and the subsequent work he conducted with his assistant Arsène d'Arsonval in the laboratories of the Collège de France, excited international interest. Sensational accounts in the popular press dubbed his extract an "elixir of life." More cautious physicians explored its possible uses in specific conditions, and branched out to try extracts of other organs and other modes of preparation. Some researchers, probably a minority, gave serious attention to Brown-Séquard's physiological theory as well. The new field of "organotherapy" received added impetus from the successful use of thyroid extracts in myxedema, a line of research with its own distinct history. Organotherapy also benefited, at least in the United States, from the prestige of the new serum therapy for diseases such as diphtheria. Although much of Brown-Séquard's work was later discredited, it played a critical role in the emergence of endocrinology.[11]

Here was a promising field of research for Hammond, whose work had often, in the past, paralleled that of Brown-Séquard. Hammond had recently published several well-received books on the subject of sexual impotence in the male and in the female, conditions for which he was frequently consulted.[12] Hammond had also been interested in myxedema at least since 1880, and was credited with the first American description of the condition. Many of the patients who were already patronizing his sanitarium in large numbers for nervous and cardiac complaints would have appeared to be suitable candidates for the extract treatments. Hammond had already dosed them with almost every other available remedy, with only moderate success. For example, in 1888 he had been treating patients with "weak heart" with digitalis, strychnine, cocaine, nitrite of amyl, and nitroglycerine, as well as physical exercise and a special diet.[13] In any case, Hammond's first experiments with animal extracts were begun within days after he first heard the news from Paris.

Hammond identified himself first and foremost as an experimental physiologist like Brown-Séquard, although nearly three decades had passed since his last important work in this field. He thus paid special attention to the interpretation of the clinical facts he felt he had established. His theory of "isopathy" was meant to account for the success of the extract treatments and apparently related phenomena. But the successful clinician also regarded highly the pecuniary rewards of his scientific labors. He had two wards added onto the sanitarium, one for men and one for women, "for the special purpose of administering the animal extracts and teaching the patient the correct method of using the extracts at home."[14] Fees for patients on these wards were lower than elsewhere in the hospital, but since Hammond and his corporate associates were manufacturing the extracts for sale, this too proved to be a profitable enterprise.

The tension between these two aspects of his work with the extracts – the entrepreneurial and the scientific – soon posed a challenge that even the resourceful Hammond was ultimately unable to resolve. His inconsistent stand on the issue of presenting his work to the public demonstrates the difficulty of drawing the fine line between serious popularization and quackish puffery. It illustrates a problem in professional self-perception with which more than a few American physicians were coming to terms toward the end of the nineteenth century.

THERAPEUTIC EXPERIMENTS WITH "ANIMAL EXTRACTS"

Hammond read with interest the reports from Paris of Brown-Séquard's early results and their confirmation by G. Variot, and began his own trials on July 24, 1889. Using very fresh material prepared according to Brown-Séquard's method, he began by injecting himself with the testicular extract. ("Not," he defensively noted, "that I thought I required the injection for any infirmity.") There were no local or systemic effects, but Hammond was happily surprised at the disappearance of a pain in his left arm from which he had suffered for over a year, since being thrown while trying to board a moving train. The second injection, two days later, resulted in a local abscess the size of a walnut. Hammond gave himself no more injections, but proceeded to administer the substance to his patients.[15]

Hammond customarily tried new remedies on patients with a wide range of complaints. Most of the nine patients on whom he first used the testicular extracts were between fifty and sixty-five years old, with a list of symptoms and diagnoses ranging from insomnia, depression, and the effects of mental overexertion, to weak heart and "cardiac asthma," to lumbago and rheumatism. The one female was a victim of melancholia and fixed delusions, and the one patient over sixty-five had recently suffered cerebral hemorrhage and was hemiplegic. The two younger men (aged thirty-four and thirty-six) had both consulted Hammond for sexual impotence. One of them was reported "cured" by the treatment and the other "improved" when he prematurely left the hospital.

Hammond found that all the patients except two had benefited from the treatment. The exceptions were the insane woman and one man who had refused a second shot after noticing the unfortunate effect of Hammond's own second injection. The investigator attempted to rule out the effects of suggestion. The rheumatic patient was given one shot of pure water in the course of his treatment without being told, and that injection had no effect although the patient was finally cured. The last patient thought his cure resulted from placebo pills Hammond had administered in addition to the injections. While many neurologists in the 1890s were moving toward psychotherapy, a technique Hammond did use on occasion, he clearly sought physiologically active remedies.

Hammond concluded that while only the newspapers would sensationalize Brown-Séquard's discovery as an "elixir of life," the preparation was a valuable addition to the materia medica. Those physicians who abused the Parisian physiologist in the "irresponsible press" were simply jealous. "If they had had the intelligence and the forethought to be the first to make use of his discovery, we should have had no such exhibitions as we have had during the last few weeks," he admonished.[16]

The first announcements of Brown-Séquard's work had been met in America with a combination of skepticism and enthusiasm. In New York, for example, such respectable physicians as Henry P. Loomis and Lewis Sayre responded to Brown-Séquard's call for further tests of the extract. The *New York Times* reported that Loomis found that "the fluid is potent to increase the strength of the human organism, presumably in old men, not by structural change, but by nutritive modification." But George Shrady, editor of the *Medical Record,* was not convinced. He deplored the premature publicity. In succeeding months, reports of deaths from infection and inflammation following the extract injections justified his caution.[17]

On the other hand, the efficacy of the thyroid extract, demonstrated by G. R. Murray in London in 1891 and quickly embraced by the American profession, gave added impetus to "organotherapy."[18] By the middle of the decade, most American physicians (homeopathic as well as regular) probably believed that there was something to be learned in this field although few shared

Hammond's confidence and enthusiasm. A *Times* correspondent treated the extracts as a remedy of last resort, noting in an obituary of Brown-Séquard in 1894 that "the scientific opinion is that until the sub-cutaneous injections recommended by Dr. Brown-Séquard have been tried it may not be affirmed that all medicinal agents have failed."

Dr. Oscar H. Merrill, writing in *American Therapist,* listed "animal extracts" with "manufacturing chemists," bacteriology, creosote, and coal tar in his peculiar catalog of "recent therapeutics" in the same year. He reported that one result of Brown-Séquard's self-rejuvenation was "a mass of literature which contains much that is premature, much that is fantastic, much that is commercial; and it is difficult not to believe that some of it is closely connected with unsoundness of mind. . . . After the boomers and the seekers after notoriety have done their worst with animal extracts," he concluded, "the final accounting will probably show some increase of positive knowledge in physiology as well as in therapeutics."[19] By the end of the century, Brown-Séquard's extracts had been eclipsed by the "thyreoxin" and the serum antitoxins with which they were originally associated.

Hammond was one of the "boomers." In a widely disseminated article, George L. Freeman reported that organopathy "has been brought into prominence – it might almost be said popularity – by Dr. William A. Hammond."[20] Hammond read his major paper on the subject at the New York Post-Graduate Medical School on January 16, 1893. It was widely reported in the medical press: according to one observer, "abstracts or reprints . . . were published in nearly all of the medical journals in the United States and Canada." A similar talk was given later that year to the Pan-American Medical Congress.[21] Hammond reported that he had abandoned the use of fresh extract preparations, partly because of technical difficulties in handling the material and partly because local abscesses appeared in about a third of the cases. After some experimentation he had settled on a procedure, which he described in detail, for making extracts of a variety of organs: bone marrow, ovaries, testes, pancreas, stomach, heart, and most importantly brain. Excretory organs were not used, since their physiological function was presumed to be elimination, not secretion.[22]

"Cerebrine," the extract of brain that he had used most extensively, gave beneficial results after a single dose. He listed these as increased pulse, increased muscular strength and endurance, improved appetite and digestion, improved vision in the elderly, and general exhilaration. Continued administration cured many cases of cerebral congestion and insomnia, migraine, hysteria, melancholia, hebephrenia, and "so-called neurasthenia." It "worked like a charm" in most cases of neuralgia, sciatica, and lumbago. Cerebrine was not a cure-all, however: it was less useful in cases of epilepsy and general paresis. "The most notable effects," Hammond emphasized, "are seen in the general lessening of the phenomena accompanying *advancing years.*"[23] A short paper a few months later detailed Hammond's results with "cardine," or heart extract. He attempted to document the action of the drug by reproducing sphygmographic tracings, although these results were disputed.[24]

Many physicians questioned the value of Hammond's extracts, and some ridiculed them. An unsigned editorial in the *Boston Medical and Surgical Journal* declared that "the notion that one may by such injections restore or make compensation for an organ diseased or destroyed is absurd." It did concede that rigorous clinical tests were needed. Wallace Wood derided the remedies of Hammond and Brown-Séquard as "sarcology and sarcotherapeutics," finding them unworthy of serious consideration.[25] Even some who were originally open to the idea came to oppose Hammond's extracts. G. Archie Stockwell of Detroit, for example, had been one of the first Americans to defend Brown-Séquard's original experiment. He had conducted his own tests with the support of the Parke-Davis pharmaceutical firm. In 1893, however, Stockwell reported that "when subjected to careful and prolonged control," the extracts "proved an utter failure aside from psychic influence." Hammond's "cerebrine," manufactured by the Columbia Chemical Company, and the "cerebrin" of Parke-Davis were no better than his own preparations. Comparing their effects with a mixture of borax, glycerin, and water in a carefully controlled series of tests, he found all three solutions to be "equally efficacious – or rather equally inert for good or evil." Hammond responded that the extract used was not actually made by his own process, and another inconclusive exchange ensued.[26]

The extract disputes had both scientific and commercial interest, and continued for several years. Frederic Coggeshall found that Hammond's extracts (among others) were "physiologically inert and therapeutically worthless."[27] Yet others who analyzed the substances came to a different conclusion. In Chicago, Dr. M. Delafontaine had analyzed a "sterilized solution of cerebrine, prepared solely by the Columbia Chemical Company, New York," packaged in a small triangular blue glass bottle with a facsimile of Hammond's signature on the seal. A Mr. Baker of the pharmaceutical concern Gale and Blocki had tried the substance and suspected from the effects that it might contain nitroglycerine. Delafontaine confirmed this. His laboratory analysis showed an absence of organic bases but positive indications of nitroglycerine. A sample of cerebrine from another firm seemed to be physiologically inert and showed no chemical reaction. Delafontaine presented these results to the Chemical Section of the Chicago Academy of Sciences.[28]

Hammond's response was equivocal. He did not question the integrity of the investigator, but thought the results improbable if the sample had actually been prepared according to his process. On the other hand, he cited his own papers in the *New York Medical Journal* to show that he had anticipated the possibility of the active agent being "analogous to nitroglycerine." He agreed that his rival's product was worthless. Soon Columbia Chemical Company advertisements appeared with the warning that dealers might be refilling their bottles with a dangerous imitation product. Delafontaine was disgusted enough to make public a fuller description of his laboratory findings and the provenance of his samples. Meanwhile the prominent chemist J. H. Long of Northwestern University independently confirmed Delafontaine's analysis. Hammond did not press the issue further.[29]

Hammond repeatedly warned against exaggerated claims for extract therapeutics, as well as against hasty and careless production. Yet he apparently remained convinced of the therapeutic value of the extracts in an astonishing array of disorders. The Hammond Animal Extract Company, whose products were made "under Dr. Hammond's supervision," boasted in 1898 that the extracts were especially useful "in some phases of disease not amenable to drugs." The carefully worded brochure promised they would "greatly add to the natural power of resistance" and "actually come to be described as rejuvenating." Cardine had a general tonic effect, and "musculine" was superior to beef tea as a tonic. "Ovarine" was "one of the most valuable" of the remedies, curing not only ovarian disease but sexual apathy, chlorosis, hysteria, amenorrhea, and insanity in women. Even thyroidine, a specific in myxedema, eczema, and other skin diseases, could probably be used in "other diseases attended with a *depraved condition of the system*."[30] While the extract remedies seemed organ-specific, they were meant to be used primarily as alteratives. This mode of therapeusis was more compatible with the traditional medical thought of the nineteenth century than with the newer concepts of the dawning "etiological era" in medicine. There is no evidence that Hammond ever lost faith in animal extract therapy.

CHEMISTRY, PHYSIOLOGY, AND "ISOPATHY"

Hammond was especially interested in the theoretical interpretation of his clinical results. He was careful to distinguish between observed clinical facts and the theory by which he proposed to explain them. His opinion was that the extracts contained "the material required for the nutrition of the corresponding organs of the body." He found this theory "physiological and plausible," while emphasizing that he was "not in the slightest degree attached" to it. Another possibility was that the chemical combination "exerts a metamorphic influence and causes the formation of a ferment having the power of restoring to the weakened brain or other viscus the lost or impaired power of assimilation." Whatever the explanation, he emphasized, "the facts remain unaltered." He considered the extract therapy a "philosophical means of combating disease," of which his own work was only a small part.[31]

Other American physicians agreed that animal extract therapeutics were especially significant because they had a scientific basis. The *Journal of the American Medical Association* editorialized that in the thyroid extract the profession had "a remedy, which was suggested by a physiological and pathological study of the thyroid gland; in other words, we have a remedy founded upon scientific deductions." Henry Hun called the field of animal extracts "the most remarkable advance that therapeutics has ever made" because it was "based on scientific methods."[32] There was sharp disagreement, however, both over the various theoretical explanations offered, and over the very nature of the science on which the new therapeutics were to be based. This debate was particularly marked by the growing rift between laboratory and clinic-oriented medical science. This was a quarrel not solely between theory and practice in medicine, but between advocates of different methods of scientific research.[33] In Hammond's case this debate is doubly interesting because it represents a return to a field of research in which he had distinguished himself nearly forty years earlier. His new perspective led him to interpret differently not only his results of the 1890s but, to some extent, those of the 1850s as well.

Hammond summarized his theory of the mechanism underlying the extract therapy as follows:

Organic beings possess the power of assimilating from the nutritious matter they absorb the peculiar pabulum which each organ of the body demands for its development and sustenance. The brain, for instance, selects that part which it requires. . . . No mistake is ever committed. . . . There are, however, diseased conditions of the various organs in which this power is lost or impaired, and, as a consequence, disturbance of function, or even death itself, is the result.

In such cases, the physician could aid nature by supplying the necessary material directly into the blood. This material could conveniently be found in an organ of the same type taken from a healthy animal. Hammond cited his successful therapeutic use of the extracts as evidence in support of this theory.[34]

Hammond's theory differed somewhat from that of Brown-Séquard, and he presented it as an essentially original contribution. He vaguely remembered having seen "the germ of the idea" in the work of a German physician who had suggested treating liver disease with beef liver some forty years earlier. John Aulde, editor of *American Therapist,* resurrected this citation as the work of a Dr. Hermann, *True Isopathy; or, The Employment of Organs of Healthy Animals as Remedies in Diseases of the Same Organs in the Human Subject* (1848). Isopathy, Aulde suggested, was a system (analogous to homeopathy) of treating diseases by administration of their own morbid products. This was a "delusion" and should not be confused with the recent work of Robert Koch, Louis Pasteur, and others whose results represented the "triumph of science over mere empiricism." But "true isopathy," or "organopathy," was the system Dr. Hermann had proposed, "an imitation of the ancient doctrine of signatures," and which Hammond had revived. This, said Aulde, required careful consideration by the profession. "Its therapeutic basis must be determined from purely scientific investigations," he insisted. "[C]linical observation should be regarded as complementary."[35]

Hammond did not accept Aulde's dichotomy between the "purely scientific" and the "clinical." He spoke directly to this question in a sharp but mutually respectful debate with William Henry Porter, professor of clinical medicine and pathology at the New York Post-Graduate Medical School and editor of the *American Medico-Surgical Bulletin*. Porter held that in "the very midst of this turmoil and expectancy" of miraculous methods for the "retention of youth and health," critical examination of extract therapy was especially necessary. Biological chemistry could supply the knowledge and methods with which to do this.

Porter gave a detailed summary of the state of knowledge of nutrition. He described three classes of nutrients and the functions of each: inorganic compounds, which served as "mechanical irritants," carbonaceous compounds, which supplied energy, and proteid molecules. These last, through a complicated series of chemical reactions, were transmuted into the tissues and the secretions. It was inconceivable to Porter that the intake of these classes of materials could be so well balanced as to prolong life indefinitely. However, there was ample room for dietary improvements that could significantly extend the life span. On the other hand, there were materials that did not fit into the nutritive process; for example, some inorganic substances, alkaloids, leucomaines, ptomaines, and toxines. These were technically irritants or poisons, although they could be used therapeutically to stimulate the system into normal, healthy functioning.

Porter asked whether Hammond's animal extracts were normal foodstuffs or poisons. He set out a rigid protocol to prove their value if they were indeed foodstuffs. A graphic formula would have to be given for a proteid that was ready to be transmuted into a particular type of tissue. The extract would have to be shown to contain this proteid, and in an appropriate quantity. Further, it would have to be demonstrated that extracts injected hypodermically moved directly and without alteration to the site at which they were to be used. Finally, the scientist would have to show that the organ would assimilate this material in preference to whatever abnormal material had accumulated at the site. If all these conditions were met, the extracts would have been proved to be of great value. But in fact not one of them had even been approached.

In addition to specifying these rigid chemical tests of efficacy, Porter explicitly criticized the clinical evidence that had been adduced in favor of the extracts. Most results, he emphasized, were claimed *"on the basis of the patient's report. The patients treated certainly seemed better, and, when questioned, declared themselves much improved."* But he considered such evidence unreliable. Controlled quantitative studies "usually prove[d] a sadly negative result except for the last possibility."[36] Porter did not absolutely deny the use of clinical evidence but he was not at all sanguine about the method.

Hammond did not question Porter's summary of the biological chemistry of digestion, but he challenged its relevance to the problem at hand. It was "unfortunate" that Porter's conditions could not be met, but not damaging to his case. Hammond pointed out that the exact chemical formulas of most foodstuffs as well as most medical remedies were unknown, but their nutritive and therapeutic properties were generally acknowledged on the basis of long experience. Besides, the nutritive value of foods or the therapeutical value of remedies could not be deduced from their chemical formulas even when these were known. In effect, Hammond rejected Porter's reductionism.

Hammond felt he could speak with authority on the chemistry of nutrition, for his own reputation as a physiologist had been built on just this work. "It is very easy for the chemist or physiologist . . . to sit in his laboratory and, from scientific principles, deduce practical results," he said a bit smugly, "but experience, which is our only guide in matters of this character, generally plays sad havoc with such conclusions." By chemical analysis alone one would suppose it possible to subsist entirely on albumen, gelatin, or some other nitrogenous substance. But his own experiments, here described as "experiences" and recounted in detail, had shown this to be false. Thus "a chemical analysis of the animal extracts or juices would not be of the slightest medical value." Only a physiological chemist would find it interesting to determine "the composition of substances which had produced certain effects upon the animal economy."[37]

Here Hammond implicitly rejected the notion that laboratory science, represented by biochemistry, was "basic" to medicine. Rather, he argued that scientific knowledge was "higher" than the facts and experiences from which it was drawn. It was to be pursued for its own sake rather than for its therapeutic impact. Both metaphors attach great significance to science, but they are nonetheless contradictory.

Hammond's interpretation of his own scientific work had changed over the decades. His original account of his self-experiments on digestion had emphasized the use of laboratory techniques of analysis. He had never counterposed physiology to chemistry. The youthful scientist had been very sure he was conducting "experimental researches," and not mere "experiences." Then, the choice had been more clear-cut. By the 1890s, however, the intellectual context of medical science had altered in important ways, and Hammond's self-perception as a scientist had changed in response.

Hammond also answered Porter's challenge to clinical methods of investigation. "There is generally no better evidence of a patient's improvement than the dicta of the patient himself," he insisted. "If he is satisfied the physician may usually be content. And, in many cases, the report of the patient is the only evidence we can obtain of improvement or cure."[38] Again this is a significant admission in view of the sophisticated diagnostic gadgetry Hammond still recommended in the latest edition of his *Treatise on the Diseases of the Nervous System,* as well as the stand he had taken in the hypnotism controversy. But Hammond was fully cognizant of the possibility of cures by the power of suggestion; accordingly, as in his experiments with hypnotism, he attempted to supplement the patient's testimony with direct observation of physical signs. Here he did use medical technology rather than unaided experience. The hemometer and the hemacytometer were used to measure increases in blood coloration and in the number of red corpuscles, to show the action of cardine in an anemic and chlorotic patient. As noted earlier, he employed the sphygmometer in other cases. But no remedy commonly in use had been as well established as Porter demanded. Efforts to obtain reliable data on the therapeutic effects of various substances were "frightfully discouraging." Extensive observations were not necessary before an agent could reasonably be used in practice. After "years of experiment and observation" a relative consensus could be reached on the value of a new medicine. Hammond was, after all, a physician of the nineteenth century. As a scientist, however, he welcomed sharp criticism. If his answers were unsatisfactory, he accurately predicted, the extracts would achieve a well-deserved obscurity. And if his theory was valid, "not all the scientific artillery of all the thinkers and workers in the world, much less the vaporings of the malicious and ignorant, can keep it down."[39]

Porter's rejoinder suggests the importance attached to the extract controversy by Hammond's contemporaries. If his conclusions differed from Hammond's, Porter declared, it was not because the material facts were in question but "because a different light has been cast upon the whole picture." He interpreted Hammond's position to be the abandonment of "the chemical side of physiology and therapeutics" in favor of exclusive reliance on "empiricism in practical medicine." This seemed to him to be "a gigantic stride backward," especially "at a time when so much is being said and written in relation to the rapid advances in the science of medicine, and . . . higher medical education." Because Hammond was "so erudite a member of the medical profession," Porter thought it necessary to respond in depth. His main point was that "precise chemical laws do govern the working of the animal economy." Therefore, "the natural base of a real science of medicine and therapeutics must be the science of chemistry."

The bulk of Porter's editorial answered Hammond's specific claims that chemistry could not play that role. Hammond had said that the numerical formula of a substance could tell little about its properties, but much more could be known. The structural formula could be established, as well as the properties of the elements and how compounds decomposed. In fact, Hammond was neglecting most of pure or theoretical chemistry. When combined with knowledge of how chemical transformations take place within the body, basic chemistry would make the medical profession "master of the clinical situation."

Porter found it unfortunate that deficiencies in medical education left most physicians ignorant of chemistry. But this was "no reason why the science of chemistry should be ignored, and empiricism given the right of way." He went so far as to say that the advance of scientific medicine would render irrelevant patients' subjective estimates of their own condition. "The physician [will have] at his hand the knowledge of the exact changes taking place within the animal economy, and can tell precisely whether the nutritive vitality is improving or retrograding." The locus of medicine – not research alone but also clinical practice – would, in this extreme view, lie ultimately in the laboratory.[40]

Porter explained that much had been learned about the digestion of foodstuffs since Hammond had made his special study. Biological chemistry had recently revealed that an exclusively proteid diet was not nutritious because carbonaceous compounds were necessary to produce heat and hence to maintain animal life. Hammond's "purely physiological experiments" had established a valid fact but did not "explain *why*." They "waited for chemistry to come forward, and explain the grand discovery, and clearly outline the remedy." Similarly, the mode of action of the extracts or other therapeutics could only be known when their structural composition was analyzed. Porter did make some deductions from Hammond's data. The doses of cardine were far too small to have produced the observed effects by supplying missing nutrients. Therefore the remedy must act like the alkaloids, as a "positive poison." Thus "true reparative action is still effected through Nature's fixed laws of chemistry," and not directly by the extracts. Porter concluded that chemical analysis would probably prove the utility of the extracts and regretted that they had so far gained only an empirical place in medicine.[41]

Porter's position was by no means universally accepted. For example, the same issue of his journal included a strong defense of clinical (as opposed to laboratory) research in medicine by Professor Semmola, of Naples.[42] But Hammond seems not to have conceptualized sharply the laboratory–clinic controversy that had begun to surface late in his own career. Rather, he was probably offended by the obscurity to which his own early research had been consigned, and by his casual exclusion from the ranks of biochemistry. The very attention to clinical specialization by which he had achieved success in neurology had shut him out of the newer specialties of laboratory medicine. Moreover, there were signs that a new "humoralist" clinical pathology was about to revolutionize the study and treatment of nervous diseases, rendering obsolete even Hammond's own special expertise. In fact, the long publishing history of Hammond's *Treatise on the Diseases of the Nervous System* ended with the appearance of the ninth edition in 1891.[43]

Hammond pursued the theoretical issue of the mode of action of the extracts in a paper published in the *Charlotte* (North Carolina) *Medical Journal* in 1896. He modified Aulde's terminology to outline his own version of "isopathy." He found "two distinct but analogous doctrines" conflated in the term. The first, that "diseases may be cured by the products of similar diseases," had recently been established by Pasteur, Koch, and Kitisato. The other was that "a diseased organ of the body may be cured by the introduction into the system of the corresponding organ of the healthy animal."[44] This linkage of antitoxins and extracts was just barely plausible even at the time. Regular nineteenth-century remedies were almost all of vegetable or mineral origin. Thus the concept of "animal therapeutics" had a measure of coherence.[45] This was especially true since the biochemical mechanisms of the thyroid extract, antitoxins, and so forth were only then being worked out. But such a broad concept lent itself to quackery of the worst sort, particularly in the absence of a careful and detailed development of the theme. Thus, for example, one Joseph R. Hawley began a *Journal of the New Animal Therapy,* superseded by the *Journal of the American Animal Therapy Association.* These puff-sheets were "devoted to the advancement of the Roberts Lymph Compound, the Roberts-Hawley Lymphs, and other Animal Derivatives prepared by the Roberts Process." Some contributors emphasized the similarity of the "lymphs" to the "Brown-Séquard Elixir" while others emphasized the differences between the two. Dr. B. F. Roberts of Missouri had apparently tried Brown-Séquard's method before developing his own remedy.[46] Hammond never descended to this sordid level, but many of his high-toned contemporaries may have feared the worst.

"Isopathy" lingered on well into the twentieth century, mainly as a straw man to be knocked down by homeopathy.[47] But a sharp distinction was quickly established between serotherapy and organotherapy. *Index Medicus,* for example, introduced both categories as subdivisions of "therapeutics" in 1896, while John V. Shoemaker distinguished between the two in his review of "Progress and Problems of Medicine To-Day" in the following year. Solomon Solis-Cohen's eleven-volume *System of Physiological Therapeutics,* published in 1905, treated the two therapeutic modalities in articles by separate authors.[48] And within the category of organotherapy, influential physicians tried to separate the well-established "thyreoid" extract from "the doubtful company in which we are meeting it lately," as S. J. Meltzer put it. Meltzer criticized not only the advertised extract remedies, but also the work of respectable researchers like Henry Hun who, "though an enthusiastic admirer of the therapeutics of the thyreoid, . . . does not hesitate to treat it under the same head with Hammond's products." Solis-Cohen pointed out that the brain and the heart, unlike the thyroid, were not secretory organs. Hence no possible benefit could be obtained from their extracts.[49]

Hammond, never one to be deterred by a hostile profession, persevered in developing what he saw as his "new system of medical practice . . . based upon sound scientific principles." He continued to insist that "one of the greatest supports which the system of Isopathy has received comes from Immunization – thus, Hydrophobia, Diphtheria, Tetanus, Cholera and many other diseases are prevented and treated on this principle." He persisted in treating cerebral hyperaemia, a disease no longer recognized by his colleagues, on principles of isopathy that his colleagues had never accepted. In his last years, as he gradually curtailed his practice because of increasing difficulty with his heart, he conducted "a series of observations" on the possible use of his extracts in the prevention (as well as cure) of disease.[50] In the calomel episode he had been out of the mainstream but retrospectively correct. With the animal extracts he was again out of the mainstream, but retrospectively in error. It is hard to say whether he would ever have come to recognize the difference.

13

"Very near being a great man"

More than Hammond's scientific reputation was at stake in the animal extract controversy, as he had invested a large part of his considerable fortune in it as well. His last years were preoccupied largely with business affairs, even as he struggled to maintain his position as a scientific leader in the medical world. But the tension between the entrepreneurial and the scientific aspects of his work proved increasingly difficult for Hammond to manage. The results were scarcely satisfactory from either standpoint.

THE ANIMAL EXTRACT BUSINESS

Only a few months after the famous Post-Graduate lecture in which he had publicly described the extracts, Hammond helped organize the Columbia Chemical Company to manufacture them. It was incorporated as a half-million-dollar enterprise, with just under half the shares taken by Hammond and another large block purchased by one James Haydon, formerly of the Health Restorative Company. Hammond legally transferred his right, title, and interest in animal extracts to the company and agreed to supervise their manufacture, in return for almost all the outstanding shares and the posts of president and director.[1]

This commercial arrangement left Hammond wide open to criticism from the medical profession. In the fall, Dr. L. Elliot, president of the Medical Society of the District of Columbia, formally accused him of violating the code of ethics. At a widely publicized and well-attended meeting of the society, Hammond was cleared of the charge of "making money from a patented medicine," apparently because the extracts had not been patented. He emerged "unscathed, as was to have been expected," reported the *New York*

Medical Journal, which "hoped that, for a time at least, persons who delight in circulating damaging rumors will be somewhat less ready with their tongues."[2] In cosmopolitan New York, Hammond was regarded as an eccentric but not as a quack.

Meanwhile Hammond locked horns with Mr. Ernest Hart, the prominent and outspoken editor of the *British Medical Journal.* The American took it upon himself to defend the propriety of commercial exploitation by physicians of nonsecret, nonpatented remedies. He also endorsed cooperation with the newspapers and other practices that Hart had attacked in a speech at the Pan-American Medical Congress.[3] Apparently still somewhat on the defensive, Hammond announced in December 1893 that "having demonstrated my right as a physician and an American citizen to hold any kind of property that the code of ethics and the law of the land permit," he had sold his stock in the Columbia Chemical Company. His only remaining connection to it, he said, was as a consulting chemist, "a post somewhat analogous to the one held in the Apollinaris Water Company by that king of medico-ethical propriety, Mr. Ernest Hart."[4] This was literally true but rather misleading. A controlling interest had actually been transferred to Mrs. Hammond as trustee, and Hammond's son-in-law Manfredi Lanza remained as secretary and treasurer of the company. The family maintained this control until August 1894, when a large block of stock was sold.[5]

Dr. Hammond then found himself in an uncomfortable position. No longer in control of the production of his extracts, he discovered that the company's practices could seriously compromise his own reputation. On the other hand, he was reluctant to sever his connection with such a highly profitable enterprise. As he described the situation, he and Mrs. Hammond had sold their stock under pressure, on "exceedingly unreasonable and exacting" terms. On orders of Vice-President Springer, production of the extracts was then moved from Hammond's house to the company office, under the charge of the general manager. Hammond therefore wished to dissociate himself from the production of the extracts, which were being made (he said) in a narrow, confined packing cellar where they were exposed to injury or even destruction through carelessness or malice. The general manager, Hammond alleged, was "entirely ignorant of chemistry, physics or physiology. To make him the superintendent . . . of the delicate processes and manipulations required," he continued, "is an act,

the fatuity of which passes comprehension." Neglect of certain
necessary precautions was likely to lead to abscesses and other
complications for the consumers, "thus causing the utter ruin of
the Company" and "bringing into public odium" all persons connected to it. Hammond apparently saw the business as a happy
conjunction of science and entrepreneurship, while his partners
had only the latter end in view.

Hammond claimed publicly that there was nothing secret about
his extracts and that they were therefore not unethical. But he
insisted privately that he alone understood the process of manufacture and that ideally no one else should know all the details. He
had worked for years to perfect the extracts, "but with all the
study and chemical and physiological knowledge I can bring to
bear . . . the laws governing the processes are not fully known to
me." He was constantly discovering "new features in the manufacture," including temperature limits, specific gravity, and the proper application of electricity at a precisely determined moment.
While some formulas had been published, those of thyroidine,
testine, ovarine, musculine, and medulline had not. He was still
experimenting with "haemine, and other extracts that will as-
suredly prove of great value." It would be "suicidal" to share the
details of the manufacturing process with others, for if they were
known "it would only be a short time before rival companies
would spring up on every side." It is impossible to know whether
these statements or those made to the public and the profession – if
either – accurately represented Hammond's opinions. It is even
difficult to say whether he was truly cynical or merely inconsistent. That there was a conflict between the official values of medical science and those of pharmaceutical manufacturing, however, is
fairly clear.[6]

In any case, Hammond had no intention of relinquishing his
interest in the remedies. "Though the discoverer of the animal
extracts and the one whose writings and lectures and influence
have given them what reputation and standing they possess," he
complained, "I have never received the slightest pecuniary reward
from their sale." He proceeded to detail the value added in production – or perhaps just the markup. "The material to make 20,000
bottles . . . costs the company less than $50. By my knowledge,
skill, labor, and professional and scientific reputation it is made so
valuable as to be sold at wholesale for $30,000 and at retail for

$50,000." Quite the exploited worker, he doubted whether "there is another such instance in the whole range of science or art of the power of knowledge to increase the value of raw material." Hammond valued his own expertise highly indeed. He thought a 10 percent royalty, such as book publishers allowed, would be reasonable compensation. As a stockholder, Hammond must have shared in the fantastic revenues generated by the company. His complaint was that he was also entitled to compensation as an inventor comparable to that which he might have received had the code of medical ethics (of which he disapproved anyway) permitted him to patent the process.

The issue of advertising was also difficult. Hard experience had taught him to keep the use of his name under his own control. Otherwise, he was certain, "in the effort to advance the business interests of the Company little regard would be paid to professional or social etiquette." His association with the company could be announced, as long as it remained a fact. But even this should not be "placarded on fences etc. and published in disreputable newspapers or periodicals."[7] Several months later he approved copy for advertisements to be placed in the New York *Evening Post* and *Herald,* the Boston *Globe,* and the Washington *Star,* although suggesting this his name be set in smaller type.[8]

Meanwhile, Hammond had received an offer from Mahlon Hutchinson, a Chicago physician who wished to purchase an interest in the Hammond Sanitarium and help the founder to manage it. The busy Washingtonian agreed. In August 1894 he sold the sanitarium and "good will" to the Illinois-based Hammond Sanitarium Company, formed mainly with his own capital. Hammond retained just under half the stock in his own name. The two doctors became resident physicians at a salary of about $500 per month apiece, and Hutchinson was the company treasurer.[9]

This arrangement left Hammond with time to begin production of the animal extracts for sale through the Hammond Sanitarium Company, in competition with the Columbia Chemical Company. The products were advertised widely through pamphlets and in both lay and medical periodicals.[10] The Sanitarium Company claimed that the extracts were "in no sense secret, proprietary, or patent medicines." They were to be taken only under the direction of a physician, and potential customers were urged to consult the family physician before writing to the sanitarium with an accurate description of their symptoms. For a $5 charge, one of the chief physicians would reply with directions for the use of the extracts. Of course, patients could still come to the sanitarium in person for the extract treatment.[11]

Now there were two Washington companies marketing the "Hammond extracts," which may account in part for the conflicting chemical analyses of the substances. The Columbia Chemical Company accused its competition of foul play. In response to a complaint from its lawyer, Hutchinson pointed out that the name of at least one extract preparation had been in common use for many years, while the names of all had been used by Hammond, in print, before the Columbia Chemical Company ever existed. In any case, as the substances were not patented, their names could not be copyrighted. "As the manufacture of the Animal Extracts is as free to the world as that of any other article of the Materia Medica," he declared, "the Hammond Sanitarium Company has begun to make them."[12] The Columbia Chemical Company took the case to court in June 1895. To Hammond's chagrin, the Supreme Court of the District of Columbia found in favor of the plaintiff, enjoining the Hammond Sanitarium Company from manufacturing the extracts for public sale.

The Hammond family attempted to circumvent this decision by forming a new "Hammond Animal Extract Company" under the name of Manfredi Lanza. For this Hammond's son-in-law was fined $10 for contempt of court, although citations against Hammond, Hutchinson, and the Sanitarium Company were discharged with costs.[13] Then Hammond made an effort at reconciliation with the Columbia Chemical Company. At issue was a final batch of extracts, about 80,000–100,000 bottles, with a retail value of close to a quarter of a million dollars. Hammond was unwilling to turn the material over to the company because "part of the organs from which they were made arrived in a frozen state and part were ruined by your own headstrong and ignorant act." He had already offered to absorb the actual loss (probably a matter of about $250) but had been turned down. Some of the material, said Hammond, had since been "made efficient," while the rest had been undergoing a reparative process when seized from him, and was consequently unfit for distribution. The scientist was now willing to resume preparation of the extracts, and to apply a new process that could shorten the preparation time from over a year to only three or four months.[14]

The scientist-entrepreneur also had serious difficulties with the Sanitarium Company. Its building had been mortgaged (mainly to Hammond himself) to pay Hammond the purchase price. Its financial affairs had since deteriorated – in Hammond's view, not by accident. In early October 1895 he sued his partner and Hutchinson's bankers, Riggs & Co., in the name of the Sanitarium Company. Hammond charged that the treasurer had stolen company funds, that he had closed the books to impede investigation, and that he had paid dividends to himself and his friends although taxes due had not been paid, nor the interest on Hammond's mortgage note, nor Hammond's salary. Hammond stated that Hutchinson had put up no bond and seemed to have neither property nor assets of his own, hardly a testimonial to the business acumen of the neurologist who had taken him on as a partner.[15]

In a countersuit filed the next day, Hutchinson retorted that the large liabilities of the company "cannot be further borne . . . unless better and more economical and prudent management is had in the administration of the affairs of said company," suggesting that the company was "at present insolvent" because of Hammond's intransigence. He found it impossible to continue to work with Hammond but was reluctant to resign as this would jeopardize the investments of himself and his friends. The Chicago-based board of directors sided with Hutchinson's request that the company be placed in receivership and asked the court to dismiss the suit brought by Hammond in the company's name. The motion for receivership was denied by the Washington court, and the sanitarium was auctioned off to meet the company's debts. Hammond bought it back and retook possession in his own name at the end of October. Hutchinson left, and all the directors except Hutchinson and Hammond resigned, leaving no quorum to transact business for the shell of a company. Hammond proceeded to run the establishment as he had in the past, "in receipt of a large and lucrative income."[16]

But that was not quite the end of the story. Hutchinson returned to Chicago and, claiming that Hammond had resigned as a director, proceeded to construct a new board. He then opened the "Central Offices of the Hammond Sanitarium Company" at Fourteenth Street and New York Avenue in Washington, only blocks from the actual sanitarium. To make matters worse, he publicized his establishment in the daily press with advertisements "quackish in character, violative of professional ethics," Hammond complained, and that "tend[ed] to cast reproach upon the standing of the plaintiff with the medical profession and the public." Hammond was in and out of court throughout January 1896 over the matter, and Hutchinson was finally enjoined from "advertising in such a way as to induce belief that he has connection with the plaintiff or the Hammond Sanitarium Company."[17]

Manfredi Lanza, who had probably handled many of Hammond's practical affairs, died in 1896. Apart from the personal tragedy this implied for Hammond's beloved daughter and his teenaged grandsons, it was a financial disaster as well. Heart problems were forcing the neurologist himself to cut back on his work. The depression of the mid-1890s was taking its toll. By 1897, Hammond was in serious financial trouble.

SCIENTIST AND ENTREPRENEUR

Hammond himself probably had little difficulty in reconciling the entrepreneurial and the scientific aspects of his role as a physician. For him, science and commerce were both inextricably linked to the progress that seemed to characterize modern America – and that simultaneously created the mental disturbances so central to his practice.[18] From its inception, his neurological practice was notorious for its businesslike and perhaps even mercenary character. Charles A. Dana recollected, for example, that "Hammond put neurology in New York on its feet economically by his amazing audacity of charging $10 as his fee and showing the bills on his table." Hammond was candid and outspoken on the question of professional remuneration. He insisted that the profession lost standing when its members treated patients for low fees or gratis, "especially when some public institution is concerned or some so-called charity with ample funds to pay good salaries to their whole staff except the medical portion."[19] Hammond apparently saw nothing wrong in endorsing other manufacturers' products as well as publicizing his own animal extracts in the popular press. His name appeared in advertisements for Comstock's Rational Food for Invalids, Infants and Dyspeptics, for Horsford's Acid Phosphate, for Aromatic Liquid Pepsin, and for something called "Mist-Niger."

But Hammond was wary of the possible repercussions to his reputation of indiscriminate advertising, recommending to the

New York Society of Medical Jurisprudence in 1887 that a committee be formed on personal rights. Its mission would be to investigate unauthorized use of physicians' signatures as endorsements of products.[20] He defended newspaper coverage of medical men and their accomplishments, and may have actively encouraged it. Accounts of the rejuvenating effects of his extracts appeared in papers from Haverhill, Massachusetts, to Columbus, Georgia. "Medical men have been charged with a reluctance to instruct the great mass of mankind in those truths which are capable of being understood and acted upon by all intelligent and moderately educated persons," he declared in 1866. "There is no doubt that if the great men of the profession had written more for the public than they have, quackery would not be so rampant and widespread as it is at the present."[21]

Nearly twenty-five years later, probably few were surprised by his article on "The Elixir of Life," a defense of animal extract research that appeared in the *North American Review.* "There are no impossibilities in nature," said Hammond, so "there is nothing inherently impossible in a so-called 'elixir of life.'" He saw nothing "unworthy in medical science in the search for such an agent."[22] He might have added that there was also nothing unworthy in physicians publicizing these facts and attempting to profit from them.

The increasing popularity of works such as Daniel A. Cathell's *The Physician Himself* and J. J. Taylor's *The Physician as Business Man* toward the end of the century suggests that Hammond's perspective on the enterprise of medicine was not unusual by then.[23] Yet some respectable physicians feared that their ancient and honorable calling was "rapidly being reduced to the level of a trade." George Shrady listed some of the temptations to "laxity of conduct": "the multitude of half-formed doctors . . . the fierceness of competition, the American passion for 'practical' and businesslike methods, the haste for success." He admonished the readers of the *Medical Record* that "the practice of medicine . . . is not, and . . . never can, by honest men, be carried on just as a trade would be."[24] Such physicians particularly deplored the successful campaign led by the New York City specialists around 1880 to reform or abolish the code of ethics of the New York State Medical Society. E. R. Squibb, for example, warned that by abrogating the code the profession would "[lower] itself from the rank of a profession to that of a trade, freed from any higher moral restraints than those of individual conviction, struggle and competition."

Squibb, a traditionalist, believed that "restrictive creeds and codes, whether in Church or State, do not obstruct progress, but are the bonds which hold society together." He considered them "the objects and results of organized civilization, and . . . the principal defenses of society against anarchy and communism."[25] But other physicians, including Hammond, saw the main danger to medicine as "trades-unionism" within the profession. Some linked this to the "cliquism" of the small coterie of New York physicians who effectively controlled the medical schools and hospitals. They invoked democratic values: all physicians were equal before the law, and therefore were proper associates in the consultations on which specialists thrived.

More emphatically they stressed freedom of choice and of trade. The main provisions of the "new code" and the logic of "no code" liberalized consultation procedures to allow specialists to accept referrals from homeopaths and to express their opinions of cases directly to the patients or their families, rather than to the attending family physician. "This entering wedge into what we may call the trades-union of the doctors of the old school," editorialized the *New York Times,* "may be fatal to the integrity and perpetuity of the existing order of things."[26] Hammond said of the "new code" that he thought it "illogical, absurd, sophistical, unsound, unwarranted, untenable, inconclusive, fallacious, evasive, irrelevant, heretical, unreasonable, unscientific, narrow-minded, visionary and futile." But, he added, the "old code" of the American Medical Association was worse, and no code would be any better.[27] He was outspoken in his denunciation of trade unions, the main theme of his 1887 novel *On the Susquehanna* and of his controversial article "On the Evolution of the Boycott."[28] Hammond also used the medium of fiction to support "free trade" in *A Strong-Minded Woman* (1885).

Hammond's own practice, most notably during his stormy later years in Washington, could serve as a graphic illustration of a very successful medical practice conducted along businesslike lines. While the energetic surgeon general of 1862 symbolized the advance of scientific medicine in America to many of Hammond's professional compatriots, the proprietor of the Hammond Sanitarium and the promoter of the Hammond Animal Extracts thirty-five years later may have seemed to many to epitomize the commercialism that was lowering the tone of a profession only barely beginning to emerge from ignorance and outright quackery. Ironically, Hammond himself was not a very good businessman. "Scheme after scheme . . . would arise in his mind, for he was optimistic almost to the verge of the visionary," recalled an associate, "but some defect that a more prudent man would have guarded against too often barred their fruition."[29]

Hammond's practice tapered off during the late 1890s, and the seventy-year-old physician suffered financial losses serious enough to jeopardize the high-toned life-style he had enjoyed for many years. In 1897 his attempts to delay payment of a promissory note led a New York attorney to ask the War Department whether a retired army officer, not collecting pay, could be charged with conduct unbecoming an officer and a gentleman.[30] Hammond's frame of mind at that time may have been reflected in a four-act play published only after his death, in which he dramatized the plight of a gentleman scientist, Mr. Coventry. The hero lives a secret life as the master of a gambling house in order to maintain the social position of his daughter, whose fortune has been lost, and to support his chemical studies. "I have enabled her to keep in the best social circles for our lineage, if backed by money, is entitled to entrance anywhere," Coventry confides to his friend Mr. Rowland.[31] Hammond's own fortune, like his scientific fame, had apparently declined as precipitously as it had risen. This must have pained him deeply.

Financial pressures led Hammond to approach Congress, through friends, seeking back pay for the years he had been excluded from the military service, or at least the pension due him as a retired officer. This he was never able to obtain, nor could his widow later – she pursued the issue at least until 1913 – in spite of strong committee recommendations and the backing of the American Medical Association.[32] The outbreak of the Spanish-American War offered Hammond a chance to recoup his fortunes – or so he thought. The seventy-year-old retired brigadier general wrote to President McKinley in March 1899 asking to be placed on active duty. "Latterly I have undergone great pecuniary losses," he confessed, and therefore needed his military pay. "There is a great deal of work in the way of medical and sanitary inspections and reports that I could perform with advantage to the service and without in the least conflicting with the Medical Department." He was promptly though politely refused. Since the war was almost over, Hammond was informed, the President did "not deem it expedient to employ retired officers."[33] Perhaps it was not only that the physician himself was a bit long of tooth; the same might have been said for some of his better-known medical doctrines as well.

Hammond seems to have lost interest in medical work as the end of the century drew near. For the first time in nearly fifty years his name was virtually absent from the pages of the nation's medical journals. He poured his literary energies instead into his last and most controversial novel, *The Son of Perdition* (1898), and then turned to the drama. But science was still a passion: Mr. Coventry, the hero of his four-act play *A Mysterious Life,* was a gentleman chemist, about to recoup his fortunes by inventing a powerful new explosive to be sold only to the United States government.

* * * * *

We can imagine how Hammond, ever the optimist and bon vivant, celebrated the coming of the new year of 1900. But on Friday, January 5, 1900, the portly physician bounded up the stairs of his elegant Washington home with characteristic disregard of his own physical limitations and immediately suffered a fatal heart attack. The cause of death was recorded as: "Primary, fatty degeneration and dilatation of the heart (some years); Immediate, sudden heart exhaustion from exertion (30 minutes)." A friend remembered that "his splendid physical endowments endured to the last, and a stranger might readily have taken him for a much younger man." He had been, another colleague declared, "one of the most attractive personalities and one of the most powerful and effective forces in American neurology." After a funeral ceremony three days later at the family residence, Brigadier General William A. Hammond, ret., was escorted to Arlington National Cemetery by a squadron of the Third U.S. Cavalry and its band, along with the Light Artillery Battery of the Washington Barracks.[34]

CONCLUSION

Hammond had scarcely been laid to rest before a professional friend reported that "since Dr. Hammond died the remark has more than once been made that he came very near being a great man." He had "committed errors, errors that a man of narrower intellect but greater worldly wisdom would be tolerably sure to avoid, and some of them led to cruel aspersions on his character." His creative imagination and ineradicable curiosity were among his greatest personal assets, but he lacked both patience and "inflexibility of purpose." He could be dogmatic and even intolerant, but was always intellectually honest, "an exceptionally fair man in argument, always ready to concede gracefully any point scored by an opponent."[35]

For Hammond there were virtually no limits to the power of the human intellect. "Man," he wrote in 1886, "may be excused for feeling some pride at having risen, though not by his own exertions, to the very summit of the organic scale." Hammond was sure that "man," as he put it, "is being developed into something better than he was originally or even than he was yesterday. . . . The forces that brought him up from a lower form are almost imperceptibly, but . . . with a power that is irresistible, carrying him to a higher one." But humanity was not merely a passive creation. "New forces that he himself has brought into action are adding their influence." Hammond predicted confidently "that the mind is destined as the brain advances in development to become infinitely more exalted than it is at this time." Science was even then proving the power of the human mind: "locked chambers full of knowledge will before long be opened to us."[36]

By the mid-1880s, enthusiasm for scientific medicine was no longer limited to a small cadre of exceptionally well educated physicians. But "scientific medicine" meant different things to different people. For some, it was virtually synonymous with laboratory work: the bacteriology of Robert Koch, perhaps, or the physiology of Michael Foster. But for others, like Hammond, it often meant clinical specialism. More than a simple division of labor, specialism meant the opportunity to collect cases of a particular type, to study and categorize them, to attempt to understand their natural history. It meant clinical experimentation (although so harsh a phrase could scarcely have been articulated) with therapeutics that might help to elucidate underlying pathology, often of a functional sort. And as laboratories were equipped with increasingly sophisticated apparatus, so too would the scientific medicine of the specialists rely heavily on hardware and metaphors drawn from the physical sciences and technology. To be sure, the limitations of this sort of medical science were readily apparent even at the time. But then so, too, were those of the laboratory. It was only in Hammond's last years that scientific medicine (in any sense) even began to impinge significantly on the therapeutic experiences of most doctors and patients.

The dramatic rise of Hammond's neurological practice and its distressing decline thirty years later coincide with the turning points of industrial capitalism in the United States. If the Civil War accelerated economic and social developments already in progress at mid-century, opening the door for the "takeoff" of the late 1860s, it did the same for Hammond's career. His brash entrepreneurial style was certainly consistent with that of the captains of industry with whom he mingled in New York society, though his high-toned science and respectable antecedents made him acceptable to those of longer-established fortunes as well. The 1890s marked the transformation of the national economy into one of finance capitalism, with the banker and the corporation supplanting the individual entrepreneur. But the individualistic Hammond and his neurological practice, which depended crucially on his personal authority, were scarcely suited to the corporate style, quite apart from his glaring inability to manage the money he amassed.

The neurologist was not literally an industrial capitalist, of course. While his career was built in a sense on his patients' misfortunes, he certainly did not exploit them as a railroad baron did his workers. But to a certain extent – suggested by his industrial metaphor for mind and brain – he may well have thought like one. Let me suggest a way in which this may have helped to shape his commitment to clinical medicine as a vehicle for science. For Hammond the entrepreneur, money was to be gotten by the transformation and sale of material goods (in particular, his extracts). For Hammond the scientist, new knowledge was to be gotten from the practical work of medicine. In both cases, the relation between the concrete or particular (commodities and patients) and the abstract or general (money and science) was clear. For the financier, in contrast, money seems to come not from production, but from other money. And for a laboratory scientist working within a relatively autonomous scientific community, new results often seem to come not from medical practice but from previous abstract science. In these cases, the relations to production or to the practice of medicine are indirect or obscured. Hammond's mode of thought, I argue, was consistently closer to that of the industrial capitalist than to that of the financier. In this sense, as in his inability to transcend the pathological and therapeutical reasoning of mid-century American medicine, he was unprepared for the epic changes of the last decades of the century.

The medical world has changed so much in the last hundred years that William Alexander Hammond, M.D., one of the best-known American physicians of his time, has been all but forgotten. Twentieth-century historians have credited him with only a few narrowly circumscribed achievements. He has been enshrined in the annals of military medicine as the efficient and energetic surgeon general whose progressive ideas and administrative talents served his country well during the Civil War. He has been mentioned, less frequently, as a patriarch of American neurology, primarily for his role as an institution builder. A few recognize his name as an eponym for athetosis. But as a scientist? No, not even as a second-rate one. Yet it was the quest for science – especially a science of brain, of mind, even of society – that motivated Hammond's entire medical career. And the informal networks he helped to form, especially those built around his preceptor William Van Buren and his young scientific friends in Philadelphia, made this career possible.

As things turned out, Hammond's particular efforts made little lasting mark on what became the institutional and intellectual traditions of scientific research in medicine. As an institution, medical science found a home in medical schools and, eventually, research institutes and hospitals, rather than within Hammond's framework of private consulting practices, specialty societies, and post-graduate schools. A laboratory rather than a clinical orientation came to dominate the American medical research tradition. Hammond's scientific work had already, by the end of his life, come to be seen not so much as mistaken as beside the point.

Part of the reason for this can be found in the way Hammond interacted with his material. His scientific outlook was bolstered by a firm philosophical commitment to materialism and the quest for a naturalistic explanation of even the most mysterious of phenomena. But it was undermined by a pervading mechanistic philosophy and a persistent adherence to aspects of traditional medical thought: his was a reductionist rather than a dialectical materialism. Science was, for him, the search for a key that would unlock chambers of knowledge, or a magic bullet against ignorance. The language of positivism was for him not simply a rhetorical device but an expression of a deeply held attitude. In a sense Hammond was impatient not only with other people but with the natural world at large. In the few instances in which his sort of work did eventually "pay off," as in his approach to localization of brain function, his own efforts were not sustained enough to break through to important results.

To grant Hammond recognition as a scientist is to question why the paths he followed – if only a short way – were not those found on modern maps of scientific discovery. It is to ask ourselves how those maps were created, and by whom, and why. Scientists (to paraphrase a famous quotation) make their own history, but they do not make it just as they please, under circumstances of their own choosing. William Alexander Hammond preserved his love for science, and the altars of expediency on which he felt compelled to sacrifice tell us a great deal about the social context of late nineteenth-century American medicine.

Notes

1 . INTRODUCTION

1   William A. Hammond (hereafter WAH), "The Proper Use of the Mind," *Quart. Jour. of Psych. Med. and Med. Jur.* 2 (1868): 137.
2   Robert E. Kohler, *From Medical Chemistry to Biochemistry: The Making of a Biomedical Discipline* (Cambridge, England, 1982), p. 324.
3   W. Bruce Fye, *The Development of American Physiology: Scientific Medicine in the Nineteenth Century* (Baltimore and London, 1987).
4   Quoted in W. Bruce Fye, "Growth of American Physiology 1850–1900," in *Physiology in the American Context 1850–1940*, ed. Gerald L. Geison (Bethesda, Md., 1987), p. 53.
5   William Henry Egle, "History of the County of Dauphin," in *History of the Counties of Dauphin and Lebanon in the Commonwealth of Pennsylvania* (Philadelphia, 1883; reprint 1977), p. 100. See also Roland Hammond, *A History and Genealogy of the Descendants of William Hammond and his Wife Elizabeth Penn, 1600–1894* (Boston, 1894); and Blanche T. Hartman, *A Genealogy of the Nesbit, Ross, Porter, Taggart Families of Pennsylvania* (Pittsburgh, 1929).
6   Egle, "History of the County of Dauphin" (see n. 5), p. 530.
7   For the context of Hammond's medical training and preparation, see William F. Norwood, *Medical Education in the United States Before the Civil War* (Philadelphia, 1944); and Kenneth M. Ludmerer, *Learning to Heal. The Development of American Medical Education* (New York, 1985).
8   WAH, "Stammering. A Few Practical Remarks, Showing How Self-Treatment May Be Employed," *The Voice* 1 (1879):31.
9   William Holme Van Buren, "[Account Book of Payments of Patients . . .] 1844–50," Rare Book Room, New York Academy of Medicine, New York City. See also William Quentin Maxwell, *Lincoln's Fifth Wheel* (New York, 1956), p. 348, and an obituary notice of Van Buren in *Med. Rec.* 23 (1883):361.
10 University of the City of New York, Medical Department, *Annual Announcement of Lectures*, sessions 1846–47 (esp. p. 10) and 1848–49 (esp. p. 5). See also the *Catalogue of the Graduates and Officers of the Medical Department of the University of the City of New York* ([New York], 1872).
11 Martyn Paine, *A Lecture, Introductory to a Course on the Institutes of Medicine and Materia Medica, for the Session of MDCCCXLVII–VIII* (New York, 1847), p. 12.
12 See Owsei Temkin, "Materialism in French and German Physiology of the Early Nineteenth Century," *Bull. Hist. Med.* 20 (1946):322–27.
13 Paul Cranefield, "The Organic Physics of 1847 and the Biophysics of Today," *Jour. Hist. Med. & All. Sci.* 12 (1957):407–23.
14 John William Draper, *Introductory Lecture to the Course of Chemistry . . . Session MDCCCXLI–XLII* (New York, 1841), esp. pp. 9–11. See also J. J. Walsh, *History of Medicine in New York* (New York, 1919), 5:413ff.
15 Martyn Paine, *A Lecture on the Improvement of Medical Education in the United States* (New York, 1843; reprinted from *N.Y. Jour. Med. & Coll. Sci.*, November 1843), p. 5.
16 Martyn Paine: *A Lecture on the Physiology of Digestion*, 4th ed. (New York, 1844); *Discourse Introductory to a Course of Lectures on the Institutes of Medicine and Materia Medica . . . Session of 1841–42* (Boston, 1842); and other papers collected in *Medical and Physiological Commentaries* (New York, 1841–44).

17 See Edwin Clarke and L. S. Jacyna, *Nineteenth-Century Origins of Neuroscientific Concepts* (Berkeley and Los Angeles and London, 1987), pp. 2–4.
18 Ibid., pp. 318–32.
19 See, for example, Martyn Paine, *Discourse on the Soul and Instinct, Physiologically Distinguished from Materialism* (New York, 1849); WAH, "On Instinct: Its Nature and Seat," *Quart. Jour. Psych. Med.* 1 (1867):1–26; and WAH, "The Seat of Instinct," *Am. Jour. Neur. & Psychiat.* 1 (1882):607–15.
20 Thomas G. Morton, *The History of the Pennsylvania Hospital, 1751–1895* (Philadelphia, 1895), pp. 507–10; G. W. Norris, *Introductory Lecture to the Course of Clinical Instruction in Surgery, at the Pennsylvania Hospital, Delivered November 1st, 1848* (Philadelphia, 1848).
21 Charles E. Rosenberg, *The Care of Strangers: The Rise of America's Hospital System* (New York, 1987), pp. 62–66.
22 William Johnston to President Taylor, 8 March 1849, in file of William A. Hammond, "Personal Papers of Medical Officers," Record Group 94/E-561, National Archives, Washington, D.C.; U.S. Census of 1850. New Mexico. Valencia County. Town of Cebolleta. William and Helen's baby daughter Helen was listed as eight months of age when the census was taken on 9 October 1850.
23 The interview was reprinted in "Justice to Surgeon-Gen. W. A. Hammond," *St. Louis Clin. Rec.* 6 (1879–80):177–78.
24 Notarized statements of J. H. Douglas, 11 August 1879, and J. B. Lippincott, 7 August 1879; and WAH to Hon. G. W. McCrary, 14 August 1879, Box 577, Record Group 94, National Archives.
25 On Hammond's role in establishing *Nation* see Frederick Law Olmsted to Henry W. Bellows, 28 July 1863, in *The Papers of Frederick Law Olmsted*, ed. Jane Turner Censer (Baltimore and London, 1986), 4:681. See also [WAH]: "The Humors of the Anthropologists," *Nation* 1 (1865):141–43; "Poisoning as a Science," *Nation* 1 (1865):242–43; "A Few Words About Cholera," *Nation* 1 (1865):306–8; and "Slaughterhouses and Health," *Nation* 3 (1866):273–74. He also wrote for the magazine *Round Table;* see "Justice to Hammond" (see n. 23).
26 "Justice to Hammond" (see n. 23).
27 George Rosen, *The Structure of American Medical Practice 1875–1941*, ed. Charles E. Rosenberg (Philadelphia, 1983), p. 35.
28 See the *Medical Register of the City of New York for the Year Commencing June 1, 1865* (New York, 1865), and subsequent editions.
29 Bonnie Ellen Blustein, "Neurology in New York: A Case Study in the Specialization of Medicine," *Bull. Hist. Med.* 53 (1979):170–83.
30 C. K. Mills, "Some Recollections of the Early Meetings and Personnel of the American Neurological Association," in the *Semicentennial Anniversary Volume of the American Neurological Association* (New York, 1924), pp. 16–46, esp. p. 20; James Herbert Morse, *Diary*, 6:90 (30 January 1883), New-York Historical Society.
31 Citizen's Committee (New York City), *Report . . . Upon the Nuisances of New York City: The Air We Breathe* (New York, 1878), esp. pp. 14–15; see also WAH, "Slaughterhouses and Health" (see n. 25); and WAH, *A Strong-Minded Woman* (New York, 1886).
32 "Sanitary Legislation," *Med. Gaz.* 4 (1870):78–79; "Health Officer of the Port," *Hosp. Gaz. & Arch. Clin. Surg.* 3 (1878):70–73.
33 Morse, *Diary* (see n. 30), 6:92 (30 January 1883).
34 WAH: "Sumptuary Laws and Their Social Influence," *Pop. Sci. Monthly* 37 (1890):33–40; "The Mischievous Ice Pitcher," *N. Am. Rev.* 148 (1889):738–42; and *Mr. Oldmixon* (New York, 1885). See also D. B. St. John Roosa, "Hammond, the Man," *Post-Graduate* 15 (1900):596, 599–600; and Morse, *Diary* (see n. 30), 6:92 (30 January 1883).
35 Mills, "Some Recollections" (see n. 30), p. 20; J. G. Hopkins, "A Spicy Letter, in Which a Georgia Doctor Tells What He Knows About Dr. Wm. A. Hammond," *Atlanta Med. & Surg. Jour.*, n.s., 1 (1884): 413–16.

36 WAH to Walter Atlee, 20 May 1888, Mayo Clinic Library, Rochester, Minn.
37 Edwin G. Zabriskie, "Graeme Monroe Hammond, M.D., 1858–1944," *Jour. Nerv. & Ment. Dis* 101 (1945):196–97; the biographical sketch in the *Semicentennial Anniversary Volume* (see n. 30), pp. 85–86; and the obituary notice in the *New York Times,* 31 October 1944, p. 19, col. 1. See also WAH, "Brains and Muscles: Their Relative Training and Development," *Union College Practical Lectures* (Butterfield Course) (New York, 1895), 1:277–78.
38 "Marriage in High Life: Fashionable Wedding at St. Thomas' Church – An Italian Marquis Marries an American Lady," *New York Times,* 11 May 1877, p. 8, col. 4; Morse, *Diary* (see n. 30); and the obituary of Clara Hammond Lanza in the *New York Times,* 15 July 1939, p. 15, col. 6. See also Clara Lanza, *Mr. Perkin's Daughter* (New York, 1881), esp. chap. 15.
39 [Frank P. Foster], "William A. Hammond, M.D., LL.D.," *N.Y. Med. Jour.* 71 (1900):64.

2. "I CAN MAKE ANY POST INTERESTING"

1   On the significance of French military medicine, see Erwin Ackerknecht, *Medicine at the Paris Hospital* (Baltimore, 1967), pp. 25–26, 141–43. See also Fielding Garrison, *History of Medicine,* 2d. ed. (Philadelphia, 1917), pp. 496–97. On Hammond's library use see the Library Register, 1842–58, Archives of the Pennsylvania Hospital, Philadelphia.
2   Harvey E. Brown, *The Medical Department of the United States Army from 1775 to 1873* (Washington, D.C., 1873), pp. 199–201.
3   Avram B. Bender, "Government Explorations in the Territory of New Mexico 1846–59," *New Mexico Historical Review* 9 (1934):1–32; Col. George Archibald McCall, *New Mexico in 1850: A Military View,* ed. Robert W. Frazer (Norman, Okla., 1968).
4   Hammond's successive assignments to different military stations can be traced through his file in "Personal Papers of Medical Officers," Record Group 94/E-561, National Archives, Washington, D.C. Information about Cebolleta, Laguna, and Fort Webster, N. Mex., can be found in Record Group 94/63 (Returns of Military Posts, filed alphabetically), available as Microcopy 617, National Archives. See also Record Group 112 (Records of the Surgeon-General's Office), Register of Letters Received, 1822–89.
5   WAH, "Brains and Muscles: Their Relative Training and Development," *Union College Practical Lectures* (Butterfield Course) (New York, 1895), 1:274.
6   McCall, *New Mexico* (see n. 3), pp. 158–60.
7   See WAH, "The American Soldier and Venereal Diseases," *N.Y. Med. Jour.* 70 (1899):181.
8   McCall, *New Mexico* (see n. 3), pp. 160–61.
9   WAH, "Observations on the Use of Potash in the Treatment of Scurvy," *Am. Jour. Med. Sci.,* n.s., 25 (1853):102–5.
10 Alfred B. Garrod, "On the Nature, Cause, and Prevention of Scurvy," *Monthly Jour. Med. Sci.,* n.s., 2 (1848):457–64. The excerpt cited by Hammond appeared in the *Am. Jour. Med. Sci.,* n.s., 16 (1848):200–3.
11 WAH, "Potash in the Treatment of Scurvy" (see n. 9), p. 103.
12 Ibid., p. 102.
13 WAH, ed., "Scurvy," in *Military Medical and Surgical Essays* (Philadelphia, 1864), pp. 175–206, esp. pp. 188–89, 193ff.
14 WAH: "The Disease of the Scythians (Morbus feminarum) and Certain Analogous Conditions," *Am. Jour. Neur. Psychiatry* 1 (1882):339–55; "The Disease of the Scythians and Certain Analogous Conditions," *Alienist and Neurologist* 4 (1883):168–69, and "The Disease of the Scythians (morbus feminarum) and Certain Analogous Conditions," *Jour. Nervous and Mental Dis.* 9 (1882):557–59. On the context of this work, see J. S. Haller and R. M. Haller, *The Physician and Sexuality in Victorian America* (Urbana, Ill., 1974); and P. L. Tylor, "'Denied the

Power to Choose the Good': Sexuality and Mental Defect in American Medical Practice, 1850–1920," *Jour. Soc. Hist.* 10 (1977):472–898.

15 Kennerly Diary, 12 November [1853], Manuscript Division, Library of Congress.

16 WAH to John L. LeConte, 5 July 1856 and 4 May 1860, the John L. LeConte Papers, American Philosophical Society, Philadelphia; WAH to Thomas Lawson, 10 February and 27 June 1852, "Personal Papers" (see n. 4).

17 Quoted in W. Bruce Fye, *The Development of American Physiology: Scientific Medicine in the Nineteenth Century* (Baltimore and London, 1987), pp. 23, 58.

18 WAH to Thomas Lawson, 18 June 1853, "Personal Papers," "Returns of Fort Meade," and "Returns of Posts" (see n. 4).

19 William F. Barry to S. Thomas, 10 June 1853, and endorsement [to Surgeon General Lawson?] on letter, A. J. Cook to WAH (copy), 20 June 1853, both filed with Hammond's "Personal Papers" (see n. 4).

20 WAH, "Statement of Asst. Surgeon Wm. A. Hammond U.S.A., as Made to the Army Medical Board, Philadelphia, Pa., April 19, 1859," and Richard H. Coolidge to General Thomas Lawson, 20 October 1857, in "Personal Papers" (see n. 4).

21 The symptoms described are consistent with DaCosta's syndrome, more recently designated the mitral valve prolapse syndrome. See Charles F. Wooley, "Where are the Diseases of Yesteryear?" *Circulation* 53 (1976):749–51.

22 WAH to Surgeon General Thomas Lawson, 18 and 26 October 1853, "Personal Papers" (see n. 4).

23 See WAH, "On Certain Dumb-Bell Forms of Crystals Found in the Urine," *Am. Jour. Med. Sci.*, n.s., 27 (1854):384–87.

24 WAH to Thomas Lawson, 15 January and 7 February 1854, "Personal Papers" (see n. 4).

25 George S. Park, "Notes of a Trip Up Kansas River," *Kansas Herald of Freedom*, 21 October 1854; reprinted in Louise Barry, *The Beginning of the West: Annals of the Kansas Gateway to the American West* (Topeka, 1972), p. 1228; WAH to John L. LeConte, 25 July 1854, LeConte Papers (see n. 16).

26 WAH to John L. LeConte, 1 February 1855, LeConte Papers (see n. 16).

27 See James C. Malin, *The Nebraska Question, 1852–54* (Lawrence, Kans., 1953).

28 Russell K. Hickman, "The Reeder Administration Inaugurated," *Kans. Hist. Quart.* 36 (1970):327; WAH to John L. LeConte, 1 February 1855, LeConte Papers (see n. 16).

29 WAH to Leidy, 18 June 1855, MS. Coll. 1, the Joseph Leidy Papers, Academy of Natural Sciences of Philadelphia.

30 See the following articles in the *Kansas Historical Collections:* James R. McClure, "Taking the Census and Other incidents in 1855," 8 (1903–4):230–33; "Kansas Experiences of Lemuel Knapp," 1–2 (1875–80):206–9; George V. Martin, "The Territorial and Military Combine and Fort Riley," 7 (1901–2):306–13. See also *Papers Relative to the Proceedings of Court Martial in the Case of Brevet Lieut. Col. Wm. R. Montgomery* (Philadelphia, 1858); and Russell K. Hickman, "The Reeder Administration" (see n. 28).

31 WAH to John L. LeConte, 29 June 1856, LeConte Papers (see n. 16).

32 Ibid.

33 WAH, "Recollections of Gen. Nathaniel Lyon," *Annals of Iowa*, 3d ser., 4 (1899–1901): 415–36; cf. WAH, "Brigadier General Nathaniel Lyon, U.S.A.: Personal Recollections," *Mag. of Am. Hist.* 13 (1885):237–48.

34 WAH, "Recollections of Gen. Nathaniel Lyon" (see n. 33), p. 433; WAH to John L. LeConte, 25 July 1854, LeConte Papers (see n. 16).

35 WAH, "Recollections of Gen. Nathaniel Lyon" (see n. 33), p. 433. See also Edward J. Pfeifer, "The Genesis of American Neo-Lamarckism," *Isis* 56 (1965):156–67; and George Stocking, "Lamarckianism in American Social Science, 1890–1915," in *Race, Culture and Evolution*, ed. George Stocking (New York, 1968), pp. 236–69.

36 See William H. Goetzmann, *Exploration and Empire: The Explorer and the Scientist in the Winning of the American West* (New York, 1966), esp. p. 232ff.

37 Ibid. See also George M. Daniels, "The Process of Professionalization in American Science: The Emergent Period, 1820–60," *Isis* 58 (1967): 151–66.

38 Edgar Erskine Hume, *Ornithologists of the United States Army Medical Corps* (Baltimore, 1942), esp. pp. 2–5.

39 Ibid., p. 550.

40 Kennerly Diary (see n. 15), 29 June and 5 August [1853].

41 Goetzmann, *Exploration and Empire* (see n. 36), p. 231.

42 WAH to John L. LeConte, 25 July 1854, LeConte Papers (see n. 16).

43 Hammond's contributions are listed in the reports of "Donations to Museum and Library," published in the *Proceedings* of the Academy for the years 1855–57. See for example the report of the Curator (Joseph Leidy) for 1857, *Proceedings* 9 (1857):224–26; and Edward Hallowell, "Description of Several New North American Reptiles," *Proceedings* 9 (1857):215–216. See also WAH to John L. LeConte, 18 January 1857, LeConte Papers (see n. 16).

44 WAH to Joseph Leidy, 22 October 1854, 18 June 1855, 7 September, 15 November and 28 December 1856, and 22 March 1857, Leidy Papers (see n. 29); WAH to John L. LeConte, 25 July 1854, 29 June 1856, LeConte Papers (see n. 16).

45 WAH to Joseph Leidy, 15 November and 28 December 1856, Leidy Papers (see n. 29). See also official report dated 23 August 1855, Ft. Kearney, Nebraska Territory, Record Group 94-E561, National Archives.

46 WAH to John L. LeConte, 25 July 1854, 1 February 1855, 29 June and 5 July 1856, LeConte Papers (see n. 16).

47 *Proceedings of the Academy of Natural Sciences of Philadelphia* 9 (1857):183; WAH to Leidy, 28 December 1856, Leidy Correspondence (see n. 29); WAH to LeConte, 23 February 1857, LeConte Papers (see n. 16).

48 WAH to John L. LeConte, 23 February 1857, LeConte Papers (n. 16).

3. "THE FIRST ORIGINAL PHYSIOLOGIST IN THE UNITED STATES"

1 WAH, "The Relations Existing between Urea and Uric Acid," *Am. Jour. Med. Sci.*, n.s., 29 (1855):119–123.

2 A list of members of the *Verein* in October 1857 (including such luminaries as Rudolf Virchow) can be found in its *Correspondenzblatt* 30 (1857):461–64; on its plan and aims, see Julius Vogel, "Was wir wollen," *Arch. f. Wiss. Heilk.* 1 (1854):1–15. Hammond's papers appear in translation in *Arch. f. Wiss. Heilk.* 2 (1858):590–608; and 4 (1860):99–122.

3 See Henry M. Madden, *Xántus: Hungarian Naturalist in the Pioneer West* (Linz, 1949); and William H. Goetzmann, *Exploration and Empire: The Explorer and the Scientist in the Winning of the American West* (New York, 1966).

4 WAH to John L. LeConte, 25 July 1854 and 1 February 1855, the John L. Le-Conte Papers, American Philosophical Society, Philadelphia; WAH to Joseph Leidy, 22 October 1854, the Joseph Leidy Papers, Academy of Natural Sciences of Philadelphia; WAH, "Relations Existing" (see n. 1).

5 WAH to Surgeon General Thomas Lawson, 20 February 1856, "Personal Papers of Medical Officers," Record Group 94/E-561, National Archives, Washington, D.C.

6 Harvey E. Brown, *The Medical Department of the United States Army from 1775 to 1873* (Washington, D.C., 1873); WAH to LeConte, 29 June 1856, LeConte Papers (see n. 4); WAH to Leidy, 15 November 1856, Leidy Papers (see n. 4).

7 WAH, "Urological Contributions," *Am. Jour. Med. Sci.*, n.s., 31 (1856):330–37.

8 James C. Whorton, "'Tempest in a Flesh-pot': The Formulation of a Physiological Rationale for Vegetarianism," *J. Hist. Med.* 32 (1977):115–39; and R. H. Shryock, "Sylvester Graham and the Popular Health Movement, 1830–70," in *Medicine in America: Historical Essays*, ed. R. H. Shryock (Baltimore, 1966), pp. 111–25.

9 WAH to John LeConte, 29 June 1856, LeConte Papers (see n. 4); WAH, "Urological Contributions" (see n. 7), p. 337; WAH, "The Physiological Effects of Alcohol and Tobacco upon the Human System," *Am. Jour. Med. Sci.*, n.s., 32 (1856):314.

10 WAH, "The Sanitary and Physiological Relations of Tobacco," *North Am. Rev.* 108 (1869):514–15. See also WAH, "Sumptuary Laws and Their Social Influence," *Pop. Sci. Monthly* 37 (1890):33–40.

11 WAH, "Brains and Muscles: Their Relative Training and Development," Union College Practical Lectures (Butterfield Course) (New York, 1895), 1:270–73.

12 WAH, "On Some of the Effects of Excessive Intellectual Exertion," *Bellevue & Charity Hosp. Reports* (New York, 1870), pp. 379–89.

13 WAH to LeConte, 29 June and 24 August 1856, LeConte Papers (see n. 4); WAH to Leidy, 7 September and 15 November 1856 and 22 March 1857, Leidy Papers (see n. 4).

14 WAH, *Experimental Researches Relative to the Nutritive Value and Physiological Effects of Albumen, Starch, and Gum, When Singly and Exclusively Used as Food* (Philadelphia, 1857), p. 12.

15 WAH, *A Treatise on Hygiene, With Special Reference to the Military Service* (Philadelphia, 1863), pp. 50–51, 55.

16 WAH, *Experimental Researches* (see n. 14), pp. 8–9, 13–17; WAH to LeConte, 18 January 1857, LeConte Papers (see n. 4).

17 WAH, *Experimental Researches* (see n. 14), passim.

18 WAH to LeConte, 23 February 1857, LeConte Papers (see n. 4); WAH to Leidy, 22 March 1857, Leidy Papers (see n. 4).

19 WAH to Leidy, 23 March 1857, Leidy Papers (see n. 4).

20 See, for example, S. W. Mitchell, "Report on the Progress of Physiology and Anatomy," *N. Am. Med.-Chir. Rev.* 2 (1858):126–28.

21 WAH, *Experimental Researches* (see n. 14), p. 70.

22 WAH to Surgeon General Lawson, 5 April 1857, "Personal Papers" (see n. 5).

23 Richard H. Coolidge to Surgeon General Lawson, endorsement to letter, WAH to Lawson, 5 April 1857, "Personal Papers" (see n. 5). The chloroform case is described in WAH, "Fatty Degeneration of the Heart – Death from the Inhalation of the Tincture of Chloroform," *Am. Jour. Med. Sci.*, n.s., 36 (1858):41–44.

24 WAH, "On the Injection of Urea and Other Substances into the Blood," *N. Am. Med.-Chir. Rev.* 2 (1858):287–93; and WAH, "On Uraemic Intoxication," *Am. Jour. Med. Sci.*, n.s., 41 (1861):55–83, summarized as "Uraemic Intoxication," *Am. Med. Times* 2 (1861):214. Both papers are reprinted in WAH, *Physiological Memoirs* (Philadelphia, 1863).

25 See Fielding M. Garrison, *History of Medicine*, 2d ed. (Philadelphia, 1917), pp. 654–56.

26 WAH, "Brigadier-General Nathaniel Lyon, U.S.A.: Personal Recollections," *Annals of Iowa*, 3d ser., 4 (1899–1901):415–36; WAH, "Statement of Asst. Surgeon Wm. A. Hammond U.S.A., as Made to the Army Medical Board, Philadelphia, Pa., April 19, 1859," in "Personal Papers" (see n. 5).

27 WAH to Lawson, 13 September 1857, "Personal Papers" (see n. 5).

28 J. Cheston Morris to Mrs. Hunt, 8 January 1897, and J. Cheston Morris to Joseph Leidy II, 24 February 1909, in Joseph Leidy II Papers, College of Physicians of Philadelphia.

29 Bonnie Ellen Blustein, "The Philadelphia Biological Society, 1857–61: A Failed Experiment?" *Jour. Hist. Med.* 35 (1980):188–202.

30 Minutes of the Biological and Microscopical Department, MS. Coll. 295, Academy of Natural Sciences of Philadelphia.

31 Some of the discussions are reported in the published *Proceedings* of the Academy as well as in the manuscript minutes. See also WAH, "Observations on the Colourless Blood-Corpuscles," *Am. Jour. Med. Sci.*, n.s., 37 (1859):348–50.

32 Minutes of the Biological and Microscopical Department (see n. 30); WAH and S. Weir Mitchell, "Experimental Researches Relative to Corroval and Vao, Two

New Varieties of Woorara, the South American Arrow Poison," *Am. Jour. Med. Sci.*, n.s., 38 (1859):13–60; and WAH, "On the Physical and Chemical Characteristics of Corroval and Vao," in *Physiological Memoirs* (see n. 24), pp. 261–70.

33 WAH and S. Weir Mitchell, "An Experimental Examination of the Toxicological Effects of Sassy Bark, the Ordeal Poison of the Western Coast of Africa," *Charleston Med. Jour. & Rev.* 14 (1859):721–40.

34 WAH to Surgeon General Thomas Lawson, 24 August 1859, "Personal Papers" (see n. 5).

35 WAH, "Experimental Researches Relative to a Supposed New Species of Upas," *Am. Jour. Med. Sci.*, n.s., 40 (1860):363–77.

36 Editorial note, *Charleston Med. Jour. & Rev.* 15 (1860):426.

37 Quoted in E. F. Cordell, *Historical Sketch of the University of Maryland School of Medicine (1807–90)* (Baltimore, 1891), pp. 115, 119–21, 131. See also *The Medical Annals of Maryland, 1799–1899* (Baltimore, 1903), pp. 426, 706.

38 WAH: "A Clinical Lecture on Scirrus, or Hard Cancer," *Maryland and Virginia Med. Jour.* 15 (1860):349–55; "A Course of Lectures on Chancre, Delivered at the Baltimore Infirmary," *Am. Med. Times* 3 (1861):1–3, 17–19, 33–35, 49–51, 65–67; *Lectures on Venereal Diseases* (Philadelphia, 1864); and "The American Soldier and Venereal Diseases," *N.Y. Med. Jour.* 70 (1899):181–87.

39 See WAH, *Physiological Memoirs* (see n. 24); also Constantin Paul, "Influence of Slow Saturnine Intoxication on the Products of Conception," ed. and trans from articles in the *Arch. Gén. de Méd.* and *Ann. d'Hygiène Publ.* by W. A. H., *Balt. Jour. Med.* 1 (1861):136–38; W. A. H., "Researches on Fermentation and Putrefaction, by G. M. Van der Broek," summarized from the *Jour. de Pharm.*, in *Balt. Jour. Med.* 1 (1861):138–39; and W. A. H., "Method of Distinguishing Spots of Blood on an Instrument Coated with Rust. By MM. Lesseur and Robin," summarized from the *Jour. de Pharm. et Ther.*, in *Balt. Jour. Med.* 1 (1861):139.

40 WAH, "Nitric Acid in Intermittent Fever," *Maryland and Virginia Med. Jour.*, n.s., 16 (1861):104–6. Cf. *Am. Jour. Med. Sci.*, n.s., 41 (1861):606–7.

41 Cited in "Appointments of Professors in the University of Maryland," *Maryland and Virginia Med. Jour.* 14 (1860):430.

42 C.-E. Brown-Séquard to S. Weir Mitchell, 20 July 1861, Mitchell Papers, Duke University Medical Center Library.

4. "THE BEST FRIEND THE SOLDIER HAS"

1 WAH to Surgeon General Thomas Lawson, 10 and 18 May 1861, in "Personal Papers of Medical Officers," File E561, National Archives, Washington, D.C.; and Lewis H. Steiner to Hon. G. W. McCrary, 7 July 1879, Box 577, Record Group 94, National Archives, Washington, D.C.

2 WAH to Hon. S. C. Pomeroy, 4 July and 7 August 1861, "Personal Papers" (see n. 1).

3 See WAH to Surgeon General Lawson, 14 and 28 October and 8 November 1861; and R. S. Satterlee to Surgeon General Lawson, 13, 19, 20, and 26 June 1861, listed in Index of Letters Received, vol. 13, Records of the Surgeon General's Office, National Archives, Washington, D.C.

4 See W. Q. Maxwell, *Lincoln's Fifth Wheel: The Political History of the U.S. Sanitary Commission* (New York: Longman's, 1956); George M. Fredrickson, *The Inner Civil War: Northern Intellectuals and the Crisis of the Union* (New York, 1965), pp. 99–105; and Bonnie Ellen Blustein, "'To Increase the Efficiency of the U.S. Army': A New Approach to Medicine in the U.S. Civil War," *Civil War History* 33 (1987):22–41.

5 Cited in Jane Turner Censer, ed., *The Papers of Frederick Law Olmsted. Defending the Union* (Baltimore, 1986), 4:312.

6 George Templeton Strong, *Diary*, ed. Allan Nevins and Milton H. Thomas (New York, 1952), 3:185 (13 October 1861).

7   Strong, *Diary* (see n. 6), 3:187 (23 October 1861); see also Maxwell, *Lincoln's Fifth Wheel* (see n. 4), p. 100.

8   See Erwin S. Bradley, *Simon Cameron, Lincoln's Secretary of War: A Political Biography* (Philadelphia, 1966).

9   Richard S. Satterlee to Surgeon General Finley, 15 January, 10 February, and 17 March 1862, Index of Letters Received (see n. 3), Vol. 14; WAH to Surgeon General Finley, 28 February 1862, "Personal Papers" (see n. 1).

10 WAH, "Two Reports on the Condition of Military Hospitals at Grafton, Va., and Cumberland, Md. (Sanitary Commission Document #41)," in *Documents of the U.S. Sanitary Commission* (New York, 1866), 1:3, 14, 16, 29, and passim.

11 See Charles E. Rosenberg, *The Care of Strangers: The Rise of America's Hospital System* (New York, 1987), p. 136.

12 See Blustein, "'To Increase the Efficiency'" (see n. 4).

13 Frederick Law Olmsted to John Olmsted, 19 April 1862, in *Papers of Frederick Law Olmsted* (see n. 5), 4:310.

14 Wolcott Gibbs to John L. LeConte, 7 March 1862, and WAH to John L. LeConte, 11 April 1861 [*sic* – 1862], the John L. LeConte Papers, American Philosophical Society, Philadelphia.

15 Robert King Stone to President Abraham Lincoln, 21 April 1862, photocopy in Autograph Case, College of Physicians of Philadelphia.

16 Editorial, *Am. Med. Times* 4 (1862):239; "The New Surgeon General," *Philadelphia Inquirer,* 24 April 1862, p. 4.

17 Frederick Law Olmsted to John Foster Jenkins, 3 May 1862, in *Papers* (see n. 5), 4:315–19.

18 Samuel Ramsay to Surgeon-General Hammond, [1863], Letters Received, Box 81, Record Group 112, Records of the Surgeon General's Office, National Archives.

19 Frederick Law Olmsted to John Foster Jenkins, 29 May 1862, and Frederick Law Olmsted to Henry Whitney Bellows, 13 June 1862, in *Papers* (see n. 5), 4:352–56, 369–72.

20 WAH to Charles S. Tripler, 19 and 22 May 1862, letterbook 30, Record Group 112, Records of the Surgeon General's Office, National Archives.

21 Frederick Law Olmsted to John Foster Jenkins, 20 May 1862, *Papers* (see n. 5), 4:338–43.

22 WAH to Charles Tripler, 22 May 1862, letterbook 30 (see n. 20).

23 Henry W. Bellows to Frederick Law Olmsted, 9 June 1862, and Frederick Law Olmsted to Henry W. Bellows, 13 July 1862, in *Papers* (see n. 5), 4:371, 405; WAH to Jonathan Letterman, 19 June 1862, letterbook 31 (see n. 20), p. 181.

24 WAH to War Secretary Stanton, 7 September 1862, in *The War of the Rebellion: A Compilation of the Official Records,* 3d ser., (Washington, D.C., 1881), 2:525.

25 Montgomery C. Meigs to Henry I. Bowditch, 30 October 1862, in *Official Records* (see n. 24), 2:697–703.

26 Strong, *Diary* (see n. 6), 3:249, 257 (29 August and 24 September 1862).

27 See notes in the *Am. Med. Times* 5 (1862): 23–24; also Index of Letters Received (see n. 3), vol. 14, passim.

28 "New Army Hospital in Philadelphia," *Am. Med. Times* 4 (1862):298; "West Philadelphia General Hospital," *Am. Med. Times* 5 (1862):294; WAH to G. E. Cooper, 15 May 1862, letterbook 30 (see n. 20).

29 WAH to G. E. Cooper, 24 May 1862, letterbook 30 (see n. 20).

30 WAH to J. J. Hayes, 2 June 1862, letterbook 30 (see n. 20); L. A. Edwards to W. S. King, 11 June 1862, letterbook 31 (see n. 20).

31 J. J. Hayes to William A. Hammond, Surgeon General, 20 July 1862, Box 42, and W. S. King to General [Hammond], 28 June 1862, Letters Received (see n. 18), Box 63.

32 William A. Hammond to General N. Arnold, House of Representatives, 16 May 1862, letterbook 30 (see n. 20).

33 WAH to H. H. Smith, 14 June 1862, letterbook 31 (see n. 20).

34 WAH to S. O. Vanderpoel, 18 June 1862, letterbook 31 (see n. 20).
35 "A Regular" to WAH, 1 August 1863, Letters Received (see n. 18), Box 81.
36 See "Female Nurses in Hospitals," *Am. Med. Times* 5 (1862):149–50; and John Brinton, *Personal Memoirs . . . 1861–65* (New York, 1914), pp. 43–45. The Surgeon General's correspondence contains numerous letters on the subject.
37 WAH to A. Lincoln, 16 July 1862, letterbook 31 (see n. 20).
38 L. D. Mott to Surgeon General Hammond, 21 September 1862, Letters Received (see n. 18), Box 64; Anne L. Austin, *The Woolsey Sisters of New York* (Philadelphia, 1971), p. 95.
39 E. J. Marsh to R. O. Abbott, 16 March 1863, and G. A. McCall to R. O. Abbott, 3 April 1863, Letters Received (see n. 18), Box 65.
40 John R. Baumgardt, ed., *Civil War Nurse: The Diary and Letters of Hannah Ropes* (Knoxville, Tenn., 1980), p. 83.
41 WAH to J. A. Armstrong, 23 May 1862, letterbook 30 (see n. 20).
42 Rosenberg, *The Care of Strangers* (see n. 11), pp. 79–83.
43 WAH to Dr. S. D. Gross, 16 May 1862, letterbook 30 (see n. 20); and WAH to H. H. Smith, 14 June 1862, letterbook 31 (see n. 20).
44 S. Weir Mitchell, "Personal Recollections of the Civil War," *Trans. & Stud. of the Coll. of Phys. of Phila.*, 3d ser., 27 (1905):91f.
45 See, for example, Theodore H. Weisenburg, "The Military History of the American Neurological Association," in the American Neurological Association *Semi-Centennial . . . Volume* (Albany, N.Y., 1924), pp. 262–309; Charles A. Dana, "Early Neurology in the United States," *Jour. Am. Med. Assoc.* 90 (1928):1421–23; and C. H. Hughes, "Address of the President of the Section [on] Neurology and Psychiatry of the First Pan-American Medical Congress," *Trans. Pan-Am. Med. Cong.*, 2, pt. 2 (1893):1791.
46 S. Weir Mitchell, "Paralysis from Peripheral Irritation, with Reports of Cases," *N.Y. Med. Jour.* 2 (1866):321–55, 401–23.
47 Mitchell, "Paralysis" (see n. 46), p. 401; and Mitchell, "Personal Recollections" (see n. 44), p. 92.
48 See letters to the surgeon general's office from John M. Cuyler, 5 November 1863 (n.s., vol. 3, #C-596) and Charles McDougall, 9 November 1863 (filed with Cuyler); from John LeConte, 22 August 1863, and John M. Cuyler, 16 September 1863 (n.s., vol. 3, #L-141, C-423); and from John Campbell, 6 October 1863 (n.s., vol. 3, #C-495), Index of Letters Received (see n. 3); and "West Philadelphia General Hospital" (see n. 28), p. 294; and *Am. Med. Times* 6 (1863):108.
49 "Specialists in Medicine," *Am. Med. Times* 6 (1863):213–14; Louis Elsberg, "On the Introduction of Specialties into Bellevue Hospital," p. 226 and "Note," p. 310.
50 *The Official Correspondence Between Surgeon General William A. Hammond, U.S.A., and the Adjutant-General of the Army, Relative to the Founding of the Army Medical Museum, and the Inauguration of the Medical and Surgical History of the War* (New York, 1883), p. 6; Mitchell, "Personal Recollections" (see n. 44), p. 88.
51 See Benjamin A. Gould, "The Sanitary Commission's Bureau of Vital Statistics," in *History of the United States Sanitary Commission*, ed. Charles J. Stillé (Philadelphia, 1866); Gould, *Investigations in the Military and Anthropological Statistics of American Soldiers* (New York, 1869); and H. J. Baxter, *Statistics, Medical and Anthropological (Report from the Provost Marshal General's Office)* (Washington, D.C., 1875).
52 "Circular #7, 7 May 1863," pp. 129–35, and "Circular, 23 March 1863," p. 170, in William Grace, *The Army Surgeon's Manual* (New York, 1865). On Coues see Index of Letters Received (see n. 3), n.s., vol. 1, #C-233; and E. E. Hume, *Ornithologists of the United States Army Medical Corps* (Baltimore, 1942).
53 WAH to Surgeon George E. Cooper, 18 May 1862, letterbook 30 (see n. 20).

54 "Standard Supply Table," reprinted in Grace, *Army Surgeon's Manual* (see n. 52), pp. 140–41.

55 See reviews in *Am. Med. Times* 6 (1863):130–31, and 7 (1863):150, 162–64, 174–76; and *Med. Gaz.* 1 (1868):330, and 4 (1870):152.

56 Thomas T. Ellis, *Leaves from the Diary of an Army Surgeon* (New York, 1863), pp. 300–302; Muir's remarks are reported in Editorial, *Am. Med. Times* 6 (1863):94; Bellows is quoted in U.S. Senate Committee on Military Affairs, *Report to Accompany Bill S.560*, 45th Cong., 2d sess., 19 February 1878, S. Rept. 102, p. 14. On Ellis, see Olmsted, *Papers* (see n. 5), 4:366.

57 Frank R. Freemon, "Lincoln Finds a Surgeon General: William A. Hammond and the Transformation of the Union Army Medical Bureau," *Civil War Hist.* 33 (1987):5–21.

58 Mitchell, "Personal Recollections" (see n. 44), p. 93; D. B. St. John Roosa, "The Coming Medical Man," in *The Old Hospital and Other Papers* (New York, 1889), pp. 95–96. See also Howard D. Kramer, "Effect of the Civil War on the Public Health Movement," *Miss. Valley Hist. Rev.* 35 (1948):449–62; Gert Brieger, "Sanitary Reform in New York City: Stephen Smith and the Passage of the Metropolitan Health Bill," *Bull. Hist. Med.* 40 (1966):407–29; Rosenberg, *Care of Strangers* (see n. 11), pp. 97–99; and Blustein, "'To Increase the Efficiency'" (see n. 4), pp. 22–41.

5. "FOGGY WITH EMBARRASSMENTS"

1 WAH to G. E. Cooper, 15 May 1862, letterbook 30, Record Group 112, Records of the Surgeon General's Office, National Archives.

2 L. A. Edwards to Mr. David Todd, July 1, 1862, letterbook 31 (see n. 1), p. 312.

3 J. J. Hayes to William A. Hammond, 4 [September] 1862, Letters Received, Box 42, Record Group 112, Records of the Surgeon General's Office, National Archives.

4 Joseph R. Smith to T. R. Azpell, 25 July 1862; to J. R. Spencer, 30 August 1862, letterbook 31 (see n. 1).

5 Griffith papers, n.d., Letters Received (see n. 3), Box 65; and Charles T. Reber to Surgeon General, 26 May 1863, Letters Received (see n. 3), Box 81.

6 S. Weir Mitchell to Genl. Hammond, 23 June 1862, Letters Received (see n. 3), Box 63.

7 A. P. Meylert to WAH, 4 December 1862, Letters Received (see n. 3), Box 64.

8 See the following letters to the Surgeon General's Office, listed in Index of Letters Received, Records of the Surgeon General's Office, National Archives: William C. Spencer, 9 September 1862 (vol. 14, #S-591); Henry Wing, 25 August 1862 (vol. 14, #W-919); J. F. Hammond, 22 August 1863 (n.s., vol. 3, #H-294); W. A. Ruckingham, Governor of Connecticut, 7 December 1863 (n.s., vol. 3, #C-720); and Alexander B. Mott, 13 November 1863 (n.s., vol. 3, #M-887).

9 S. Weir Mitchell, "Personal Recollections of the Civil War," *Trans. & Stud. of the Coll. of Phys. of Phila.*, 3d ser., 27 (1905):88.

10 On the origin of the museum see Frank R. Freemon, "Lincoln Finds a Surgeon General: William A. Hammond and the Transformation of the Union Army Medical Bureau," *Civil War Hist.* 33 (1987):11; and *The Official Correspondence Between Surgeon General William A. Hammond, U.S.A., and the Adjutant-General of the Army, Relative to the Founding of the Army Medical Museum, and the Inauguration of the Medical and Surgical History of the War* (New York, 1883).

11 The best account is that in John H. Brinton, *Personal Memoirs . . . 1861–65* (New York, 1914), pp. 257ff. See also Charles H. Alden, "The Special Training of the Medical Officer," *Proc. of the Fourth Annual Meeting of the Assoc. of Military Surgeons of the U.S.* (St. Louis, 1894), pp. 675–89; and "An Army Medical School," *Am. Med. Times* 5 (1862):262–63 and 6(1863):10, 12. See also WAH's annual

report for the fiscal year ending 30 June 1862, in *The War of the Rebellion: A Compilation of the Official Records,* 3d ser., 2:749–54.

12 For example, see Joseph B. Brown to Surgeon General Hammond, Index of Letters Received (see n. 8), n.s., vol. 3, #B-405.

13 Joseph R. Smith to Richard Yates, 11 September 1862, letterbook 32 (see n. 1); William T. Collins to Surgeon General's Office, 19 October 1863, Index of Letters Received (see n. 8).

14 J. M. Howard to [Secretary of War] Stanton, 30 October 1862, Letters Received (see n. 3), Box 42.

15 These examples are drawn from the Index of Letters Received (see n. 8), vols. 14 and n.s., 1–4.

16 George Templeton Strong, *The Diary of George Templeton Strong,* ed. Allan Nevins and Milton H. Thomas (New York, 1952), 3:304 (11 March 1863); WAH to Lincoln, 13 February 1863, in *Collected Works of Abraham Lincoln,* ed. Roy P. Basler (New Brunswick, N. J., 1953), 5:445.

17 These examples are drawn from the Index of Letters Received (see n. 8), vol. 14. The consuls' suggestions are listed as #S-1138-40.

18 See the following letters listed in Index of Letters Received (see n. 8): Warren Webster, 1 December 1862 (vol. 14, #W-554-557); Richard S. Satterlee, 3 and 21 February, 9, 11, 14, and 17 March, 26 May 1863, and n.d. (vol. 14, #S-21, 28, 33, 35, 38, 39, 74); J. H. Bill, 18 and 31 July, 24 August, 16 September 1863 (n.s., vol. 1, 3, #B-198, 234, 376, 467); A. K. Smith, 10, 11, and 13 June 1863 (n.s., vol. 4, #S-53, 66, 73). Also L. A. Edwards to Elisha Harris, 22 May 1862, letterbook 30 (see n. 1). See also George Winston Smith, ed., "The Squibb Laboratory in 1863," *Jour. Hist. Med. & All. Sci.* 13 (1958):382–84.

19 L. A. Edwards to R. S. Satterlee, 17 June 1862, letterbook 30 (see n. 1).

20 S. H. Melcher to William A. Hammond, 1 November 1862, Letters Received (see n. 3), Box 64.

21 H. S. Hendee to [Joseph Weiss?], Editor of the *Chronicle,* 20 May 1863, Letters Received (see n. 3), Box 43.

22 See "William A. Hammond, M.D., LL.D.," *N.Y. Med. Jour.* 71 (1900):64.

23 John R. McClurg to William A. Hammond, 6 August 1863, Letters Received (see n. 3), Box 66.

24 John S. Haller, Jr., *American Medicine in Transition, 1840–1910* (Urbana, Ill., 1981), pp. 86–88.

25 John Harley Warner, *The Therapeutic Perspective: Medical Practice, Knowledge, and Identity in America, 1820–1855* (Cambridge, Mass., 1986), p. 221.

26 Mitchell, "Personal Recollections" (see n. 9), p. 89. See also Gert Brieger, "Therapeutic Conflicts and the American Medical Profession," *Bull. Hist. Med.* 41 (1967):215–22.

27 Bellows is quoted in U.S. Senate Committee on Military Affairs, *Report to Accompany Bill S.560,* 45th Cong., 2d sess., 19 February 1878, S. Rept. 102, p. 14; see also Strong, *Diary* (see n. 16), 3:306, 314 (17 March and 25 April 1863). Correspondence between Hammond and George Bellows and F. L. Olmsted is cited in William Q. Maxwell, *Lincoln's Fifth Wheel: The Political History of the U.S. Sanitary Commission* (New York, 1956), p. 234. See also Saul Jarcho, "Edwin Stanton and American Medicine," *Bull. Hist. Med.* 45 (1971): 153–58.

28 Strong, *Diary* (see n. 16), 3:353 (31 August 1863).

29 F. J. Hayden to Joseph Leidy, 11 September 1863; and typescript of letter, J. Leidy to Dr. Hayden, 24 September 1863, in the Joseph Leidy Papers, Academy of Natural Sciences of Philadelphia.

30 Editorial, *N.Y. Med. Jour.* 1 (1865):246–48.

31 *Am. Med. Times* 7 (1863):283; see also "Progress of the Medical Bureau," pp. 137–38.

32 Strong, *Diary* (see n. 16), 3:353, 358–59 (31 August and 25 September 1863); see also H. A. Warriner, "Surgeon General Hammond at Memphis," *U.S. Sanit. Comm. Bull.* 1 (1863–64):28.

33 Strong, *Diary* (see n. 16), 3:385 (23 December 1863). The "Circular in Behalf of the Surgeon General" was published in the *Am. Med. Times* 8 (1864):10–11, without the signatures; see also the letter, "U.S. Sanitary Commission, to his excellency the President of the United States," pp. 23–24.

34 "Republican," [letter to the editor], *U.S. Sanitary Comm. Bull.* 1 (1863–64):146–47; [editorial response], pp. 147–48.

35 Strong, *Diary* (see n. 16), 3:393–94 (16 January 1864). See also "Surgeon General Hammond," *Am. Med. Times* 8 (1864):58, and "Medical Service in the Federal Army," p. 96.

36 "Position of the Surgeon General," *Am. Med. Times* 8 (1864):8–10.

37 Extracts from the *London Med. Times & Gaz.* were published in "The Surgeon General and the Profession," *Am. Med. Times* 8 (1864):116–17; and "The Hammond Court-Martial," pp. 92–93.

38 Strong, *Diary* (see n. 16), 3:394 (16 January 1864).

39 Nathan Reingold, "Science in the Civil War: The Permanent Commission of the Navy Department," *Isis* 49 (1958):307–18; typescript of letter, Joseph Leidy to Dr. Haydon, 7 June 1863, Leidy Papers (see n. 29).

40 For a detailed legal discussion of the charges see Henry C. Friend, "Abraham Lincoln and the Court Martial of Surgeon General William A. Hammond," *Commercial Law Jour.* 62 (1957):71–80.

41 See WAH, *Statement of the Causes which led to the Dismissal of Surgeon General William A. Hammond from the Army, with a Review of the Evidence Adduced Before the Court* (New York, 1864).

42 Strong, *Diary* (see n. 16), 3:396 (22 January 1864).

43 The manuscript trial record is available in the National Archives. The best published account of the case is Mark D. Miller, "William A. Hammond: Restoring the Reputation of a Surgeon General," *Mil. Med.* 152 (1987):452–57. See also Lewis C. Duncan, "The Days Gone By: The Strange Case of Surgeon General Hammond," *Mil. Surg.* 64 (1929):98–110, 252–61; John Brinton, *Personal Memoirs . . . 1861–65* (New York, 1914), p. 256; and Maxwell, *Lincoln's Fifth Wheel* (see n. 27), pp. 239–47.

44 Joseph Henry to Alexander Dallas Bache, 21 August 1864, Joseph Henry Papers, Smithsonian Institution, Washington, D.C.; Samuel Jackson to Brig. Gen. W. A. Hammond, 18 May 1864, Autograph Case, College of Physicians of Philadelphia.

45 "Case of Surgeon General Hammond," *Am. Med. Times* 9 (1864):118–19; "Variétés. De l'organization du service médical dans l'Armée Americaine," *Arch. gén. de Méd.*, 6th ser., 5 (1864):245–47; Henry to Bache (see n. 44).

46 WAH to George B. Moore, 23 August 1864, Autograph Case, College of Physicians of Philadelphia.

47 See U.S. Senate Committee on Military Affairs, S. Rept. 102 (see n. 27); and Miller, "Restoring the Reputation" (see n. 43).

48 See letter, Larrey to Hammond, 16 March 1867, in *N.Y. Med. Jour.* 5 (1867):165–66.

49 W. A. H., "Abraham Lincoln," *N. Y. Med. Jour.* 1 (1865):163–64.

6. "A NEW YORK MEDICAL MAN"

1 Spencer F. Baird to Hon. G. W. McRary [*sic* – McCrary], 30 July 1879, Box 577, Record Group 94, National Archives; "Personals," *Va. Med. Monthly* 14 (1887–88):421.

2 [C. E. Nelson], "Professional Advertising," *Planet* 1 (Feb. 1883):10; cf. *Planet* 2 (March 1883):15; "Mens Conscia Recti," "Advertising by Specialists," *Am. Med. Times* 8 (1864):168; "Advertising Specialists," *Med. Rec.* 7 (1872):376; "The Advertising Rights of General Practitioners and Specialists," *Med. Rec.* 24 (1883):658; and "Chloral Hydrate," [letter to the editor], *Med. Rec.* 18 (1880):476.

3 L. C. McHenry, *Garrison's History of Neurology* (Springfield, Ill., 1969), pp. 270–310, 316; M. G. Echeverría, "Lectures on Diseases of the Nervous System, Delivered at the University Medical College," *Am. Med. Times* 2 (1861):299–302, 315–17, 331–33, 346–50, 363–66.

4 "Outdoor Department of Bellevue Hospital," *N.Y. Med. Jour.* 4 (1866):31–38; see also *N.Y. Med. Jour.* 5 (1867):87.

5 *Annual Circular and Catalogue of the Bellevue Hospital Medical College, City of New York, 1867–68* (New York, 1867), esp. pp. 5–7; James B. Burnet, "Letter from New York," *West. Jour. Med.* 3 (1868):31–38; Frederick A. Castle, *Second Decennial Catalogue . . . of the Bellevue Hospital Medical College of the City of New York; together with a History of the College . . .* (New York, 1884).

6 *Annual Circular and Catalogue of the Bellevue Hospital Medical College . . . 1872–73* (New York, 1872), p. 4.

7 Charles L. Dana, "Hammond, the Teacher," *Post-Graduate* 15 (1900):621–22.

8 Notice, *N.Y. Med. Jour.* 10 (1869):328. See also *Med. Rec.* 4 (1869):432; *Phys. & Pharm.* 2 (1870):18; and "Clinics for Mental Diseases in Great Britain," *N.Y. Med. Jour.* 11 (1870):443–44.

9 "New York State Hospital for Diseases of the Nervous System," *N.Y. Med. Jour.* 11 (1870):327–28; *Second Annual Report of the Board of Trustees of the New York State Hospital for Diseases of the Nervous System* (New York, 1872); "Private Hospital for Diseases of the Brain and Nervous System," *Med. Gaz.* 1 (1868):128; Notice, *Med. Gaz.* 4 (1870):224.

10 G. M. Beard, "Hospital for the Paralyzed and Epileptic," *Med. Rec.* 4 (1869):358–59. See also M. Critchley, "Hughlings Jackson, the Man; and the Early Days of the National Hospital," *Proc. Amer. Phil. Soc.* 53 (1960):613–18; and McHenry, *Garrison's History* (see n. 3), p. 305.

11 *First Annual Report of the Board of Trustees of the New York State Hospital for Diseases of the Nervous System* (New York, 1871); *Second Annual Report* (see n. 9).

12 *Annual Circular . . . 1872–73* (see n. 6), p. 5.

13 *Annual Catalogue of the Bellevue Hospital Medical College . . . 1874–75* (New York, 1874); *Annual Circular of the Bellevue Hospital Medical College . . . 1875* (New York, 1875). See also Castle, *Second Decennial Catalogue* (see n. 5).

14 D. B. St. John Roosa, "Hammond, the Man," *Post-Graduate* 15 (1900):600. See also *Catalogue of the Graduates and Officers of the Medical Department of the University of the City of New York*, 3d ed. (New York, 1890); and Robert J. Carlisle, "The University and Bellevue Hospital Medical College," in *New York University 1832–1932* (New York, 1933), pp. 281–304.

15 Thomas L. Stedman, "Our New York Letter," *New Eng. Med. Monthly* 2 (1882–83):19.

16 See typescript of letter, Joseph Leidy to [Carson], 29 October 1879, the Joseph Leidy Papers, Academy of Natural Sciences of Philadelphia. Remarks on this topic can be found in the pages of almost any American medical journal from mid-century onward. See also, "Two Proposed Bills Regulating the Practice of Medicine in this State," *New York Times*, 10 March 1882, p. 8, col. 3; Editorial, *New York Times*, 11 March 1882, p. 4, col. 6; and esp. "The Medical Standard: Discussing the Proposed New Bills," *New York Times*, 13 March 1882, p. 5, cols. 5–6, which includes the comments of the prominent New York physicians Abraham Jacobi, F. R. Sturgis, John C. Peters, O. D. Pomeroy, and George F. Shrady.

17 "The Resignation of the Post-Graduate Faculty of the University Medical College – What They Propose to Do," *Med. Gaz.* 8 (1882):205.

18 Thomas L. Stedman, "Our New York Letter," *New Eng. Med. Monthly* 1 (1881–82):410–13, 501–4. For general discussions of educational reform during this period, see Robert P. Hudson, "Abraham Flexner in Perspective: American Medical Education 1865–1910," *Bull. Hist. Med.* 46 (1972):545–61; and Howard Berliner, "A Larger Perspective on the Flexner Report," *Int. Jour. Health Serv.* 5 (1975):573–92.

19 Roosa, "Hammond, the Man" (see n. 14), p. 601.

20 WAH, "On Certain Animal Extracts: Their Mode of Preparation and Physiolog-
    ical and Therapeutical Effects," *Post-Graduate* 8 (1893):97.
21 For a detailed discussion of postgraduate medical education in the United States
    in the late nineteenth century, see Steven J. Peitzman, "'Thoroughly Practical':
    America's Polyclinic Medical Schools," *Bull. Hist. Med.* 54 (1980):166–187.
22 "Resignation of the Post-Graduate Faculty" (see n. 17); see also Notice, *Med. Rec.*
    22 (1882):558; and Stedman, "Our New York Letter" (see n. 15), p. 131.
23 Letter, *Med. Rec.* 10 (1875):686–87.
24 Notice, *Med. Rec.* 22 (1882):558.
25 See advertisements in *Quart. Bull. Clin. Soc.* 1 (1885):204; *N.Y. Med. Jour.* 43
    (1886):303; and *N.Y. Med. Jour.* 47 (1888):411.
26 Notice, *Quart. Bull Clin. Soc.* 2 (1886–87):[ii].
27 Editorial, *New York Times,* 22 April 1882, p. 4, col. 7; New York Post-Graduate
    Medical School, *Announcement of the Second Year, Sessions of 1883–84* (New York,
    1883); Illinois State Board of Health, *Medical Education and Medical Colleges in the
    United States and Canada, 1765–1891* (Springfield, Ill., 1891). See also Peitzman,
    "'Thoroughly Practical' " (see n. 21).
28 See Charles E. Rosenberg, "Social Class and Medical Care: The Rise and Fall of
    the Dispensary," *Jour. Hist. Med.* 29 (1974):32–54. For a thoughtful contempo-
    rary discussion, see J. West Roosevelt, "Concerning the Advice-Gratis System,"
    Med. Rec. 25 (1884):137–38.
29 Data on the faculty of the Post-Graduate were compiled from its *Announcement of
    the Second Year* (see n. 27); comparative data came from a very interesting statis-
    tical study of the *Medical Register* made by "F," an opponent of "medical cliques,"
    in 1875. See "Medical Appointments," *Med. Rec.* 10 (1875):687.
30 "Itis," "Polyclinics, Post-Graduate Schools, etc., and Their Relation to the Medi-
    cal Profession," *Med. Rec.* 23 (1883):696–97. For another point of view, see
    Thomas E. Satterthwaite, "The New York Post-Graduate School and the Abuse
    of Medical Charity," *Med. Rec.* 23 (1883):23.
31 Illinois State Board of Health, *Medical Education* (see n. 27), pp. 8–9, 22.
32 Abraham Flexner, *Medical Education in the United States and Canada* (New York,
    1910), p. 174; cf. Charles Carroll Lee, "The Necessity for Post-Graduate Instruc-
    tion in the Present State of American Medical Education," *Post-Graduate* 4
    (1889):114–18.
33 Flexner, *Medical Education* (see n. 32), p. 174.
34 New York Post-Graduate Medical School and Hospital, *34th Annual Announce-
    ment, 1915–16* (New York, 1915), p. [9].
35 New York Post-Graduate Medical School and Hospital, *27th Annual Announce-
    ment, 1908–9* (New York, 1908), p. [9].
36 New York Post-Graduate Medical School and Hospital, *28th Annual Announce-
    ment, 1909–10* (New York, 1909), p. [9].
37 See, for example, WAH, "Rabies in the Human Subject," *Quart. Bull. Clin. Soc.*
    1 (1886):293–97, with report of the discussion at a special meeting, 25 January
    1886, pp. 297–304.
38 New York Post-Graduate Medical School, *34th Annual Announcement* (see n. 34),
    p. [9].
39 See Russell C. Maulitz, "Physician Versus Bacteriologist: The Ideology of Sci-
    ence in Clinical Medicine, " *The Therapeutic Revolution,* ed. Maurice J. Vogel and
    Charles E. Rosenberg (Philadelphia, 1979), pp. 91–108.
40 National Institute of Letters, Arts and Science, New York, "Report of the Pro-
    ceedings of the First Regular Meeting, . . .12 June 1868," Manuscript Collec-
    tion, New-York Historical Society, pp. 78ff.
41 Ibid., pp. 44ff, 107, 9–10, 48–49.
42 See *N.Y. Med. Jour.* 8 (1869):557–58.
43 George Templeton Strong, *Diary,* 4:216ff. (New York, 1952); National Institute,
    "Proceedings" (see n. 40), p. 44ff. See also Austin Flint to Joseph Leidy II, 23 June
    1909, and E. O. Hovey to Joseph Leidy II, 21 June 1909, Joseph Leidy II Papers,

College of Physicians of Philadelphia; and reports in *Med. Gaz.* 1 (1868):305, and 2 (1869):417.

44 See Gardner Murphy, *Historical Introduction to Modern Psychology*, 2d ed. (New York, 1949); Gregory Zilboorg, *A History of Medical Psychology* (New York, 1941); and McHenry, *Garrison's History* (see n. 3).

45 Quoted in Zilboorg, *History of Medical Psychology* (see n. 44), p. 435.

46 Owsei Temkin, "Materialism in French and German Physiology of the Early Nineteenth Century," *Bull. Hist. Med.* 20 (1946):322–27.

47 See *The Coca Leaf and Cocaine Papers*, ed. George Andrews and David Solomon (New York, 1975); WAH, "Coca – Its Preparations and Their Therapeutical Qualities with Some Remarks on the So-Called Cocaine Habit," *Va. Med. Monthly* 14 (1887–88):598–612. On Hammond and Charcot, see Editorial and "An Accusation Successfully Met," *Hosp. Gaz.* 6 (1879):633–35.

48 See John Albert Pitts, "The Association of Medical Superintendents of American Institutions for the Insane, 1844–1892: A Case Study of Specialism in American Medicine" (Ph.D. diss., University of Pennsylvania, 1979).

49 Bonnie Ellen Blustein, "'A Hollow Square of Psychological Science': American Neurologists and Psychiatrists in Conflict," in *Madhouses, Mad-Doctors, and Madmen*, ed. Andrew T. Scull (Philadelphia, 1981), pp. 241–70.

50 [WAH], review of John P. Gray, *The Dependence of Insanity on Physical Disease* (Utica, N.Y., 1871), in *Jour. Psych. Med.* 5 (1871):567–69, 576.

51 "To the Reader," *Psych. & Med.-Leg. Jour.*, n.s., 1 (1874):71.

52 WAH, "The Effects of Alcohol Upon the Nervous System," *Psych. & Med.-Leg. Jour.*, n.s., 1 (1874):1.

53 The manuscript minute books of the New York Neurological Society are on deposit in the Rare Book Room, New York Academy of Medicine. I am grateful to Dr. Fletcher H. McDowell for permission to consult these records, and to Mrs. Alice Weaver for her assistance in locating them. Reports of the meetings were frequently published in various New York medical journals. On asylum reform, see Blustein, "'A Hollow Square'" (see n. 49).

54 See the American Neurological Association, *Semicentennial Anniversary Volume* (Albany, N.Y., 1924). Reports of A.N.A. meetings were frequently published and often contain more detail than the laconic minute books, on deposit at the New York Academy of Medicine.

55 "Medico-Legal Society," *Med. Rec.* 22 (1882):55, 420; "The Medico-Legal Society," *N.Y. Med. Jour.* 35 (1882):268–69; E. S. G[aillard], "Medico-Legal Society," *Am. Med. Weekly* 14 (1882):226–31, 454–56; Thomas L. Stedman, "Our New York Letter," *N. Eng. Med. Monthly* 2 (1882):73–76; "Transactions of the Medico-Legal Society," *Med.-Leg. Jour.* 1 (1883–84):106–7, 116–18, 440–42, 570–73, 651–53; [Note], *Med. Rec.* 23 (1883):18; "New York Society of Medical Jurisprudence," *N.Y. Med. Jour.* 37 (1883):123; "The Medico-Legal Society," *N.Y. Med. Jour.* 39 (1884):44; "Medico-Legal Science in New York City," *Med. Rec.* 26 (1884):712.

56 "A Medical Song from 'Patience,'" *Med. Rec.* 20 (1881):643.

57 [Frank Foster], "William A. Hammond, M.D., LL.D.," *N.Y. Med. Jour.* 71 (1900):64.

58 For a full account see Mark D. Miller, "William A. Hammond: Restoring the Reputation of a Surgeon General," *Mil. Med.* 152 (1987):452–57.

59 WAH to Hon. G. W. McCrary, 14 August 1879, and related papers, Box 577, Record Group 94, National Archives.

7. "A LABORIOUS AND SKILFUL OBSERVER"

1 WAH, *A Treatise on the Diseases of the Nervous System* (New York, 1871); 2d ed. (1872); 3d ed. (1873); 4th ed. (1874); 5th ed. (1876); 6th ed. (1876); 7th ed (1881); 8th ed. (1886); 9th ed. with G. M. Hammond (1891). Translations include a French edition by F. Labadie-Lagrave (1879); a Spanish edition by Federico

Toledo y Cueva (1887), and an Italian edition by A. Rubino (1887). Major changes were made in the sixth, seventh, and eighth editions. Those in the ninth edition were largely the work of the author's son. References here are to the first edition, unless otherwise noted.

2   New York State Hospital for Diseases of the Nervous System, *First Annual Report . . . for the year ending April 20, 1871* (New York, 1871); and *Second Annual Report . . . for the year ending April 1, 1872* (New York, 1872).

3   Spencer F. Baird to G. W. McRary [*sic* – McCrary], 30 July 1879, Box 577, Record Group 94, National Archives.

4   "Cures for Seasickness," *Med. Rec.* 19 (1881):728.

5   WAH, "Pott's Disease Simulating Spinal Irritation, a Clinical Lecture," *Med. Gaz.* 8 (1881):260; WAH, "A Clinical Lecture on the Differential Diagnosis of Antero-Lateral Sclerosis and Posterior Sclerosis on the Spinal Cord," *Jour. Nerv. & Ment. Dis.* 15 (1888):496–509.

6   WAH, *Treatise* (see n. 1), p. [xi].

7   George Rosen, *The Specialization of Medicine, with Particular Reference to Ophthalmology* (1944; reprint ed., New York, 1972).

8   Unsigned review (probably by WAH) of X. Galezowski, *Etude ophthalmoscopique sur les alterations due nerf optique, et sur les maladies cérébrales dont elles dépendent* (Paris, 1865), and E. Bouchut, *Du diagnostic des maladies du système nerveux par ophthalmoscopie* (Paris, 1866), in *N.Y. Med. Jour.* 3 (1866):140–41.

9   WAH, *Treatise* (see n. 1), p. xiii.

10 WAH, "The Dynamometer and Dynamograph of Mathieu," *Quart. Jour. Psych. Med.* 2 (1868):139–46.

11 WAH, *Treatise* (see n. 1), pp. 90–91. See also WAH, "Clinical Lectures Delivered at the Bellevue Hospital Medical College," *Jour. Psych. Med.* 6 (1872):625–51.

12 See, for example, L. C. McHenry, ed., *Garrison's History of Neurology* (Springfield, Ill., 1969), pp. 327, 411. For a history of athetosis see Malcolm B. Carpenter, "Athetosis and the Basal Ganglia," *Arch. Neur. & Psychiat.* 63 (1950):875–901.

13 WAH, *Treatise* (see n. 1), pp. 654–61.

14 WAH, "Athetosis," *Med. Rec.* 8 (1873):309–11.

15 Charles E. Rosenberg, "The Therapeutic Revolution: Medicine, Meaning and Social Change in Nineteenth-Century America," *Perspectives in Biology and Medicine* 20 (1977):485–506; John Harley Warner, *The Therapeutic Perspective: Medical Practice, Knowledge, and Identity in America, 1820–1885* (Cambridge, Mass., 1986).

16 WAH, "A Clinical Lecture on Cerebral Embolism," *Am. Med. Bi-Weekly* 12 (1881):217–29.

17 WAH, "On Convulsive Tremor," *N.Y. Med. Jour.* 5 (1867):185–98.

18 WAH, "A Clinical Lecture on Glosso-labio-laryngeal Paralysis – Syphilitic Brain Tumor – Idiocy – Mysophobia," *Hosp. Gaz.* 6 (1879):113–16.

19 WAH, *Treatise* (see n. 1), pp. 513–16. See also WAH, "Clinical Lecture on the Differential Diagnosis of Antero-Lateral Sclerosis and Posterior Sclerosis of the Spinal Cord," *Jour. Nerv. & Ment. Dis.* n.s., 15 (1888):496–509.

20 WAH, "Elongation of the Sciatic Nerve in Locomotor Ataxia," *Jour. Nerv. & Ment. Dis.* 8 (1881):553–59. See also "American Neurological Association," *Med. Rec.* 19 (1881):17–22; and L[andon] C[arter] G[ray], "Nerve Stretching," *Am. Jour. Neur. & Psychiat.* 1 (1882):198–220.

21 WAH, "The Treatment of Locomotor Ataxia and other Diseases of the Nervous System by Suspension," *N.Y. Med. Jour.* 49 (1889):510–12.

22 See the following articles in the *N.Y. Med. Jour.*: "An Accident with the Suspension Apparatus," 49 (1889):549; "The Suspension Apparatus," 49 (1889):607; W. H. Dewitt, "Correspondence," 49 (1889):690; Winslow W. Skinner, "A Danger to be Avoided in the Treatment of Nervous Affections by Suspension," 49 (1889):715–16; "New York Neurological Society," 50 (1889):525–27; L. C. Gray, "The Curability of Locomotor Ataxia," 50 (1889):533–42; "The Mechanical

Treatment of Locomotor Ataxia," 51 (1890):265–66; and "The Adverse Possibilities of Suspension," 51 (1890):352.

23 On attempts to use animal extracts in the treatment of locomotor ataxia, see C. E. Brown-Séquard, "Remarques à l'occasion du fait de guérison d'ataxie locomotrice, communiqué par M. Depous," *Comp. Rend. Soc. Biol.*, 9e ser., 3 (1891):405–7; and "Remarques sur l'influence du liquide testiculaire dans plusieurs cas nouveaux d'ataxie locomotrice. . . , " *Comp. Rend. Soc. Biol.*, 9e ser., 4 (1892):551–52.

24 Unsigned review of WAH, *Treatise on the Diseases of the Nervous System*, 8th ed., in *Neur. Rev.* 1 (1886):249–50.

25 WAH, "On the Treatment of Chorea with Hypodermic Injections of Arsenic," *St. Louis Clin. Rec.* 6 (1879):193.

26 WAH, "On Obscure Abscess of Liver," *St. Louis Clin. Rec.* 7 (1880):294–302; see also WAH, "On Obscure Abscesses of the Liver, their Association with Hypochondria, and Other Forms of Mental Derangement, and Their Treatment," *St. Louis Clin. Rec.* 5 (1878):49–58. This paper was read before the New York Neurological Society on 3 June 1878 and was widely reported in the medical press. See WAH, "Hepatic Abscess," *Med. Rec.* 15 (1879):691–20; J. Marion Sims, "Diagnosis of Abscess of the Liver by Symptoms of Cerebral Hyperaemia; With Some Remarks on Treatment of Hepatic Abscess by Aspiration," *Med. Gaz.* 7 (1880):74–75; and "Enlargement of Liver," *Post-Graduate* 3 (1888):34–40.

27 C. L. Dana, "Therapeutics and Neurological Therapeutics," *Quart. Bull. Clin. Soc.* 1 (1886):244.

28 J. W. Holland, review of WAH, *A Treatise on the Diseases of the Nervous System*, in *Am. Pract.* 4 (1871):232; unsigned review of *Treatise* in *Med. Rec.* 6 (1871):354.

29 Rosen, *Specialization* (see n. 7). This review has generally been accepted by historians; see Rosemary Stevens, *American Medicine and the Public Interest* (New Haven, Conn., 1971); and Stanley J. Reiser, *Medicine and the Reign of Technology* (Cambridge, England, 1978), esp. pp. 146–47.

30 McHenry, *Garrison's History of Neurology* (see n. 12), p. 279.

31 "Proceedings of Societies. New York Obstetrical Society," *N.Y. Med. Jour.* 1 (1865):146.

32 "On the Treatment of Bedsores," *Am. Pract.* 5 (1872):244–45; WAH, "A Clinical Lecture on Chronic Myelitis," *Am. Med. Times* 2 (1861):379–80; Becquerel et al., "The Application of Electricity to Therapeutics," trans. E. S. Dunster, *Quart. Jour. Psych. Med. & Med. Jur.* 1 (1867):283–316. See also *Med. Gaz.* 2 (1869):398.

33 [WAH], "Contemporary Literature," *Quart. Jour. Psych. Med. & Med. Jur.* 2 (1868):164.

34 Charles E. Morgan, *Electrophysiology and Therapeutics, Being a Study of the Electrical and Other Physical Phenomena of the Muscular and Other Systems during Health and Disease, Including the Phenomena of the Electric Fishes*, with a Preface by WAH (New York, 1868), p. [v]; review in *N.Y. Med. Jour.* 7 (1868):122–27; and review by J. F. H[ibbard] in *West. Jour. Med.* 3 (1868):424–26.

35 George M. Beard, "Study of Nervous Diseases in Germany," *Med. Rec.* 4 (1869):380; review of Moritz Meyer, *Electricity in Its Relations to Practical Medicine*, trans. WAH (New York, 1869), in *Med. Rec.* 4 (1869):326; review of Meyer, *Electricity*, in *Med. Gaz.* 3 (1869):190–91. See also "List of Some Recent Publications," *N. Am. Rev.* 109 (1869):620; review in *Phys. & Pharm.* 2 (1869):6–7; and review by J. W. H[olland] in *Am. Pract.* 2 (1870):110–12.

36 Review of Meyer, *Electricity* (see n. 35) in *N.Y. Med. Jour.* 10 (1870):499–500; review of W. B. Neftel, *Galvanotherapeutics* (New York, 1870) in *Med. Gaz.* 6 (1870):61.

37 "The New York Neurological Society," *Arch. Elect. & Neurol.* 1 (1874):119–21; "The New York Society of Neurology and Electrology," *Arch. Elect. & Neurol.* 1 (1874):116–19.

38 "Sweet Peace," *Med. Rec.* 22 (1882):531; *Cincinnati Lancet & Clinic* 9 (1882):501; *New England Medical Month.* 2 (1883):143.

39 Review of G. M. Beard and A. D. Rockwell, *A Practical Treatise on the Medical and Surgical Uses of Electricity*, 2d ed. (New York, 1875), in *Med. Rec.* 10 (1875):210. Contrast this with a favorable notice of the first edition in *Med. Rec.* 6 (1871):326–28. Also, A. D. Rockwell, "The Relation of Electro-Therapeutics to Electrophysiology," *Med. Rec.* 10 (1875):121–24.

40 J. D. S. Smith, "Electrotherapeutics and the American Neurological Association," A. D. Rockwell, "Reply to Dr. J. D. S. Smith," and L. C. Gravy, "Electrotherapeutics and the American Neurological Association," *Med. Rec.* 16 (1879):118, 166–67, 237–38.

41 The first quotation is from Iago Galdston, "The Natural History of Specialism in Medicine," *J. Am. Med. Assn.* 170 (1959):296; the second from B. J. Stern, *American Medical Practice in the Perspective of a Century* (New York, 1945), p. 45.

42 Joseph Collins, "Hammond the Physician and Neurologist," *Post-Graduate* 15 (1900):605; unsigned review of WAH, *A Treatise on the Diseases of the Nervous System*, 6th ed. (New York, 1876), in *Jour. Nerv. & Ment. Dis.* 3 (1876):461.

43 J. Leonard Corning, review of WAH, *A Treatise on the Diseases of the Nervous System*, 8th ed. (New York, 1886), in *Gaillard's Med. Jour.* 43 (1886):211; Louis J. Casamajor, "Notes for an Intimate History of Neurology and Psychiatry in the United States," *Jour. Nerv. & Ment. Dis.* 98 (1943):605; Charles L. Dana, "Early Neurology in the United States," *Jour. Am. Med. Assoc.* 90 (1928):1421.

8. "SO GREAT HER SCIENCE"

1 "Practitioners and Scientists," *Therapeutic Gazette* 2 (1886):834.

2 "The Specialist," poem read at the Annual Dinner of the Faculty of the New York Post-Graduate Medical School, 11 March 1886, *Quart. Bull. Clin. Soc.* 1 (1886):270.

3 The best source on the history of polio is Morris Fishbein, *A Bibliography of Infantile Paralysis 1789–1949, With Selected Abstracts and Annotations . . .* , 2d ed. (Philadelphia, 1951). Only 123 entries represent the years 1789–1870. See also Arthur Bloomfield, *A Bibliography of Internal Medicine: Communicable Diseases* (Chicago, 1958).

4 Charles Fayette Taylor, *Infantile Paralysis and Its Attendant Deformities* (Philadelphia, 1867), p. 6.

5 Fishbein, *Bibliography* (see n. 3), pp. 1–10.

6 J. M. Paul, "Case of Paralysis Occurring in a Child," *N. Am. Med. & Surg. Jour.* 8 (1829):70; G. Colman, "Medical Notes . . . Paralysis in Teething Children," *Am. Jour. Med. Sci.* 5 (1843):248.

7 Taylor, *Infantile Paralysis* (see n. 4), p. iii.

8 Abraham Jacobi, "Critical Examination of All Recent Works Relating to Infantile Pathology and Therapeutics," *N.Y. Med. Jour.* 6 (1858):108. On Jacobi, see Abt-Garrison, *History of Pediatrics* (Philadelphia, 1965), pp. 105–6.

9 Charles Fayette Taylor, "Neglected Cases. Infantile Paralysis," *Am. Med. Times* 5 (1862):189, 215–17. On Taylor, see A. R. Shands, Jr., *The Early Orthopaedic Surgeons of America* (St. Louis, 1970).

10 M. G. Echeverría, "Remarks on Atrophic Fatty Palsy in Infancy," *Am. Med. Times* 3 (1861):22–23; and M. G. Echeverría, "Treatment of Paralysis by Hypodermic Infections of Strychnine, with Remarks in Infantile Palsy," *Proc. Connecticut State Med. Soc.* 3 (1868):132–44.

11 WAH, "On the Treatment of a Certain Form of Paralysis Occurring in Children," *N.Y. Med. Jour.* 2 (1865):169, 173.

12 WAH, "The Pathology and Treatment of Organic Infantile Paralysis," *Quart. Jour. Psych. Med. & Med. Jur.* 1 (1867):51–52. Cf. WAH, "Lecture on the Pathology and Treatment of Infantile Paralysis," *Med. & Surg. Reporter* 16 (Philadelphia, 1867):369–71; and WAH, "Further Remarks on Organic Infantile Paralysis," *Quart. Jour. Psych. Med. & Med. Jur.* 2 (1868):531–54.

13 WAH, "Pathology and Treatment" (see n. 12), p. 51; WAH, "Lecture" (see n. 12), p. 369.

14 WAH, *A Treatise on the Diseases of the Nervous System* (New York, 1871), pp. 692–93.

15 For a review of the vast literature on aphasia, see Alfred Meyer, "The Frontal Lobe Syndrome, the Aphasias and Related Conditions. A Contribution to the History of Cortical Localization," *Brain* 97 (1974):565–600. Perhaps the most useful general introduction is still the historical section of Henry Head, *Aphasia and Kindred Disorders of Speech* (Cambridge, England, 1926).

16 Head, *Aphasia* (see n. 15), 1:25.

17 WAH, *Treatise* (see n. 14), pp. 196, 199.

18 "Proceedings of Societies. Medical Society of the County of New York. Aphasia," *Med. Gaz.* 6 (1870):65. Cf. "On Aphasia," *Med. Rec.* 6 (1871):3–6; and "Report of Special Meeting of the New York County Medical Society," *N.Y. Med. Jour.* 13 (1871):304–26. This material appeared in almost identical form in WAH, *Treatise* (see n. 14), pp. 166–218. See also T. M. B. Cross, "Amnesic and Ataxic Aphasia," *Am. Pract.* 5 (1872):193–202, which describes the case of "Captain D," who was seen by Cross and Hammond at the New York State Hospital for Diseases of the Nervous System and who appeared regularly at Hammond's clinical lectures at the Bellevue Hospital Medical College.

19 WAH, *Treatise* (see n. 14), p. 217.

20 Samuel H. Greenblatt, "The Development of Hughlings Jackson's Approach to Diseases of the Nervous System, 1863–66: Unilateral Seizures, Hemiplegia and Aphasia," *Bull. Hist. Med.* 51 (1977):412–30.

21 Quoted in Head, *Aphasia* (see n. 15), 1:50.

22 See Otto H. Marx, "Aphasia Studies and Language Theory in the Nineteenth Century," *Bull. Hist. Med.* 40 (1966):328–49.

23 Greenblatt, "Jackson's Approach" (see n. 20), pp. 415, 430. For a different view see W. Riese, "The Sources of Hughlings Jackson's View on Aphasia," *Brain* 88 (1965):811–22, which considers philosophical aspects of Jackson's position.

24 *Med. Rec.* 6 (1871):20–21.

25 Head, *Aphasia* (see n. 15), 1:vii, 31.

26 *Med. Rec.* 6 (1871):19.

27 Greenblatt, "Jackson's Approach" (see n. 20), p. 412; J. D. Spillane, "1874–84: A Memorable Decade in the History of British Neurology," *Trans Am. Neur. Assn.* 99 (1974):88–94.

28 WAH, "Unilateral Hallucinations," *N.Y. Med. Jour.* 42 (1885):682. This paper was also published in *Med. News* 47 (1885):687–88. For reports of the discussion at the meeting see *N.Y. Med. Jour.* 42 (1885):697–98, and *Med. News* 47 (1885):688–89.

29 WAH, "Mysterious Disappearances," *Forum* 3 (1887):76.

30 Clara Lanza, *Mr. Perkin's Daughter* (New York, 1881). For medical notices and reviews, see *Med. Rec.* 19 (1881):339, and 20 (1881):45; and *Am. Med. Biweekly* 12 (1881):94, and 13 (1881):17.

31 WAH, *A Mysterious Life: A Four-Act Drama* (New York, 1901).

32 WAH, review of Frederick Bateman, *Darwinism Tested by Language* (London, 1877), in *Jour. Nerv. & Ment. Dis.* 5 (1877):362–70, 744–52.

33 "New York College of Veterinary Surgeons," *Med. Rec.* 13 (1878):197–98; cf. *Hosp. Gaz. & Arch. Clin. Surg.* 3 (1878):128–29.

34 WAH, "On Sleep and Insomnia. Part I. Physiology of Sleep," *N.Y. Med. Jour.* 1 (1865):88–101; and WAH, "Physiology of Sleep," *N.Y. Lancet: A Family Med. Jour.* 1 (1866):43–45. For a fuller treatment of Hammond's work on sleep, see Bonnie Ellen Blustein, "The Brief Career of 'Cerebral Hyperaemia': William A. Hammond and His Insomniac Patients, 1854–90," *Jour. Hist. Med. & All. Sci.* 41 (1986):24–51.

35 WAH, "On Sleep" (see n. 34).

36 Lorraine J. Daston, "British Responses to Psycho-Physiology, 1860–1900," *Isis* 169 (1978):192–208. See also Leon S. Jacyna, "The Physiology of Mind, the Unity of Nature, and the Moral Order of Victorian Thought," *Brit. Jour. Hist. Sci.* 7 (1981):109–32; and Karl M. Figlio, "Theories of Perception and the Physiology of Mind in the Late Eighteenth Century," *Hist. Sci.* 13 (1975):177–212.

37 Nathaniel S. Shaler, "Sleep and Dreams," *Internat. Rev.* 6 (1879):234–47.
38 Arthur E. Durham, "The Physiology of Sleep," *Guy's Hosp. Reports*, 3d ser., 6 (1860):149–173; *Report of the Thirteenth Meeting of the B.A.A.S. held at Oxford in June and July 1860* (London, 1861).
39 WAH, "On Sleep" (see n. 34).
40 Durham, "Physiology of Sleep" (see n. 38); see also William H. Byford, "On the Physiology of Repose or Sleep," *Am. Jour. Med. Sci.*, n.s., 31 (1856):357–68. Hammond almost certainly saw this article, as his own paper on the effects of tea and coffee appeared in the same number of the *Journal*.
41 WAH, "On Sleep" (see n. 34). See also WAH, *On Wakefulness: with an Introductory Chapter on the Physiology of Sleep* (Philadelphia, 1866), and subsequent revisions of this book.
42 J. Leonard Corning, "Sleep," *Med. Rec.* 22 (1882):10–11; J. Milner Fothergill, "The Causes and Treatment of Sleeplessness," *Pract.* 16 (1876):103–17; see also extract of this article, "Causes and Treatment of Insomnia," *Med. Rec.* 11 (1876):205–6; E. Colon Angell, "Lectures on the Therapeutical Uses of the Turkish Bath," *Med. Gaz.* 1 (1868):177–80; "The Physiology of Sleep," *N.Y. Med. Jour.* 38 (1883):210–11; "Book Notices. Insomnia and Other Disorders of Sleep. By Henry Lyman . . . ," *N.Y. Med. Jour.* 44 (1886):277; George W. Rachel, "Tissue Metamorphosis and Sleep," *Med. Rec.* 23 (1883):65–67; and a review of WAH, *Sleep and Its Derangements* (Philadelphia, 1869), in *Med. Rec.* 4 (1870):518–19.
43 Henry Wurtz, "The Chemistry of Sleep," *Pop. Sci. Monthly* 46 (1894):230–39; cf. "Physiology of Sleep," *Westminster Rev.*, n.s. 25 (1864):203–17.
44 Henry Charleton Bastian, "The Theory of Sleep," *Appleton's Jour.* 1 (1869):279–80.
45 Shaler, "Sleep and Dreams" (see n. 37). Cf. "The Mystery of Sleep," *Eclectic Mag.*, n.s., 3 (1866):452–58.
46 Samuel Henry Dickson, "Wakefulness; Sleep; Anaesthesia," *Am. Jour. Med. Sci.*, n.s., 56 (1868):87–100.
47 E[dward] C. S[eguin], review of James Cappie, *The Causation of Sleep* (Edinburgh, 1872), in *Arch. Sci. Pract. Med.* 1 (1873):373–74.
48 See Frank K. Freemon, *Sleep Research: A Critical Review* (Springfield, Ill., 1972), esp. p. 146.
49 Review of WAH, *On Wakefulness* (see n. 41), in *N.Y. Med. Jour.* 2 (1866):311.
50 See "Physiology of Sleep" (see n. 43).
51 Russell C. Maulitz, "Physician Versus Bacteriologist," in *The Therapeutic Revolution*, ed. Maurice J. Vogel and Charles E. Rosenberg (Philadelphia, 1979), pp. 91–108; Gerald L. Geison's discussion of British neurophysiology in *Michael Foster and the Cambridge School of Physiology* (Princeton, 1978), pp. 31–35; Donna J. Haraway, "Animal Sociology and a Natural Economy of the Body Politic, Part I," *Signs* 4 (1978):21–23.

9. "SYSTEMS OF CURES AND WONDERFUL REMEDIES"

1 See Russell C. Maulitz, *Morbid Appearances* (Cambridge, England, 1988).
2 WAH, *A Treatise on the Diseases of the Nervous System* (New York, 1871), p. 275.
3 Ibid., pp. 612, 614 (emphasis added).
4 Ibid., p. 709 (emphasis added).
5 Review of WAH, *A Treatise on the Diseases of the Nervous System* (7th ed., New York, 1881), in *Med. Rec.* 20 (1881):16–17.
6 Many of the sections of Hammond's *Treatise* that are devoted to specific conditions indicate the numbers of patients of each type the author claimed to have seen. Although this information is incomplete and probably not entirely reliable, it is the only available basis for plausible quantitative estimates.
7 See Barbara Sicherman, "The Uses of a Diagnosis: Doctors, Patients and Neurasthenia," *Jour. Hist. Med.* 32 (1977):33–54; and F. G. Gosling, *Before Freud: Neurasthenia and the American Medical Community, 1870–1910* (Urbana, Ill., 1987).

8   WAH, "Chlorosis a Disease of the Nervous System," *Quart. Jour. Psych. Med. & Med. Jur.* 2 (1868):417–41.
9   WAH, "Can We Diagnosticate Hyperaemia or Anemia of the Brain and Cord?" *Va. Med. Month.* 17 (1890):678–680.
10 WAH, "Insomnia and Recent Hypnotics," *N. Am. Rev.* 156 (1893):18–26. See also Bonnie Ellen Blustein, "The Brief Career of 'Cerebral Hyperaemia': William Hammond and His Insomniac Patients, 1854–90," *Jour. Hist. Med. & All. Sci.* 41 (1986):24–51.
11 WAH, "On Sleep and Insomnia. Part II. The Pathology and Treatment of Insomnia," *N.Y. Med. Jour.* 1 (1865):182–204.
12 WAH, *Robert Severne: His Friends and His Enemies* (Philadelphia, 1867), pp. 44, 56.
13 WAH, "The Therapeutics of Wakefulness," *Det. Rev. Med. Pharm.* 4 (1869):26–30. See also "Abstract of a Lecture on the Therapeutics of Wakefulness Delivered at Bellevue Hospital Medical College," *Med. Rec.* 3 (1868):436–37; "Bromide of Potassium for the Sleeplessness of Infants. [Medical Times and Gazette, December 12, 1868]," *N.Y. Med. Jour.* 9 (1869):85–86; and "Sleep-Producing Agents," *Phys. & Pract.* 1 (1869):10.
14 WAH, *Sleep and Its Derangements* (Philadelphia, 1869), pp. 223, 230.
15 WAH, *Cerebral Hyperaemia the Result of Mental Strain or Emotional Disturbance* (New York, 1878).
16 WAH, *A Treatise on the Diseases of the Nervous System* (New York, 1871), pp. 33–37. See also n. 6 above.
17 "W. A. Hammond, *Cerebral Hyperaemia*" [book review], *Am. Med. Bi-weekly* 12 (1881):36.
18 WAH, *Cerebral Hyperaemia* (see n. 15), p. 68.
19 Ibid., p. 10.
20 Ibid. See also WAH: "The Proper Use of the Mind," *Quart. Jour. Psych. Med. & Med. Jur.* 2 (1868):660–97; "Brain-Forcing in Childhood," *Pop. Sci. Monthly* 30 (1886–87):721–32; and "How to Rest," *N. Am. Rev.* 153 (1891):215–19. See also George M. Beard, *American Nervousness* (New York, 1881).
21 WAH, *Cerebral Hyperaemia* (see n. 15); cf. review of WAH, *Treatise* (see n. 16) in *Med. Rec.* 20 (1881):16–17.
22 WAH, *Cerebral Hyperaemia* (see n. 15), pp. 83–84; cf. comments of William M. Leszynsky in "New York Neurological Society," *N.Y. Med. Jour.* 51 (1890):636–38.
23 WAH, *Cerebral Hyperaemia* (see n. 15), pp. 77, 81, 98–99, 102.
24 *AMA Drug Evaluations*, 3d ed. (Littleton, Mass., 1977).
25 J. G. Hopkins, "A Spicy Letter, in which a Georgia Doctor Tells What He Knows About Dr. Wm. A. Hammond, of New York, and His Treatment of a Georgia Patient," *Atlanta Med. & Surg. Jour.*, n.s., 1 (1884–85):413–16; WAH, "Dr. Hammond's Reply to Dr. Hopkins," *Atlanta Med. & Surg. Jour.*, n.s., 1 (1884–85):484–87.
26 Charles L. Dana, "Hammond, the Teacher," *Post-Graduate* 15 (1900):620.
27 Hopkins, "A Spicy Letter" (see n. 25); WAH, "Dr. Hammond's Reply" (see n. 25).
28 WAH, "Records of Practice. III. A Case of Hysterical Deception," *Neur. Cont.* 1, #1 (1879):72–79.
29 "American Neurological Association," *Jour. Nerv. & Ment. Dis.* 1 (1876):429–34, esp. 431.
30 WAH, *On Certain Conditions of Nervous Derangement* (New York, 1881), p. 255.
31 WAH, "False Hydrophobia," *N. Am. Rev.* 151 (1890):167–72; see also WAH, "Rabies in the Human Subject," *Quart. Bull. Clin. Soc.* 1 (1886):293–305.
32 See, for example, "Normal and Hypnotic Sleep the Results of Inhibition of Mental Activity," *N.Y. Med. Jour.* 50 (1889):304, for a report of Brown-Séquard's research contradicting the sleep theory of Hammond and Arthur Durham.
33 Toby A. Appel, "Biological and Medical Societies and the Founding of the American Physiological Society," in *Physiology in the American Context 1850–1940*, ed. Gerald L. Geison (Bethesda, Md., 1987), pp. 155–76.

34 "New York Neurological Society," *N.Y. Med. Jour.* 51 (1890):636–38.
35 WAH, "Can We Diagnosticate Hyperaemia?" (see n. 9), pp. 678–80.
36 Ibid.; see also "New York Neurological Society," *N.Y. Med. Jour.* 52 (1890):553–57.

10. "A POSITIVE MENTAL SCIENCE"

1 WAH, "Brains and Muscles: Their Relative Training and Development," *Union College Practical Lectures* (Butterfield Course) (New York, 1895), 1:266.
2 See Edwin Clarke and L. C. Jacyna, *Nineteenth Century Origins of Neuroscientific Concepts* (Berkeley and Los Angeles and London, 1987).
3 [WAH], review of Henry Maudsley, *The Physiology and Pathology of the Mind,* in *Nation* 5 (1867):85–86.
4 [WAH], review of Henry Maudsley, *The Physiology and Pathology of the Mind,* in *Quart. Jour. Psych. Med. & Med. Jur.* 1 (1867):330. See also Michael J. Clark, "Rejection of Psychological Approaches to Mental Disorder in Late Nineteenth-Century British Psychiatry," in *Madhouses, Mad-Doctors, and Madmen: The Social History of Psychiatry in the Victorian Era,* ed. Andrew Scull (Philadelphia, 1981), pp. 271–312.
5 Editorial, *N. Eng. Med. Monthly* 1 (1881):41.
6 J. C. Bucknill, "Another Word for Dr. Beard," *Med. Rec.* 20 (1881):695–96; J. Crichton Browne, "A Word for Truth," *Med. Rec.* 21 (1882):23–26. See also J. Crichton Browne, "Dr. Beard's Experiments in Hypnotism," *Brit. Med. Jour.* 2 (1881):378–79; and "The Controversy Concerning Hypnotism," *Med. Rec.* 21 (1882):73.
7 See G. M. Beard, "The Moral Character of Trance Subjects," *Med. Rec.* 21 (1882):81–82.
8 WAH, "A Word for Dr. Beard," *Med. Rec.* 20 (1881):446–47.
9 H. Donkin, "Dr. Beard's Trained Subject," *Med. Rec.* 20 (1881):641–42; see also J. H. Girdner, "Concerning Hypnotism," *Med. Rec.* 20 (1881):472.
10 "Mesmerism and Crime. How Patients Might Be Led to Commit Crimes by Unscrupulous Persons," *New York Times,* 7 April 1881, p. 2, col. 7. See also "Crime Committed in the Mesmeric State," *Med. Rec.* 19 (1881):438; and "Startling Acts in Syggnosticism – Manifestations of an Extraordinary Kind Produced by Dr. W. A. Hammond," *Am. Med. Bi-Weekly* 12 (1881):112–14, reprinted from the *New York Times,* 28 January 1881.
11 WAH, "The Medico-Legal relations of Hypnotism or Syggignoscism [*sic*]," *N.Y. Med. Jour.* 45 (1887):115–21.
12 WAH, "Hypnotism," *Med. & Surg. Reporter* 45 (1881):649–54; G. M. Beard, "The Terminology of Trance," *Med. Rec.* 19 (1881):584–85.
13 WAH, *Insanity in Its Medico-Legal Relations:. Opinion Relative to the Testamentary Capacity of the Late James C. Johnson, of Chowan County, N.C.* (New York, 1866), p. 5; WAH, "A Medico-Legal Study of the Case of Daniel McFarland," *Jour. Psych. Med.* 4 (1870):458.
14 WAH, *A Treatise on Insanity in Its Medical Relations* (New York, 1883), p. 266.
15 WAH, "The Physiology and Pathology of the Cerebellum," *Quart. Jour. Psych. Med. & Med. Jur.* 3 (1869):209–44.
16 WAH, *A Treatise on the Diseases of the Nervous System* (New York, 1871), p. 324; and WAH, "The Brain Not the Sole Organ of the Mind," *Jour. Nerv. & Ment. Dis.,* n.s., 1 (1876):1–19.
17 WAH, *A Treatise on the Diseases of the Nervous System,* 6th ed. (New York, 1876), pp. 312, 325–28.
18 WAH, "On Thalamic Epilepsy," *Neur. Cont.* 1, no. 3 (1881):1–24. This paper was widely reprinted in medical journals. See also WAH, *Treatise on Insanity* (see n. 14), p. 33; WAH, "Thalamic Epilepsy," *Va. Med. Monthly* 13 (1886–87):447–83.

19 WAH, "The Relations Between the Mind and the Nervous System," *Pop. Sci. Monthly* 26 (1884):1–20.

20 WAH, *Treatise on Insanity* (see n. 14), pp. 33, 285–93.

21 WAH, "Mysophobia," *Neur. Cont.* 1, #1 (1879):40–54; and WAH, "Hebephrenia – Mental Derangement of Puberty," *Va. Med. Monthly* 19 (1892–93):1–9.

22 Among the many reviews of Hammond's *Treatise of Insanity* are those in *Jour. Nerv. & Ment. Dis.* 10 (1883):537–47; *Med. Rec.* 24 (1883):164–65; *N.Y. Med. Jour.* 37 (1883):687; *N. Eng. Med. Monthly* 2 (1883):415–16; *Va. Med. Monthly* 10 (1883):427–29; *Am. Jour. Neurol. & Psychiat.* 2 (1883):322–33.

23 Nancy Tomes, "A Generous Confidence: Thomas Story Kirkbride's Philosophy of Asylum Construction and Management," in *Madhouses, Mad-Doctors, and Madmen* (see n. 4), pp. 121–43.

24 See John Albert Pitts, "The Association of Medical Superintendents of American Institutions for the Insane, 1844–1892: A Case Study of Specialism in American Medicine" (Ph.D. diss., University of Pennsylvania, 1979).

25 Gray is quoted in "Medical Psychology" [editorial], *Med. Rec.* 5 (1870–71):541–43; see also "T," "Psychology in Our Medical Schools," *Med. Rec.* 5 (1870–71):550–51.

26 See Bonnie Ellen Blustein, "'A Hollow Square of Psychological Science': American Neurologists and Psychiatrists in Conflict," in *Madhouses, Mad-Doctors, and Madmen* (see n. 4), pp. 241–70.

27 Edward C. Spitzka, "Reform in the Scientific Study of Psychiatry," *Jour. Nerv. & Ment. Dis.* 5 (1878):200–29. See also New York Neurological Society, Minutes, on deposit in the Rare Book Room, New York Academy of Medicine (hereafter cited as NYNS Minutes), 4 March 1878.

28 Eugene Grissom, "True and False Experts," *Am. Jour. Insanity* 35 (1878–79):1–36; WAH, *An Open Letter to Eugene Grissom*, 2d ed. (New York, 1878); WAH, *A Second Open Letter to Eugene Grissom* (New York, 1878); WAH, *To The Medical Profession. January 15, 1879* (New York, 1879). For a recent account favorable to Grissom, see D. S. Werman, "True and False Experts: A Second Look" *Am. Jour. Psychiat.* 130 (1973):1351–54.

29 See E. A. Gaillard, review of Grissom, "True and False Experts," *Am. Med. Bi-Weekly* 9 (1878):56; review and analysis of the controversy in *St. Louis Clin. Rec.* 5 (1878):158–65; and editorial note, *Am. Jour. Insanity* 35 (1878–79):480–83.

30 See U.S. Senate Committee on Military Affairs, *Report to Accompany Bill S. 560*, 45th Cong., 2d sess., 19 February 1878, S. Rept. 102.

31 E. C. Spitzka, "Merits, Motives and Progress of the Reform in Asylum Abuses," *Jour. Nerv. & Ment. Dis.* 5 (1878):694–714.

32 WAH, "The Non-Asylum Treatment of the Insane," *Transactions of the Medical Society of New York* (1879), pp. 280–97; also published in *Neur. Cont.* 1, no. 1 (1879):1–22.

33 WAH, *Robert Severne: His Friends and His Enemies* (Philadelphia, 1867), p. 100.

34 WAH, *Diseases of the Nervous System* (see n. 16), pp. 383–84.

35 WAH, *Diseases of the Nervous System*, 6th ed. (see n. 17), p. 376.

36 WAH, *Treatise on Insanity* (see n. 14), pp. 720–21.

37 James Herbert Morse, *Diary*, 6:92 (30 January 1883), New-York Historical Society.

38 WAH, "The Construction, Organization and Equipment of Hospitals for the Insane," *Neur. Cont.* 1, #2 (1880):1–25.

39 See Blustein, "A Hollow Square" (see n. 26), for a fuller description of these events, which are reported in the NYNS Minutes (see n. 27).

40 "Treatment of the Insane," *New York Times*, 14 November 1879, p. 3, col. 1; see also [Editorial], *New York Times*, 9 March 1879, p. 4, cols. 6–7.

41 L. C. Gray, "Lunacy Reform," *Medical Record* 17 (1880):132–33. On NAPIPI see Barbara Sicherman, "The Quest for Mental Health in America" (Ph.D. diss., Columbia University, 1967).

42 Editorial, "Discussing Lunacy Reform," *Medical Record* 17 (1880):124; in the same issue, see also "A Petition Against Lunacy Reform," p. 192, and W. C. Church et al., "Lunacy Reform," p. 246.

43 WAH, "General Paralysis of the Insane, with Special Reference to the Case of Abraham Gosling," in "Proceedings of Societies," *Gaillard's Med. Jour.* 29 (1880):652–55, with report of discussion in the Medico-Legal Society, pp. 655–63. See also "The Case of Abraham Gosling," *Med. Rec.* 17 (1880):444; and "Medical News," *Am. Med. Biweekly* 13 (1881):286.

44 "Insane Asylum Methods, Alleged Abuses Laid Before the Senate Committee," *New York Times,* 2 December 1880, p. 8, col. 1.

45 NYNS Minutes (see n. 27), 7 December 1880.

11. "ALL MEN ARE INSANE"

1 [WAH], review of William Murray, *A Treatise on Emotional Disorders of the Sympathetic System of Nerves,* in *Quart. Jour. Psych. Med. & Med. Jur.* 1 (1867):336–37; quotation from S. W. Francis, *Biographical Sketches of Distinguished Living New York Physicians* (New York, 1867), p. 213; WAH, dedication to S. Weir Mitchell in *A Treatise on the Diseases of the Nervous System,* 6th ed. (New York, 1876); "A Treatise on Insanity in its Medical Relations" (unsigned review), *Alienist & Neurol.* 4 (1883):533.

2 University of the City of New York, Medical Department, *Fifth Annual Reunion Dinner of the Alumni* (New York, 1876), p. 58.

3 WAH, "A Few Words About the Nerves," *Galaxy* 6 (1868):183.

4 "A Treatise on Insanity in Its Medical Relations," anonymous review in *Am. Jour. Neurol. & Psychiat.* 2 (1883):322.

5 WAH, *A Treatise on Insanity* (New York, 1883), pp. [v], vi.

6 WAH, *Insanity in Its Medico-Legal Relations: Opinion Relative to the Testamentary Capacity of the Late James C. Johnston, of Chowan County, N.C.* (New York, 1866), pp. 2ff, 9ff, 21ff. See also "Johnston Will Case," *Quart. Jour. Psych. Med. & Med. Jur.* 1 (1867):157–59, which reprints the judge's charge to the jury; and an anonymous book review in *Med. Rec.* 2 (1867):206.

7 WAH, *Robert Severne: His Friends and His Enemies* (Philadelphia, 1867); Charles A. Lee, "Remarks on the Trial of Calvin M. Northrup, Esq., Indicted for the Crime of Administering Belladonna to His Wife, with Intent to Kill," *Quart. Jour. Psych. Med. & Med. Jur.* 2 (1868):28–47; [WAH], "Poisoning as a Science," *Nation* 1 (1865):243.

8 WAH, "The Medico-Legal Value of Confession as an Evidence of Guilt," *Jour. Psych. Med.* 5 (1871):359. See also "New York Medico-Legal Society," *Med. Rec.* 5 (1871):871–72.

9 WAH, *Doctor Grattan* (New York, 1885).

10 "Dr. Hammond's Suit Dismissed," *New York Times,* 24 June 1881, p. 3, cols. 1–2.

11 "Dr. Hammond's Novel," *Lit. World* 16 (1885):23, see also "Novels of the Week," *Athenaeum* (London), #3013 (1885):107–8.

12 WAH, "Abnormal Condition of Uncertainty," *N.Y. Med. Jour.* 44 (1886):509–10.

13 WAH, "Mysophobia," *Neur. Cont.* 1, no. 1 (1879):40–54.

14 WAH, "Abnormal Condition" (see n. 12), p. 510.

15 WAH, "Society versus Insanity," *Putnam's Magazine* 16 (1870):326ff; WAH, *Insanity in Its Relation to Crime: A Text and a Commentary* (New York, 1873), esp. pp. 49, 71.

16 WAH, "The Punishability of the Insane," *International Rev.* 11 (1881):448.

17 Charles E. Rosenberg, *The Trial of the Assassin Guiteau: Psychiatry and Law in the Gilded Age* (Chicago, 1968).

18 WAH, "Reasoning Mania; Its Medical and Medico-Legal Relations, with Special Reference to the Case of Charles J. Guiteau," *Jour. Nerv. & Ment. Dis.* 9 (1882):1–26; also published in *Sanitarian* 10 (1882):205–19; and see *N. Eng. Med. Monthly* 1

(1882):306. For reports on the discussion at the Medico-Legal Society see *Jour. Nerv. & Ment. Dis.* 9 (1882):375–82; Thomas L. Stedman, "Our New York Letter," *N. Eng. Med. Monthly* 1 (1882):310–14; and "Meeting of the New York Medico-Legal Society, March 1st 1882," *Med. Gaz.* 9 (1882):123–30.

19 WAH, "A Problem for Sociologists," *N. Am. Rev.* 135 (1882):423.

20 Cited in Rosenberg, *The Assassin Guiteau* (see n. 17), p. 157.

21 WAH, "Problem for Sociologists" (see n. 19), p. 423; "Madness and Murder," *N. Am. Rev.* 147 (1888):626.

22 WAH, "Problem for Sociologists" (see n. 19), pp. 431–32.

23 WAH, "A New Substitute for Capital Punishment and Means for Preventing the Propagation of Criminals," *N.Y. Med. Exam.* 1 (1892):190–94.

24 Ibid., pp. 422ff.; see also WAH, "Self-Control in Curing Insanity," *N. Am. Rev.* (1891):311–18.

25 "Guiteaumania," reprinted from *Brit. Med. Jour.*, in *Med. Gaz.* 9 (1882):356–58; "Progress in Neurology – Appendix," *Am. Jour. Neurol. & Psychiat.* 1 (1882):325. See also A. J. Spencer, "The Insanity of Guiteau," *N. Eng. Med. Monthly* 1 (1882):198–203.

26 Editorial, *Med. Gaz.* 4 (1870):222–23. See also review of M. G. Echeverría, *The Trial of John Reynolds, Medico-Legally Considered*, in *Med. Gaz.* 5 (1870):69–71.

27 "The Case of McFarland," *Phys. & Pharm.* 3 (1870):10. See also WAH, "A Medico-Legal Study of the Case of Daniel McFarland," *Jour. Psych. Med.* 4 (1870):449–81 (reprinted, New York, 1870); and New York County Courts, Court of General Sessions, *The Trial of Daniel McFarland . . . By a practical law reporter* (New York, 1870).

28 Thomas L. Stedman, "Our New York Letter," *N. Eng. Med. Monthly* 1 (1882):228.

29 WAH, *Robert Severne* (see n. 7), p. 358.

30 WAH, "Is Drunkenness Curable?" *N. Am. Rev.* 153 (1891):346–52. See also "Aberrations of the Sexual Instinct," excerpt from *London Med. Times & Gaz.*, in *Quart. Jour. Psych. Med. & Med. Jur.* 1 (1867):66–90.

31 C. H. Hughes, "Erotopathia; Morbid Erotism," *Proc. Pan-Am. Med. Cong.* 2, pt. 2 (1893), pp. 1845–46.

32 Whitelaw Reid, "The Press," in *Fifth Reunion* (see n. 2), p. 59. See also the remarks of George J. Fisher, p. 35, and A. E. MacDonald, p. 41.

33 WAH: "Woman," in *Fifth Reunion* (see n. 2), pp. 61–62; *Lal; a Novel* (New York, 1884); and *A Strong-Minded Woman; or, Two Years After* (New York, 1885).

34 WAH, "Woman," in *Fifth Reunion* (see n. 2), pp. 54–65.

35 WAH, "The Brain Not the Sole Organ of the Mind," *Jour. Nerv. & Ment. Dis.* 1 (1876):4.

36 WAH, "Woman," in *Fifth Reunion* (see n. 2), p. 65. See Steven Shapin and Barry Barnes, "Head and Hand: Rhetorical Resources in British Pedagogical Writing, 1770–1850," *Oxford Rev. of Ed.* 2 (1976):321–54, esp. p. 235.

37 WAH, "Woman in Politics," *N. Am. Rev.* 137 (1883):137–46. See also *Med.-Leg. Jour.* 1 (1884):635; and *N. Eng. Med. Monthly* 2 (1883):557.

38 WAH, "Woman in Politics" (see n. 37), passim. See also WAH, "How Shall Women Dress," *N. Am. Rev.* 140 (1885):565–68.

39 L. D. Blake et al., "Dr. Hammond's Estimate of Woman," *N. Am. Rev.* 137 (1883):495–519. On Blake and Lozier see entries in *Notable American Women 1607–1950: A Biographical Dictionary* (Cambridge, Mass., 1971).

40 See, for example, "Life Insurance and the Perils of Childbirth," *N.Y. Med. Jour.* 38 (1883):127.

41 James Herbert Morse, *Diary*, 7:9 (3 March 1884), in the collection of the New-York Historical Society.

42 WAH, "Slaughterhouses and Health," *Nation* 3 (1866):273–74.

43 WAH, "Brain-Forcing in Childhood," *Pop. Sci. Monthly* 30 (1886–87):722ff. See also WAH, "The Relations Between the Mind and the Nervous System," *Pop. Sci. Monthly* 26 (1884):1–20.

44 Morse, *Diary* (see n. 41); H. H. Gardener, "Sex and Brain Weight," *Pop. Sci. Monthly* 31 (1887):266–68, 698–700. See also A. Washburn, "Helen H. Gardener," in *Notable American Women* (see n. 39).

45 WAH, "Men's and Women's Brains," *Pop. Sci. Monthly* 31 (1887):554–58; also his brief note, p. 846.

46 [WAH], review of S. B. Brittan, *Man and His Relations*, in *N.Y. Med. Jour.* 1 (1865):64; WAH, *On Certain Conditions of Nervous Derangement* (New York, 1881), pp. 18–20. See also Joseph Czermak, "Hypnotism in Animals," trans. Clara Hammond, in *Pop. Sci. Month.* 3 (1873):618–27. The translator, the neurologist's daughter, was fourteen years old.

47 WAH, *Certain Conditions* (see n. 46), pp. 95–113. See also "He Wouldn't Stand the Test," *Med. Gaz.* 7 (1880):79; "Tanner," p. 517; and note, p. 543.

48 WAH, *Certain Conditions* (see n. 46), p. 59; WAH, "Merlin and His Influence on the English Character and Literature," *Quart. Jour. Psych. Med. & Med. Jur.* 1 (1867):27–49.

49 See "Physiology and Materialism – Some New Philosophical Views," *Med. Rec.* 20 (1881):127–28; J. Richardson Parke, "Does Medical Science tend to Materialism?" *N.Y. Med. Jour.* 53 (1891):29–31; and S. S. Turner, "Death from Brain Disease without Symptoms," *N.Y. Med. Jour.* 53 (1891):299–300.

50 [WAH], "The Hygienic Relations of Celibacy," *Nation* 5 (1867):357–58; WAH, *Certain Conditions* (see n. 46), pp. 43–47; see also [WAH], review of Henry C. Lea, *The Psychology of Celibacy*, in *Quart. Jour. Psych. Med. & Med. Jur.* 1 (1867):317–26.

51 WAH, *Certain Conditions* (see n. 46), pp. 120–21; see also Polydore Vergil, *Polydori Virgilii de Rerum Inventoribus*, trans. into English by John Langley [1663] with an account of the author and his works by WAH (New York, 1868).

52 WAH, *Certain Conditions* (see n. 46), p. 123.

53 WAH, "On the Evolution of the Boycott," *Forum* 1 (1886):369–76; Henry A. Brann, "Dr. Hammond as an Amateur Theologian," *Cath. World* 43 (1886):651–59.

54 WAH, *The Son of Perdition* (Chicago, 1898); review in *Nation* 68 (1899):167; and review in *Lit. World* 30 (1899):7.

55 "Medical Novelists," *Med. Rec.* 26 (1884):103; C. K. Mills, "Some Recollections of the Early Meetings and Personnel of the American Neurological Association," in American Neurological Association, *Semicentennial Anniversary Volume* (Albany, N.Y., 1924), pp. 20–21.

12. "I SAID THAT I WOULD BE BACK"

1 WAH to [Walter F.] Atlee, 20 May 1888, Mayo Clinic Library, Rochester, Minn.

2 "Letter from Washington," *N.Y. Med. Jour.* 48 (1888):599.

3 *The Hammond Sanitarium for Diseases of the Nervous System, Diseases of the Skin and for those Diseases Generally in which the Hammond Animal Extracts are Especially Useful* (Washington, D.C., 1894), pp. 47–48. A copy of this advertisement is in the file of In Equity #17,060, Record Group 21 (U.S. Supreme Court of the D. of C., Law Cases 1863–1934), National Archives. See also WAH, "Bill of Complaint," in the same file.

4 *The Hammond Sanitarium* (see n. 3); WAH, "Brains and Muscles: Their Relative Training and Development," *Union College Practical Lectures* (Butterfield Course) (New York, 1895), 1:274–77.

5 WAH, "Bill of Complaint" (see n. 3). See also the "Personal" column, *Buffalo Med. and Surg. Jour.* 28 (1888–89):421.

6 WAH, "Brain Surgery," *North Am. Rev.* 156 (1893):390–96.

7 WAH, "A Case of Brain Surgery and Its Relations to Cerebral Localization," *N.Y. Med. Jour.* 52 (1890):337–40; see also a note in *N.Y. Med. Jour.* 50 (1889):672; WAH, "Merycism," *N.Y. Med. Jour.* 60 (1894):109–11. For a report of the discus-

sion following presentation of this paper before the American Neurological Association see *N.Y. Med. Jour.* 61 (1895):27.

8 WAH, "Seven Recent Cases of Brain Surgery," *Med. News* 59 (Philadelphia, 1891):501–5.

9 WAH, "The Fetichism of Antisepsis," *Am. Medico-Surgical Bull.* 7 (1894):70–73.

10 Merriley Borrell, "Organotherapy, British Physiology, and the Discovery of the Internal Secretions," *Jour. Hist. Biol.* 9 (1976):235–68. See also J. M. D. Olmsted, *Charles-Edouard Brown-Séquard: A Nineteenth-Century Neurologist and Endocrinologist* (Baltimore, 1956).

11 Merriley Borrell, "Brown-Séquard's Organotherapy and Its Appearance in America at the End of the Nineteenth Century," *Bull. Hist. Med.* 50 (1976):309–20; Diana Long Hall and Thomas F. Glick, "Endocrinology: A Brief Introduction," *Jour. Hist. Biol.* 9 (1976):229–33; and A. F. W. Hughes, "A History of Endocrinology," ed. Margaret Wells Egar, *Jour. Hist. Med.* 32 (1977):292–313.

12 WAH, *Sexual Impotence in the Male* (New York, 1883; reprint 1886); and WAH, *Sexual Impotence in the Male and Female* (Detroit, 1887). Excerpts were reprinted in several medical journals and the works were translated into Italian, German, French, and Russian.

13 WAH, "On Myxoedema, with Special Reference to Its Cerebral and Nervous Systems," *Neur. Cont.* 1, no. 3 (1881):36–43; also published in *Boston Med. & Surg. Jour.* 103 (1880):14–15. The discussion of this paper before the June 1880 meeting of the American Neurological Association is reported in *Med. Rec.* 18 (1880):240–46. See also WAH, "Weak Heart and Its Treatment," *Ther. Gaz.*, 3d ser., 6 (1890):667–73; also published in *N.Y. Med. Jour.* 49 (1889):218–19.

14 *Hammond Sanitarium* (see n. 3).

15 WAH, "Experiments Relative to the Therapeutical Value of the Expressed Juice of the Testicles when Hypodermically Introduced into the Human System," *N.Y. Med. Jour.* 50 (1889):232–34. The title of this paper is strikingly similar to that of Hammond's A.M.A.-prize essay of 1857, suggesting that he may have expected comparable recognition for it. A Wisconsin physician suggested that Hammond had tried to rejuvenate not only himself but his mother-in-law. See J. F. Pember, "Serotherapy," *Trans. Wisc. State Med. Soc.* 35 (1901):145.

16 WAH, "Experiments Relative to the Therapeutical Value" (see n. 15).

17 "Doctors Who Disagree," *New York Times*, 23 August 1889, p. 2., col. 4; "Another Victim of the Elixir," *New York Times*, 3 September 1889, p. 1., col. 4. See also R. Harvey Reed, "The Use of Pulverized Testicle Juice as a Therapeutic Agent," *Jour. Nat. Assoc. Railway Surgeons* 2 (1889):161–64.

18 Borrell, "Brown-Séquard's Organotherapy" (see n. 11).

19 "Dr. Brown-Séquard," *New York Times*, 3 April 1894, p. 5, col. 5; Oscar H. Merrill, "Notes on Recent Therapeutics," *Am. Ther.* 2 (1894):193–94.

20 George L. Freeman, "Organic Extracts in the Treatment of Disease," *N.Y. Med. Times* 21 (1893):199–203. A note in this homeopathic journal suggests that the article had appeared previously in other periodicals, including *Am. Ther.*, *Medical Age*, and the prestigious *Bost. Med. & Surg. Jour.*

21 G. Archie Stockwell, "A Study of the 'Organic Extracts' 'Cerebrine' and 'Cerebrin,' " *Med. News* (Philadelphia) 63 (1893):231—34. See WAH, "On Certain Organic Extracts: Their Preparation and Physiological and Therapeutical Effects," *N.Y. Med. Jour.* 57 (1893):93–96. The same article, with varying titles, also appeared in the *Va. Med. Monthly* 19 (1893):993–1003; the *Am. Med.-Surg. Bull.* 6 (1893):179–84; and the *Post-Graduate Med. Jour.* 8 (1893):97–105. Cf. WAH, "A New Process for Extracting the Essential Principles of Certain Animal Organs, and on their Physiological and Therapeutic Properties," reported in the *N.Y. Med. Jour.* 58 (1893):359.

22 WAH, "On Certain Organic Extracts" (see n. 21), pp. 94–95; see also *Method of Administration of the Animal Extracts, Prepared According to the Formula of Dr. William A. Hammond, and Under His Supervision* (Washington, D.C.: Columbia Chemical Company, 1894).

23 WAH, "On Certain Organic Extracts" (see n. 21), pp. 95–96.
24 WAH, "Cardine; the Extract of the Heart. Its Preparation and Physiological and Therapeutical Effects," *N.Y. Med. Jour.* 57 (1893):429–31; J. S. Leonhardt, "Organic Juices in Therapeutics," *N.Y. Med. Jour.* 57 (1893):641–43; WAH, "A Further Contribution to the Subject of 'Animal Extracts,'" *N.Y. Med. Jour.* 58 (1893):14–15; J. S. Leonhardt, "The Sphygmograph as an Instrument of Precision," *N.Y. Med. Jour.* 58 (1893):225–26; and WAH, "The Sphygmograph as an Instrument of Precision (with Apologies to Dr. Leonhardt)," *N.Y. Med. Jour.* 58 (1893):588–89.
25 "The Injections of Organic Liquids and Their Utility in Therapeutics," *Boston Med. & Surg. Jour.* 128 (1893):46–47; Wallace Wood, "Sarcology and Sarcotherapeutics," *N.Y. Med. Jour.* 57 (1893):457–58; see also "Sarcology," *Am. Ther.* 1 (1893):290.
26 G. Archie Stockwell, "Historical, Critical and Scientific Aspects of Brown-Séquard's Discovery – The So-Called 'Elixir,'" *Ther. Gaz.*, 3d ser., 5 (1889): 812–19, and 6 (1890):14–19; Stockwell, "A Study of the Organic Extracts" (see n. 21); G. A. Stockwell, "Wants Cerebrine," *Jour. Am. Med. Assoc.* 21 (1893):395; and WAH, "Can Get All the Cerebrine He Wants," *Jour. Am. Med. Assoc.* 21 (1893):464. See also A. Jacobi, "Thyreoid Extract," *N.Y. Med. Jour.* 61 (1895):21.
27 "A Clinical Test of Some of the So-called Organic Extracts," reported from the *Boston Med. & Surg. Jour.*, in *N.Y. Med. Jour.* 63 (1896):160–61.
28 M. Delafontaine, "Analysis of 'Cerebrine,'" *Jour. Am. Med. Assoc.* 21 (1893):323.
29 WAH, "Dr. Hammond Replies to His Critics," *Jour. Am. Med. Assoc.* 21 (1893):428; Delafontaine, "Cerebrin Again," *Jour. Am. Med. Assoc.* 21 (1893):868 (reprinted in *Med. News* 63 [1893]:672); J. H. Long, "Analysis of 'Cerebrine' and 'Medulline,'" *Jour. Am. Med. Assoc.* 21 (1893):1015.
30 The Hammond Animal Extract Co., *The Hammond Animal Extracts. Isopathy or, the Treatment of Diseased Organs of the Body by Extracts of the Corresponding Organs . . .* (New York, 1898). It is interesting that "sexual apathy" in women was by this time considered pathological rather than a sign of natural delicacy.
31 WAH, "On Certain Organic Extracts" (see n. 21), pp. 93, 96.
32 "Editorial," *Jour. Am. Med. Assoc.* 20 (1893):162; Henry Hun, "The Uses and Abuses of Animal Extracts as Medicine," *N.Y. Med. Jour.* 61 (1895):33–37.
33 Russell C. Maulitz, "'Physician versus Bacteriologist': The Ideology of Science in Clinical Medicine," in *The Therapeutic Revolution*, ed. Maurice J. Vogel and Charles E. Rosenberg (Philadelphia, 1979), pp. 91–108. See also Knud Faber, *Nosography: The Evolution of Clinical Medicine in Modern Times*, 2d ed. (New York, 1930).
34 WAH, "On Certain Organic Extracts" (see n. 21), p. 93.
35 John Aulde, "True Isopathy" and "Organopathy," *Am. Ther.* 1 (1893):192–93 and 193–94; see also "'Organopathy'" and "'True Isopathy,'" *N.Y. Med. Jour.* 57 (1893):247 and 359–60. See also "Animal Extracts in Early Medical Annals," *Jour. Am. Med. Assoc.* 21 (1893):315–16, which cites allegedly parallel examples from Nicholas Culpeper's *Dispensatory* (1650) and other sources.
36 [William Henry Porter], "Animal Extracts," *Am. Med.-Surg. Bull.* 6 (1893):593–98.
37 WAH, "Animal Extracts," *Am. Med.-Surg. Bull.* 6 (1893):811–17.
38 Ibid., p. 815.
39 Ibid., pp. 816–17; WAH, "Cardine" (see n. 24).
40 [William Henry Porter], "Animal Juices," *Am. Med.-Surg. Bull.* 6 (1893):907–13.
41 Ibid., pp. 910–13.
42 M. Semmola, "On the Therapeutic Antagonism of Natural Diseases," *Am. Med.-Surg. Bull.* 6 (1893):930–34.
43 C. L. Dana, "Modern Pathology and the Pathology of Nervous Diseases, with Some Therapeutic Deductions and Experiments with Organic Extracts," *Boston Med. & Surg. Jour.* 128 (1893):486–90; also the report of the discussion of this paper in the Boston Medico-Psychological Association, 16 March 1893, *Boston*

Med. & Surg. Jour. 128 (1893):500; and "Organic Extracts: The New Departure in Neurological Therapeutics," *Boston Med. & Surg. Jour.* 129 (1893):19–20.

44 WAH, "Animal Therapeutics in the Treatment of Cerebral Hyperaemia," *Charlotte Med. Jour.* 8 (1896):158.

45 See, for example, H. Baillon and A. Zuccarelli, "Animal Juices and Artificial Serums," *Am. Med.-Surg. Bull.* 6 (1893):954–59; J. N. Baskett, "Some Observations on Nuclein Therapy," *Am. Ther.* 4 (1895):81–84; and F. Kraus, "The Present Status of Animal Therapeutics," translated from *Therapeutische Wochenschrift,* in *Jour. Am. Med. Assoc.* 26 (1896):528–32.

46 Frank C. Wilson, "Early Experience with Brown-Séquard's Elixir and Recent Experience with the Roberts-Hawley Lymph," *Jour. Am. Animal Ther. Assoc.* 1 (1900):3–12; cf. Joseph R. Hawley, *The New Animal Cellular Therapy* (Chicago, 1901).

47 See, for example, W. W. Young, "Isopathy and Homeopathy: Their Relationship," *Jour. Am. Inst. Homeopathy* 28 (1935):741–43; and G. W. Mackenzie, "The Comparative Merits of Isopathy and Homeopathy," *Hahneman. Month.* 71 (1936):788–92.

48 John V. Shoemaker, "Progress and Problems of Medicine Today," *N.Y. Med. Jour.* 66 (1897):549–50; Joseph McFarland, "Serum Therapy," and Oliver T. Osborne, "Organotherapy," in *A System of Physiological Therapeutics,* ed. S. Solis-Cohen (Philadelphia, 1905), 11:17–65, 69–122.

49 S. J. Meltzer, "On the Thyreoid Therapy: Its History and Use in Internal Medicine," *N.Y. Med. Jour.* 61 (1895):651–56; S. Solis-Cohen, "The Possibilities and Uses of Organic Extracts," reprinted from *The Polyclinic* in *Med. News* (Philadelphia) 63 (1893):696. Cf. "Animal Extracts Again," editorial, *Am. Med.-Surg. Bull.* 7 (1894):833–37; J. Lindsay Porteous, "Myxedema, Its History, Etiology, Pathology and Treatment," *Am. Ther.* 2 (1893):1–9; and "The Thyroid Treatment of Myxedema," *Am. Ther.* 2 (1893):97–100.

50 Hammond Animal Extract Co., *The Hammond Animal Extracts* (see n. 30).

13. "VERY NEAR BEING A GREAT MAN"

1 Documentation of the history of the Columbia Chemical Company can be found in the records of *Columbia Chemical Co.* v. *Hammond Sanitarium Company, William A. Hammond and Mahlon Hutchinson,* In Equity #16,448, Record Group 21 (U.S. Supreme Court of the D. of C., Law Cases 1863–1934), National Archives. See esp. the "Amended Bill of Complaint."

2 See "An Unsuccessful Attempt at Discipline" and "Medical Ethics," *N.Y. Med. Jour.* 58 (1893):603, 614–15.

3 Ernest Hart, [Address on the American Medical Profession], *Trans. Pan-Am. Med. Cong.* 2 (1893, pt. 2):132–35. Cf. the stenographic abstract published as "Mr. Ernest Hart on the Profession, the Public, and the Code," *N.Y. Med. Jour.* 58 (1893):420–24. See also WAH, "Mr. Ernest Hart and the American Medical Profession," *N.Y. Med. Jour.* 58 (1893):325–27; and Ernest Hart, "Dr. Hammond and the Medical Profession," *N.Y. Med. Jour.* 58 (1893):395, also published in *Jour. Am. Med. Assoc.* 21 (1893):508–9 and *Med. News* (Philadelphia) 63 (1893):339–40. See also Ernest Hart, "A Distinguished English Visitor on the American Medical Profession," *N.Y. Med. Jour.* 58 (1893):442–43; "A House Divided Against Itself," *N.Y. Med. Jour.* 58 (1893):127; Medicas (pseud.), "Personal Ethics for Visiting Foreigners," *Jour. Am. Med. Assoc.* 21 (1893):746. For a vivid sketch of Ernest Hart, see "Letter from London," *N.Y. Med. Jour.* 44 (1886):353.

4 "Dr. Hammond Explains His Relations to the Columbia Chemical Company," *Jour. Am. Med. Assoc.* 21 (1893):1023.

5 See *Columbia Chemical Co.* v. *Hammond* records (see n. 1).

6 See Jonathan Liebenau, *Medical Science and Medical Industry* (Baltimore, 1987).

7 The preceding paragraphs are summarized from WAH to Board of the Columbia Chemical Co., 6 September 1894, filed with *Columbia Chemical Co.* v. *Hammond* records (see n. 1).
8 Copy for these advertisements is included as an exhibit in the *Columbia Chemical Co.* v. *Hammond* records (see n. 1).
9 Documentation of the history of the Hammond Sanitarium, Inc., can be found in the records of *William A. Hammond, plaintiff* v. *Mahlon Hutchinson, defendant*, In Equity #17,060, Record Group 21 (U.S. Supreme Court of the D. of C., Law Cases 1863–1934), National Archives. See esp. the "Bill of Complaint."
10 See W. C. Boteler to Columbia Chemical Co., 7 May 1895, and "Exhibit #7," filed with *Columbia Chemical Co.* v. *Hammond* records (see n. 1).
11 The Hammond Sanitarium Co., *Animal Extracts Prepared According to the Process of Dr. William A. Hammond* (Washington, D.C., [1895]).
12 Mahlon Hutchinson to W. P. Springer, Esq., 9 May 1895, filed with *Columbia Chemical Co.* v. *Hammond* records (see n. 1).
13 See *Columbia Chemical Co.* v. *Hammond* records (see n. 1); also Supreme Court of the District of Columbia, *The Columbia Chemical Company vs. the Hammond Sanitarium Company . . . Opinion by Mr. Justice Hagner* (Washington, D.C., 1895). The restraining order against Hammond was dissolved in May 1897; see *Columbia Chemical Co.* v. *Hammond* records (see n. 1), Equity Minutes, vol. 49, pp. 98, 102.
14 WAH to William P. Springer, 22 July 1895, filed with *Columbia Chemical Co.* v. *Hammond* records (see n. 1).
15 See the records of *The Hammond Sanitarium Co., plaintiff* v. *Mahlon Hutchinson, and E. Francis Riggs, Charles C. Glover, Thomas Hyde and James M. Johnston*, In Equity #16,849, Record Group 21 (U.S. Supreme Court of the D. of C., Law Cases 1863–1934), National Archives.
16 See the records of *Mahlon Hutchinson* v. *Wm. A. Hammond and the Hammond Sanitarium Co.*, In Equity #6850 [*sic* – probably #16,850]. Record Group 21 (see n. 1); see also "Bill of Complaint" (see n. 9).
17 "Bill of Complaint" (see n. 9); Supreme Court of the District of Columbia, In Equity #17,060. *William A. Hammond* v. *Mahlon Hutchinson* (Washington, 1896). Hammond also took pains to disassociate himself from another establishment, the "Institute for the Administration of the Animal Extracts," which advertised in the New York newspapers in 1895; see WAH, "Animal Extracts," *N.Y. Med. Jour.* 61 (1895):54.
18 WAH, *Cerebral Hyperaemia* (New York, 1877), pp. 5–6.
19 Charles L. Dana, "Early Neurology in the United States," *Jour. Am. Med. Assoc.* 90 (1928):1422; cf. J. G. Hopkins, "A Spicy Letter, in which a Georgia Doctor Tells What He Knows About Dr. Wm. A. Hammond, of New York, and His Treatment of a Georgia Patient," *Atlanta Med. & Surg. Jour.*, n.s., 1 (1884–85):413–16; WAH, "What Should a Doctor be Paid?" *N. Am. Rev.* 158 (1894):660–67; cf. WAH, "Medico-legal Points in The Case of David Montgomery," *Jour. Psych. Med.* 6 (1872):62–76, in which he defended the propriety of accepting a $500 fee.
20 See "Unwarrantable Use of Physicians' Names," *N.Y. Med. Jour.* 46 (1887):701.
21 WAH, Introduction to *Notes on Epidemics for the Use of the Public*, by Francis Edmund Anstie (1st Am. ed., Philadelphia, 1866), p. iii.
22 WAH, "The Elixir of Life," *N. Am. Rev.* 149 (1889):257–64.
23 D. A. Cathell, *The Physician Himself, and What He Should Add to the Strictly Scientific* (Baltimore, 1882); J. J. Taylor, *The Physician as Business Man* (Philadelphia, 1891).
24 [George Shrady], "The Moral Danger of the American Medical Profession," *Med. Rec.* 28 (1885):264. Similar expressions of sentiment abound in the medical literature of the period.
25 [E. R. Squibb], "The Codes of Medical Ethics," *Ephemeris* 1 (1883):179, 195.

26 "Ethics and Medicine," *New York Times*, 19 February 1882, p. 8, col. 6. See also John S. Haller, Jr., *American Medicine in Transition, 1840–1910* (Urbana and Chicago, Ill., 1981), pp. 263–265.

27 Hammond's remarks were reported in several journals; see, for example, *Am. Med. Weekly* 15 (1882):649.

28 WAH, "On the Evolution of the Boycott," *Forum* 1 (1886):369–76.

29 [Frank P. Foster], "William A. Hammond, M.D., LL.D.," *N.Y. Med. Jour.* 71 (1900):64.

30 Arthur A. Michell to War Department, November 1897, in Box 577, Record Group 94, National Archives.

31 WAH, *A Mysterious Life; A Four-Act Drama* [New York, 1901], p. [4].

32 Mark D. Miller, "William A. Hammond: Restoring the Reputation of a Surgeon General," *Mil. Med.* 152 (1987):452–57.

33 WAH to His Excellency, the President, 8 March 1899, in Box 577, Record Group 94, National Archives; see also Miller, "William A. Hammond" (see n. 32), p. 456.

34 H. C. McLean to Col William H. Carter, 1 March 1900, File E-561, Record Group 94, National Archives; [Foster], "William A. Hammond" (see n. 29), p. 64; Charles L. Dana, "Hammond, the Teacher," *Post-Graduate* 15 (1900):622. Documents regarding funeral arrangements are contained in Box 577, Record Group 94, National Archives.

35 [Foster], "William A. Hammond" (see n. 29).

36 WAH, "The Coming Man," *Forum* 1 (1886):76–78.

Note on sources

There is evidence that Hammond kept detailed notes on his patients and engaged in an extensive correspondence, but the bulk of these and other papers, personal and professional, including his doctoral thesis on "The Etiological and Therapeutical Influence of the Imagination," have most likely been destroyed. His career must therefore be reconstructed primarily from his own extensive published work, listed below, and from other materials in contemporary medical journals. These often included "news and notes" items as well as editorial comments and formal articles. Contemporary and retrospective biographical essays on Hammond have been cited in the text where appropriate, and will not be listed here. One of the more useful sources is a collection of obituary essays in *Post-Graduate* 15 (1900):2–40. Hammond's early scientific endeavors in Kansas and Philadelphia are documented in excellent collections of letters preserved in the John L. LeConte Papers, American Philosophical Society, Philadelphia; and in the Joseph Leidy Papers and the Minutes and Correspondence of the Academy of Natural Sciences of Philadelphia.

The classic study of Civil War medicine is George Washington Adams, *Doctors in Blue: The Medical History of the Union Army in the Civil War* (New York: Schumann, 1952), complemented by W. Q. Maxwell, *Lincoln's Fifth Wheel: The Political History of the U.S. Sanitary Commission* (New York, 1956). For more recent analyses, see Bonnie Ellen Blustein, "'To Increase the Efficiency of the Medical Department': A New Approach to Medicine in the U.S. Civil War," *Civil War History* 33 (1987):22–41; and Frank R. Freemon, "Lincoln Finds a Surgeon General: William A. Hammond and the Transformation of the Union Army Medical Bureau," *Civil War History* 33 (1987):5–21. The National Archives contain large quantities of valuable material on medicine in the Civil War era, most of which has not been examined carefully. The correspondence of the surgeon general's office has been preserved in Record Group 112, which also includes indexes of letters received and letterpress copies of letters and telegrams sent. In some cases, endorsements on letters indicate the disposition of the matter. All the records were carefully cross-referenced by index number, but users should be warned that it is not always easy to locate an original letter in this way. Files on individual physicians can be found in Record Group 94 (Records of the Adjutant General's Office) in two categories: "Personal Papers of Medical Officers" and "Appointments, Commissions and Promotions" (the ACP file).

The voluminous manuscript record of Hammond's court-martial is available, indexed, in the National Archives. This episode has been studied in some detail: the best account is Mark D. Miller, "William A. Hammond: Restoring the Reputation of a Surgeon General," *Military Medicine* 152 (1987):452–57. For a detailed legal discussion of the charges, see Henry C. Friend, "Abraham Lincoln and the Court Martial of Surgeon General William A. Hammond," *Commercial Law Journal* 62 (1957):71–80. See also Lewis C. Duncan, "The Days Gone By: The Strange Case of Surgeon General Hammond," *Military Surgeon* 64 (1929):98–110, 252–61.

For a general overview of the context of Hammond's neurological career, see Charles E. Rosenberg, "The Practice of Medicine in New York a Century Ago," *Bulletin of the History of Medicine* 41 (1967):223–53; George Rosen, *The Structure of American Medical Practice 1875–1941,* edited by Charles E. Rosenberg (Philadelphia, 1983); and Bonnie Ellen Blustein, "Neurology in New York: A Case Study in the Specialization of Medicine," *Bulletin of the History of Medicine* 53 (1979):170–83. Records of the American Neurological Association and the New York Neurological Society are housed at the New York Academy of Medicine. See also the *Centennial Anniversary Volume* (New York: Springer, 1975) and the *Semi-Centennial Anniversary Volume* (Albany, N.Y.: American Neurological Association, 1924) of the American Neurological Association. The diaries of James Herbert Morse and the records of the National Institute of Letters, Arts and Sciences, both at the New-York Historical Society, were also useful.

268   *Note on sources*

On Hammond's Washington sanitarium and his work there on the animal extracts, much information not available in the published record can be found in federal court records of the District of Columbia, in the National Archives (Record Group 21). The specific cases are In Equity #16,448, #16,849, #16,850, and #17,060. These files include correspondence and copies of brochures and advertisements.

For a bibliography of published primary and secondary materials relating to Hammond, see Bonnie Ellen Blustein, "A New York Medical Man: William Alexander Hammond, M.D. (1828–1900), Neurologist" (Ph.D. diss., University of Pennsylvania, 1979). For an annotated bibliography of Hammond's works, arranged chronologically, see Jack D. Key and Bonnie Ellen Blustein, *William A. Hammond, M.D. (1828–1900): The Publications of an American Neurologist* (Rochester, Minn.: Davies, 1983).

Bibliography of William Alexander Hammond, M.D.

MONOGRAPHS

Cerebral Hyperaemia the Result of Mental Strain or Emotional Disturbance. New York: Putnam, 1878. 2d. ed., Washington: Brentano, 1895.

Clinical Lectures on Diseases of the Nervous System. Reported, edited, and histories of the cases prepared, with notes, by T. M. B. Cross. New York: Appleton, 1874.

Fasting Girls; Their Physiology and Pathology. New York: Putnam, 1879.

Insanity in Its Medico-Legal Relations. Opinion Relative to the Testamentary Capacity of the Late James C. Johnston, of Chowan County, N.C. New York: Baker, Voorhis & Co., 1866.

Insanity in Its Relations to Crime. A Text and a Commentary. New York: Appleton, 1873.

Lectures on Venereal Diseases. Philadelphia: Lippincott, 1864.

On Certain Conditions of Nervous Derangement. New York: Putnam, 1881. Rev. ed., 1883.

On Wakefulness: With an Introductory Chapter on the Physiology of Sleep. Philadelphia: Lippincott, 1866.

The Physics and Physiology of Spiritualism. New York: Appleton, 1871.

Physiological Memoirs. Philadelphia: Lippincott, 1863.

Sexual Impotence in the Male. New York: Birmingham, 1883. Detroit: Warren, 1886.

Sexual Impotence in the Male and Female. Detroit: Davis, 1887. Reprint ed., New York: Arno Press, 1974.

Sleep and Its Derangements. Philadelphia: Lippincott, 1869. Reprint eds., 1878, 1883.

Sleep, Sleeplessness and the Derangements of Sleep; Or, the Hygiene of the Night. London: Simpkin, 1892.

Spinal Irritation (Posterior Spinal Anaemia). Detroit: Davis, 1886. 2nd ed., 1891.

Spiritualism and Allied Causes and Conditions of Nervous Derangement. New York: Putnam, 1876. London: Lewis, 1876.

A Treatise on Hygiene, with Special Reference to the Military Service. Philadelphia: Lippincott, 1863.

A Treatise on Insanity in Its Medical Relations. New York: Appleton, 1883. Reprint eds., 1891; Arno Press, 1973.

A Treatise on the Diseases of the Nervous System. New York: Appleton, 1871. 2d ed., 1872. 3d ed., 1873. 4th ed., 1874. 5th ed., 1876. 6th ed., 1876. 7th ed., 1881. 8th ed., 1886. 9th ed. (With G. M. Hammond), 1891. Rev. eds., 1892, 1893, 1898.

PAMPHLETS AND BROADSIDES

Defence of Brigadier General William A. Hammond, Surgeon-General, U.S. Army. With His Statement of the Causes Which Led to His Dismissal. Washington, D.C.: Printed for the author, 1864.

Disease of the Scythians: Morbus Feminarum and Certain Analogous Conditions. N.p., 1882.

Experimental Researches Relative to the Nutritive Value and Physiological Effects of Albumen, Starch, and Gum, When Singly and Exclusively Used as Food, being the Prize Essay of the American Medical Association for 1857. Philadelphia: Collins, 1857.

A Medico-Legal Study of the Case of Daniel McFarland. Read before the Medico-Legal Society of the City of New York, May 12, 1870. New York: Appleton, 1870.

Memorial to the U.S. Senate, Concerning the Withdrawal of His Commission as Surgeon-General. New York, 1864. Broadside.

The Official Correspondence Between Surgeon-General William A. Hammond, U.S.A., and the Adjutant-General of the Army, Relative to the Founding of the Army Museum and the Inauguration of the Medical and Surgical History of the War. New York: Appleton, 1883.

An Open Letter to Eugene Grissom, M.D. New York: Trow's, 1878. 2d ed., 1878.

Personal Recollections of General Nathaniel Lyon. Washington, D.C.: Military Order of the Loyal Legion of the United States, 1900.

Report on the Subject of Scurvy with Special Reference to Practice in the Army and Navy. (By William A. Hammond et al.) Washington, D.C.: Government Printing Office, 1862.

A Second Open Letter to Dr. Eugene Grissom. New York: Trow's, 1878.

Spinal Irritation: Its Pathology and Treatment. New York: Putnam, 1876.

A Statement of the Causes Which Led to the Dismissal of Surgeon-General William A. Hammond from the Army, with a Review of the Evidence Adduced Before the Court. New York: Printed for the author, 1864.

To the Medical Profession. New York: Trow's, 1879.

WORKS EDITED

Electricity in Its Relations to Practical Medicine, by Moritz Meyer. Translated from the 3d. German ed., with notes and additions by William A. Hammond. New York: Appleton, 1869. Reprint ed., 1874.

Electrophysiology and Therapeutics: Being a Study of the Muscular and Other Systems During Health and Disease, Including the Phenomena of the Electric Fishes, by Charles E. Morgan. New York: Wood, 1868.

Journal of Nervous and Mental Diseases, 1876–83.

Journal of Psychological Medicine, 1870–72.

Maryland and Virginia Medical Journal, 1860–61.

Military Medical and Surgical Essays Prepared for the U.S. Sanitary Commission. Philadelphia: Lippincott, 1864.

Neurological Contributions, 1879–81.

New York Medical Journal, 1865–67.
Polydori Virgilii de Rerum Inventoribus, by Polydore Virgil. Translated by John Langley, with an account of the author and his works by William A. Hammond. New York: Agathynian Club, 1868.
Psychological and Medico-Legal Journal, 1874–75.
Quarterly Journal of Psychological Medicine and Medical Jurisprudence, 1867–69.

ARTICLES IN PROFESSIONAL JOURNALS

"Abnormal Condition of Uncertainty." *New York Medical Journal* 44 (1886):509–10.
"Abraham Lincoln." *New York Medical Journal* 1 (1865):163–64.
"Abstract of a Lecture Upon the Therapeutics of Wakefulness." *Medical Record* 3 (1868):436–37.
"Abstracts of Lectures on the Therapeutics of Pain." *Medical Gazette* 1 (1868):203–4, 210–12, 219–21, 226–28, 243–46.
"Allochiria: Its Nature and Seat." *New York Medical Journal* 37 (1883):35–37; *Journal of Nervous and Mental Diseases,* n.s., 8 (1883):263–70.
"The American Soldier and Venereal Diseases, a Refutation of Some of the Statements of Edward Atkinson." *New York Medical Journal* 70 (1899):181–87.
"Animal Extracts." *American Medico-Surgical Bulletin* 6 (1893):811–17.
"Animal Extracts." *New York Medical Journal* 61 (1895):54.
"Animal Therapeutics in the Treatment of Cerebral Hyperaemia." *Charlotte Medical Journal* 8 (1896):156–61.
"Aphasia." *Quarterly Journal of Psychological Medicine* 5 (1871):311–36.
"An Appeal to the Medical Profession." *Medical Record* 9 (1874):488–91.
"Athetosis." *Medical Record* 8 (1873):309–11.
"Bell's Paralysis." *Medical and Surgical Reporter* 5 (1881):515–16.
"The Brain Not the Sole Organ of the Mind." *Journal of Nervous and Mental Diseases,* n.s., 1 (1876):1–19.
"Bromide of Calcium." *American Journal of the Medical Sciences,* n.s., 63 (1872): 283–84.
"Bromide of Calcium in the Treatment of Syphilitic Neuralgia." *American Journal of Syphilology and Dermatology* 4 (1873):306–9.
"Can Get All the Cerebrin He Wants." *Journal of the American Medical Association* 21 (1893):464.
"Can We Diagnosticate Hyperaemia or Anaemia of the Brain and Cord?" *Virginia Medical Monthly* 17 (1890–91):675–96.
"Canned Tomatoes and Chloride of Zinc." *New York Medical Journal* 43 (1886):370–72.
"Cardine: The Extract of the Heart, Its Preparation and Physiological and Therapeutical Effects." *New York Medical Journal* 57 (1893):429–31.
"A Case of Brain Surgery and Its Relations to Cerebral Localization." *New York Medical Journal* 52 (1890):337–40.
"A Case of Convulsive Tremor Cured by Arsenic Administered Hypodermically in Large Doses." *Quarterly Bulletin of the Clinical Society* 1 (1886):234–38.

"A Case of Epilepsy due to Cerebral Anemia." *Quarterly Journal of Psychological Medicine and Medical Jurisprudence* 2 (1868):368–71.

"A Case of Hysterical Deception." *Neurological Contributions* 1, no. 1 (1879):72–79.

"A Case of Intellectual Monomania, with Mental Depression." *Illustrated Medicine and Surgery* 2 (1883):131–36; *American Journal of Neurology and Psychiatry* 2 (1883):110–28.

"A Case of Locomotor Ataxia, Cured." *Journal of Nervous and Mental Diseases* 10 (1883):507–9.

"A Case of Progressive Facial Atrophy with Remarks on the Pathology of the Disease." *Journal of Nervous and Mental Diseases*, n.s., 5 (1880):250–57.

"Cases of Certain Menstrual Neuroses." *Medical Gazette* 8 (1881):334–35.

"Cerebral Softening." *Medical and Surgical Reporter* 45 (1881):540–44; *Medical Herald* 3 (1883):361–68.

"Cerebral Symptoms from Impacted Cerumen in the Ear." *Medical Record* 14 (1878):414–15; *Hospital Gazette* 5 (1879):26–29.

"Certain Animal Extracts: Their Mode of Preparation, and Physiological and Therapeutical Effects." *American Medico-Surgical Bulletin* 6 (1893):179–84; *Virginia Medical Monthly* 19 (1893):993–1003.

"Certain Railway Injuries of the Spine in their Medico-Legal Relations." *Journal of the National Association of Railway Surgeons* 2 (1890):409–24.

"Chlorosis a Disease of the Nervous System." *Quarterly Journal of Psychological Medicine and Medical Jurisprudence* 2 (1868):418–41.

"Circular to Physicians." *American Medical Times* 6 (1863):119.

"A Clinical Lecture on Arrest of Development." *Neurological Contributions* 1, no. 1 (1879):23–39.

"A Clinical Lecture on Cerebral Embolism." *American Medical Bi-Weekly* 12 (1881):217–19; *Gaillard's Medical Journal* 31 (1881):385–87.

"A Clinical Lecture on Chronic Myelitis." *American Medical Times* 2 (1861):379–81.

"A Clinical Lecture on Epilepsy." *New York Medical Journal* 37 (1883):337–40.

"A Clinical Lecture on Facial Paralysis." *Boston Medical and Surgical Journal* 99 (1878):485–88.

"A Clinical Lecture on Glosso-labio-laryngeal Paralysis – Syphilitic Brain Tumor – Idiocy – Mysophobia." *Hospital Gazette* 6 (1879):113–16.

"A Clinical Lecture on Scirrhus, or Hard Cancer." *Maryland and Virginia Medical Journal* 15 (1860):349–55.

"A Clinical Lecture on the Differential Diagnosis of Antero-lateral Sclerosis and Posterior Sclerosis of the Spinal Cord." *Journal of Nervous and Mental Diseases*, n.s., 15 (1888):496–509.

"A Clinical Lecture on the Treatment of Locomotor Ataxia: Operation for Elongation of the Sciatic Nerve Performed." *St. Louis Clinical Record* 8 (1881–82):193–95.

"Clinical Lectures Delivered at the Bellevue Hospital Medical College, Session of 1870–71." *Journal of Psychological Medicine* 5 (1871):1–53, 311–46, 534–50, 625–51.

"Coca; Its Preparations and Their Therapeutical Qualities, with Some Remarks on the So-Called Cocaine Habit." *Transactions of the Medical Society of Virginia for 1887*, pp. 212–26; *Virginia Medical Monthly* 14 (1887–88):598–612.

"The Conditions of the Arteries After Death." *Medical Record* 20 (1881):668–69.

"The Constringing Influence of Ergot on the Capillary Blood-Vessels." *Medical Record* 6 (1871):429.

"The Construction, Organization and Equipment of Hospitals for the Insane." *Neurological Contributions* 1, no. 2 (1880):1–25.

"A Contribution to the Study of the Nature and Consequences of Malarial Poisoning." *Cincinnati Medical News* 6 (1877):701–8; *St. Louis Clinical Record* 4 (1877–78):129–33.

"A Course of Lectures on Chancre." *American Medical Times* 3 (1861):1–3, 17–19, 33–35, 49–51, 65–67.

"Description of a Large Permanent Galvanic Battery for Medical Use." *New York Medical Journal* 14 (1871):486–90.

"Diffused Cerebral Sclerosis." *New York Medical Journal* 13 (1871):129–44.

"The Disease of the Scythians (Morbus feminarum) and Certain Analogous Conditions." *American Journal of Neurology and Psychiatry* 1 (1882):339–55.

"Dr. Hammond Explains His Relations to the Columbia Chemical Company." *Journal of the American Medical Association* 21 (1893):1023.

"Dr. Hammond Replies to His Critics." *Journal of the American Medical Association* 21 (1893):428.

"Dr. Hammond's Reply to Dr. Hopkins." *Atlanta Medical and Surgical Journal* 1 (1884):484–87.

"Dr. Ryerson on the French Language and on Wounds of the Abdomen." *Medical Gazette* 9 (1882):208–9.

"The Dynamometer and Dynamograph of Mathieu." *Quarterly Journal of Psychological Medicine and Medical Jurisprudence* 2 (1868):139–46.

"Eccentricity and Idiosyncrasy." *New York Medical Journal* 36 (1882):350–58.

"The Effects of Alcohol upon the Nervous System." *Psychological and Medico-Legal Journal*, n.s., 1 (1874):1–33.

"The Effects of Alcohol upon the Nervous System." *Neurological Contributions* 1, no. 2 (1880):29–60.

"Elongation of the Sciatic Nerve in Locomotor Ataxia." *Journal of Nervous and Mental Diseases*, n.s., 8 (1891):553–59.

"Emotional Morbid Impulses – Suicide." *New England Medical Monthly* 2 (1883):291–94.

"Epilepsy." *Medical and Surgical Reporter* 44 (1881):568–71.

"Experimental Researches Relative to a Supposed New Species of Upas." *American Journal of the Medical Sciences*, n.s., 40 (1860):363–77.

"Experimental Researches Relative to the Nutritive Value and Physiological Effects of Albumen, Starch, and Gum, When Singly and Exclusively Used as Food." *Transactions of the American Medical Association* 10 (1857):511–87.

"Experiments Relative to the Therapeutical Value of the Expressed Juice of the Testicles When Hypodermically Introduced into the Human System." *New York Medical Journal* 50 (1889):232–34.

"Experiments with Bibron's Antidote to the Poison of the Rattlesnake." *American Journal of the Medical Sciences*, n.s., 35 (1858):94–96.

"Fatty Degeneration of the Heart – Death From the Inhalation of the Tincture of Chloroform." *American Journal of the Medical Sciences*, n.s., 36 (1858):41–44.

"The Fetichism of Antisepsis." *American Medico-Surgical Bulletin* 7 (1894):70–73.

"A Few Practical Remarks on Some of the So-Called Reflex Diseases of the Nervous System, Peculiar to Women." *American Journal of Surgery and Gynecology* 8 (1895–96):54–56.

"Functions of the Cerebellum." *Medical Record* 3 (1869):523.

"A Further Contribution to the Subject of 'Animal Extracts.' " *New York Medical Journal* 58 (1893):14–15.

"Further Remarks on Organic Infantile Paralysis." *Quarterly Journal of Psychological Medicine and Medical Jurisprudence* 2 (1868):531–34.

"General Paralysis of the Insane, with Special Reference to the Case of Abraham Gosling." *Gaillard's Medical Journal* 29 (1880):652–55.

"Glonoine in Migraine or Sick Headache." *The Medical Brief* 14 (1886):330–32.

"Hebephrenia – Mental Derangement of Puberty." *Virginia Medical Monthly* 19 (1892–93):1–9.

"Hemiplegia from Cerebral Hemorrhage. A Clinical Lecture." *Medical Gazette* 8 (1881):405–6.

"Hepatic Abscess." *Medical Record* 15 (1879):620.

"Hereditary Tendency." *Journal of Nervous and Mental Diseases*, n.s., 9 (1882):695–711.

"Hypnotism." *Medical and Surgical Reporter* 45 (1881):649–54.

"Hysterical Muscular Contractions." *Journal of Nervous and Mental Diseases*, n.s., 2 (1877):54–67.

"Hysterical Paralysis." *Medical and Surgical Reporter* 45 (1881):513–15.

"Incontinence of Urine as a Pre-ataxic Sign of Locomotor Ataxia." *New England Medical Monthly* 1 (1881–82):289–91.

"The Influence of Age upon the Mind and Body in Relation to Mental Derangement." *Alienist and Neurologist* 4 (1883):220–35.

"The Influence of the Disulphate of Quinine on the Intracranial Circulation." *Psychological and Medico-Legal Journal*, n.s., 1 (1874):230–40; *American Journal of the Medical Sciences*, n.s., 69 (1875):295–96.

"Insane Asylum Investigation." *Neurological Contributions* 1, no. 3 (1881):59–60.

"Insanity of Malarial Origin." *Neurological Contributions* 1, no. 1 (1879):55–61; *American Medical Bi-Weekly* 11 (1879):164–65.

"Insanity of Malarial Origin." *Quarterly Bulletin of the Clinical Society* 2 (1886):11–16.

"Instruments for the Study of Nervous Affections." *Medical Record* 3 (1868):187.

"Katatonia." *Alienist and Neurologist* 3 (1882):558.

"Lard as an Antidote to Strychnia." *American Journal of the Medical Sciences*, n.s., 33 (1857):273.

"A Lecture on Sleep." *Gaillard's Medical Journal* 29 (1880):125–57.

"Lecture on the Pathology and Treatment of Infantile Paralysis." *Medical and Surgical Reporter* 16 (1867):369–71.

"Lectures. On Infantile Convulsions." *Medical Gazette* 1 (1867):83–85.

"Lectures on Public Hygiene." *New York Medical Journal* 15 (1872):506–22.

"Medico-legal Points in the Case of David Montgomery." *Journal of Psychological Medicine* 6 (1872):62–76.

"The Medico-legal Relations of Hypnotism or Syggignoscism [*sic*]." *New York Medical Journal* 45 (1887):115–21.

"A Medico-legal Study of the Case of Daniel McFarland." *Journal of Psychological Medicine* 4 (1870):449–81.

"The Medico-legal Value of Confession as an Evidence of Guilt." *Journal of Psychological Medicine* 5 (1871):357–70.

"Merlin and His Influence on the English Character and Literature." *Quarterly Journal of Psychological Medicine and Medical Jurisprudence* 1 (1867):27–49.

"Merycism." *New York Medical Journal* 60 (1894):109–11.

"Method of Distinguishing Spots of Blood on an Instrument Coated with Rust. By MM. Leseur and Robin." *Baltimore Journal of Medicine* 1 (1861):139.

"Miryachit, a Newly Described Disease of the Nervous System, and Its Analogues." *New York Medical Journal* 39 (1884):191–92; *Aesculapian* 1 (1884):57–60.

"Mr. Ernest Hart and the American Medical Profession." *New York Medical Journal* 58 (1893):325–27, 409–11.

"Morbid Impulse." *Psychological and Medico-Legal Journal*, n.s., 1 (1874):73–97; *Papers Read Before the Medico-Legal Society of New York*, 2d ser. (1882), pp. 427–68.

"Multiple Cerebral Sclerosis." *American Practitioner* 3 (1871):129–50.

"Mysophobia." *Neurological Contributions* 1, no. 1 (1879):40–54; *Independent Practitioner* 1 (1880):115–25.

"Myxoedema: With Special Reference to Its Cerebral and Nervous Symptoms." *Boston Medical and Surgical Journal* 103 (1880):14–15.

"Neuralgia of the Testis." *Neurological Contributions* 1, no. 3 (1881):25–35.

"A New Process for Extracting the Essential Principles of Certain Animal Organs, and on their Physiologic and Therapeutic Properties." *New York Medical Journal* 58 (1893):359.

"A New Substitute for Capital Punishment and Means for Preventing the Propagation of Criminals." *New York Medical Examiner* 1 (1892):190–94.

"Nitric Acid in Intermittent Fever." *American Journal of the Medical Sciences*, n.s., 41 (1861):606–7.

"Nitric Acid in Intermittent Fever." *Maryland and Virginia Medical Journal* 16 (1861):104–6.

"The Non-Asylum Treatment of the Insane." *Transactions of the Medical Society of the State of New York for the Year 1879*, pp. 280–97; *Neurological Contributions* 1, no. 1 (1879):1–22.

"Note Relative to the Bromide of Potassium." *New York Medical Journal* 14 (1871):594–95.

"Note Relative to the Monobromide of Camphor." *New York Medical Journal* 15 (1872):522–23; *American Journal of the Medical Sciences*, n.s., 64 (1872):292.

"Observations on the Colourless Blood-Corpuscles." *American Journal of the Medical Sciences*, n.s., 37 (1859):348–50.

"Observations on the Use of Potash in the Treatment of Scurvy: With Cases." *American Journal of the Medical Sciences*, n.s., 25 (1853):102–5.

"The Odor of the Human Body, as Developed by Certain Affections of the Nervous System." *Transactions of the American Neurological Association* 2 (1876–77):17–23; *Neurological Contributions* 1, no. 1 (1879):3–9.

"On a Hitherto Undescribed Form of Muscular Incoordination." *Transactions of the American Neurological Association* 2 (1876–77):154–58.

"On an Improved Method of Treating Facial Paralysis." *St. Louis Clinical Record* 5 (1878):25–27.

"On Aphasia." *Medical Record* 6 (1871):3–6.

"On Certain Animal Extracts; Their Mode of Preparation and Physiological and Therapeutical Effects." *Post-Graduate Medical Journal* 8 (1893):97–105; *Ontario Medical Journal* 1 (1892–93):273–77.

"On Certain Dumb-bell Forms of Crystals Found in the Urine." *American Journal of the Medical Sciences*, n.s., 27 (1854):384–87.

"On Certain Organic Extracts: Their Preparation and Physiological and Therapeutical Effects." *New York Medical Journal* 57 (1893):93–96.

"On Convulsive Tremor." *New York Medical Journal* 5 (1867):185–99.

"On Instinct: Its Nature and Seat." *Quarterly Journal of Psychological Medicine and Medical Jurisprudence* 1 (1867):1–27.

"On Melancholia and Facial Paralysis." *Medical Gazette* 8 (1881):291.

"On Myxoedema, With Special Reference to Its Cerebral and Nervous Symptoms." *Neurological Contributions* 1, no. 3 (1881):36–43; *St. Louis Clinical Record* 7 (1880):97–100.

"On Obscure Abscesses of the Liver, Their Association with Hypochondria, and Other Forms of Mental Derangement, and Their Treatment." *Neurological Contributions* 1, no. 3 (1881):68–107.

"On Obscure Diseases of the Liver; their Association with Hypochondria, and Their Treatment." *St. Louis Clinical Record* 5 (1878):49–58 and 7 (1880–81):294–302.

"On Pigmentary Deposits in the Brain Resulting from Malarial Poisoning." *Transactions of the American Neurological Association* 1 (1875):142–56.

"On Sleep and Insomnia." *New York Medical Journal* 1 (1865):89–101, 182–204.

"On Some of the Effects of Excessive Intellectual Exertion." *Bellevue and Charity Hospital Reports* (1870), pp. 379–89; *American Journal of the Medical Sciences*, n.s., 59 (1870):455–56.

"On Some of the Effects of the Bromide of Potassium When Administered in Large Doses." *Quarterly Journal of Psychological Medicine and Medical Jurisprudence* 3 (1869):46–60.

"On Thalamic Epilepsy." *Neurological Contributions* 1, no. 3 (1881):1–24; *Archives of Medicine* 4 (1880):1–23; *Boston Medical and Surgical Journal* 103 (1880):36–37; *Medical Record* 18 (1880):243–44.

"On the Action of Certain Vegetable Diuretics." *American Journal of the Medical Sciences*, n.s., 37 (1859):275–78; *Proceedings of the Academy of Natural Sciences of Philadelphia for 1858*, pp. 17–21.

"On the Alterations Induced by Intermittent Fever in the Physical and Chemical Qualities of the Urine, and on the Action of the Disulphate of Quinine." *American Journal of the Medical Sciences*, n.s., 35 (1858):322–26.

"On the Cause of Vice-President Wilson's Death." *Boston Medical and Surgical Journal* 93 (1875):693–704.

"On the Influence of the Maternal Mind Over the Offspring During Pregnancy and Lactation." *Quarterly Journal of Psychological Medicine and Medical Jurisprudence* 2 (1868):1–28; *Detroit Review of Medicine and Pharmacy* 3 (1868):137–43, 189–94, 244–50.

"On the Injection of Urea and Other Substances into the Blood." *North American Medico-Chirurgical Review* 2 (1858):287–93; *Charleston Medical Journal* 13 (1858):835–36.

"On the Occurrence of Amyloid Bodies in the Blood of Persons Affected with Epilepsy." *Maryland and Virginia Medical Journal* 16 (1861):271–74.

"On the Physiological Effects and Therapeutical Uses of the Hydrate of Chloral." *Medical Record* 4 (1870):498–99; *New York Medical Journal* 10 (1870):469–75.

"On the Proper Method of Using the Iodide of Potassium in Syphilis of the Nervous System." *New England Medical Monthly* 4 (1884–85):150–52.

"On the Secondary Formation of Blood-Crystals." *Proceedings of the Academy of Natural Sciences of Philadelphia for 1858*, pp. 15–17.

"On the Treatment of a Certain Form of Paralysis Occurring in Children." *New York Medical Journal* 2 (1865):168–74.

"On the Treatment of Chorea with Hypodermic Injections of Arsenic." *St. Louis Clinical Record* 6 (1879):389–93.

"On the Use of Opium in the Treatment of Hypochondria." *Gaillard's Medical Journal* 28 (1879):389–93.

"On Uraemic Intoxication." *American Journal of the Medical Sciences*, n.s., 41 (1861):55–83.

"Our Friends Who Have Passed Away." *Proceedings of the American Philosophical Society* 18 (1880):541–43.

"The Pathology and Treatment of Organic Infantile Paralysis." *Quarterly Journal of Psychological Medicine and Medical Jurisprudence* 1 (1867):49–66.

"Petition to the Senate of the United States." *Boston Medical and Surgical Journal* 71 (1864–65):527–28.

"The Physiological Effects of Alcohol and Tobacco upon the Human System." *American Journal of the Medical Sciences*, n.s., 32 (1856):305–20.

"The Physiology and Pathology of the Cerebellum." *Quarterly Journal of Psychological Medicine and Medical Jurisprudence* 3 (1869):209–44; *American Journal of the Medical Sciences*, n.s., 58 (1869):293.

"Pott's Disease Simulating Spinal Irritation, a Clinical Lecture." *Medical Gazette* 8 (1881):260.

"The Proper Use of the Mind." *Quarterly Journal of Psychological Medicine and Medical Jurisprudence* 2 (1868):125–39.

"The Question of Lucid Intervals in Insanity." *Journal of Nervous and Mental Diseases*, n.s., 10 (1883):253–60.

"Rabies in the Human Subject." *Quarterly Bulletin of the Clinical Society* 1 (1886):293–305.

"Reasoning Mania; Its Medical and Medico-Legal Relations, with Special Reference to the Case of Charles J. Guiteau." *Journal of Nervous and Mental Diseases*, n.s., 9 (1882):1–26; *Sanitarian* 10 (1882):205–19.

"The Relations Existing Between Urea and Uric Acid." *American Journal of the Medical Sciences*, n.s., 29 (1855):119–23.

"A Remarkable Case of Cerebral Hemorrhage." *Psychological and Medico-Legal Journal*, n.s., 1 (1874):396–400.

"Remarks on Cases of Katatonia." *New York Medical Journal* 37 (1883):481–84.

"Remarks on Cocaine and the So-Called Cocaine Habit." *Journal of Nervous and Mental Diseases*, n.s., 11 (1886):754–59; *New York Medical Journal* 44 (1886):637–39. Reprinted in *The Coca Leaf and Cocaine Papers*, edited by George Andrews and David Solomon (New York and London: Harcourt, Brace, Jovanovich, 1975).

"Remarks on Paralytic Insanity or General Paralysis of the Insane with Special Reference to the Case of Abraham Gosling." *Medical Gazette* 7 (1880):289–91.

"Researches on Fermentation and Putrefaction, by G. M. Van der Broek." *Baltimore Journal of Medicine* 1 (1861):138–39.

"The Scientific Value of the Results of the Post-Mortem Examination in the Case of William McCormick, Dead of Hydrophobia." *Psychological and Medico-Legal Journal*, n.s., 1 (1874):194–202; *New York Medical Journal* 20 (1874):261–69.

"Scurvy." In *Military Medical and Surgical Essays*, edited by William A. Hammond (Philadelphia: Lippincott, 1864).

"Seven Recent Cases of Brain Surgery." *Medical News* 59 (1891):501–5.

"A Simple Aesthesiometer." *Quarterly Journal of Psychological Medicine and Medical Jurisprudence* 2 (1868):830.

"The So-Called Family or Hereditary Form of Locomotor Ataxia." *Medical Record* 22 (1882):19.

"Some of the Therapeutical Uses of Nitroglycerine." *Virginia Medical Monthly* 8 (1881–82):525–31.

"Some Points in the Pathology and Treatment of Hepatic Abscess." *St. Louis Medical and Surgical Journal* 35 (1878):72–76.

"Some Remarks on Sexual Excesses in Adult Life as a Cause of Impotence." *Virginia Medical Monthly* 10 (1883):145–50.

"Spasmodic Stricture of the Urethra as a Cause of Impotence." *Medical Gazette* 10 (1883):265–67.

"The Sphygmograph as an Instrument of Precision (With Apologies to Dr. Leonhardt)." *New York Medical Journal* 58 (1893):588–89.

"Spinal Irritation." *Journal of Psychological Medicine* 4 (1870):225–64.

"The State of the Mind During Sleep." *Quarterly Journal of Psychological Medicine and Medical Jurisprudence* 2 (1868):660–97.

"Suggestions for Improvements in the Management of the Insane and of Hospitals for the Insane in the State of New York." *Neurological Contributions* 1, no. 3 (1881):61–67.

"Syphilitic Aphasia." *Neurological Contributions* 1, no. 1 (1879):62–71.

"Tetany." *New England Medical Monthly* 5 (1885–86):479–81.

"Thalamic Epilepsy." *Virginia Medical Monthly* 13 (1886–87):477–83.

"The Therapeutic Use of the Magnet." *Medical Gazette* 7 (1880):679–80.

"The Therapeutical Use of the Magnet." *Neurological Contributions* 1, no. 3 (1881):44–58; *Gaillard's Medical Journal* 30 (1881):85–86; *New York Medical Journal* 32 (1880):449–60.

"The Therapeutics of Wakefulness." *Detroit Review of Medicine and Pharmacy* 4 (1869):26–30.

"Thomsen's Disease." *Gaillard's Medical Journal* 41 (1886):614–17.

"Three Cases of the Successful Treatment of Vascular Tumors by Injection with the Fluid Extract of Ergot." *Archives of Clinical Surgery* 1 (1876):123–24.

"To the Medical Profession." *Psychological and Medico-Legal Journal,* n.s., 1 (1874):202–12; *Medical Record* 9 (1874):488–91.

"The Treatment of Locomotor Ataxia and Other Diseases of the Nervous System by Suspension." *New York Medical Journal* 49 (1889):510–12.

"The Treatment of Migraine." *New York Medical Journal* 38 (1883):544–46.

"Two Cases of Chorea Treated Efficiently with Sulphate of Manganese." *Medical Gazette* 1 (1868):45.

"Two Reports on the Condition of Military Hospitals at Grafton, Va., and Cumberland, Md." In *Documents of the U.S. Sanitary Commission,* vol. 1, no. 41 (New York, 1866).

"Unilateral Hallucinations." *Medical News* 47 (1885):687–88; *Boston Medical and Surgical Journal* 114 (1886):14–15; *New York Medical Journal* 42 (1885):649–52.

"Upon a Hitherto Undescribed Form of Muscular Incoordination." *Medical Record* 11 (1876):460–61.

"Urological Contributions." *American Journal of the Medical Sciences,* n.s., 31 (1856):330–37.

"Weak Heart and Its Treatment." *Therapeutic Gazette,* 3d ser., 6 (1890):667–73; *New York Medical Journal* 49 (1889):218–19.

"William Hammond on Hysteria." *Bulletin of the New York Academy of Medicine* 47 (1971):1551–54.

"A Word for Dr. Beard." *Medical Record* 20 (1881):446–47.

With Silas Weir Mitchell. "An Experimental Examination of the Toxicological Effects of Sassy Bark, the 'Ordeal Poison' of the Western Coast of Africa." *Charleston Medical Journal and Review* 14 (1859):721–40; *Proceedings of the Academy of Natural Sciences of Philadelphia.* Suppl. (1859), pp. 13–16.

With Silas Weir Mitchell. "Experimental Researches Relative to Corroval and Vao, Two New Varieties of Woorara, the South American Arrow Poison." *American Journal of the Medical Sciences,* n.s., 38 (1859):13–60; *Proceedings of the Academy of Natural Sciences of Philadelphia* (1860), pp. 4–9; *Charleston Medical Journal* 14 (1859):675–77.

TRANSLATIONS OF WORKS BY HAMMOND

"De la paralysie du bras, chez les nouveau-nés." *Paris Médical* 6 (1881):373–75.

"De l'emploi de l'aimant dans la thérapeutique." *Annales de psychiatrie et d'hypnologie* 4 (1894–95):327–35, 375–88.

"De l'épilepsie thalamique." *Annales de psychiatrie et d'hypnologie* 4 (1894–95):33–48, 68–77.

L'impuissance sexuelle chez l'homme et la femme. Paris: Lecrosnier & Babé, 1890.

Manuale clinico terapeutico sulla impotenza sessuale nell' uomo. Translated by A. Rubino. Naples: Jovene, 1884.

"Miryachit, nouvelle maladie du système nerveux." Translated from *Medicina contemporanea* in *Union médicale* (Paris), 3.s., 37 (1884):706–8.

"Miryachit, nuova malattia del sistema nervoso." *Medicina contemporanea* (Napoli) 1 (1884):126–30.
"L'odore del corpo umano in alcune malattie del sistema nervoso." *Giornale internazionale di scienze mediche*, n.s., 5 (1883):193–97.
"Die physiologischen Wirkungen des Alkohol und Tabak auf den menschlichen Organismus." *Archiv für wissenschaftliche heilkunde* 2 (1858):590–608.
Polovoye bezslïe u mezhchin i zhenshtshis. Translated by A. G. Feinberg. St. Petersburg: Prakt. Med., 1889.
"Le scorbut." In *Essais d'hygiène et de thérapeutique militaire*, edited by T. W. Evans (Paris, 1865), pp. 71–109.
Sexuelle Impotenz beim männlichen und weiblichen Geschlecht. Translated by Leo Salinger. Berlin: Steinitz, 1889. 3d ed., 1904.
"Sul giusto uso della mente." *Medicina contemporanea* (Napoli) 2 (1885):13–17.
Traité des maladies du système nerveux. Translated and edited by F. Labadie-Lagrave. Paris: Baillière, 1879.
Tratado de las enfermedades del sistema nervioso. Translated by Federico Toledo y Cueva. Madrid: Revista de medicina y cirugía prácticas, 1887.
Trattato delle malattie del sistema nervoso. Translated and edited by Alfredo Rubino. Naples: Detken, 1887.
"Über die Ausscheidung der Phosphorsaüre durch die Nieren." *Archiv für wissenschaftliche Heilkunde* 4 (1860):108–16.
"Über die Einspritzung von Harnstoff und andern Substanzen in das Blut." *Archiv für wissenschaftliche Heilkunde* 4 (1860):99–107.
"Über die physikalischen und chemischen Veränderung des Urins bei Intermittens und über die Wirkung des schwefelsauren Chinins." *Archiv für wissenschaftliche Heilkunde* 4 (1860):117–22.
With Silas Weir Mitchell. "Recherches expérimentales sur le corroval et le vao, deux nouvelles variétés de curare ou poison des flèches dans l'Amérique du Sud." *Journal de la physiologie de l'homme et des animaux* (Brown-Séquard) 2 (1859):707–9.

ARTICLES WRITTEN FOR THE GENERAL PUBLIC

"Brain Forcing in Childhood." *Popular Science Monthly* 30 (1886–87):721–32.
"Brain Surgery." *North American Review* 156 (1893):390–97.
"Brains and Muscles: Their Relative Training and Development." *Union College Practical Lectures* (Butterfield Course). Schenectady, N.Y.: Union College, 1895. 1:263–82.
"Brigadier-General Nathaniel Lyon, U.S.A.; Personal Recollections." *Magazine of American History* 13 (1885):237–48.
"The Coming Man." *Forum* 1 (1886):75–82.
"The Elixir of Life." *North American Review* 149 (1889):257–64.
"The Evolution of the Boycott." *Forum* 1 (1886):369–76.
"An Explanation of the 'Joint-Snake.'" *Popular Science Monthly* 30 (1887):841–42.
"False Hydrophobia." *North American Review* 151 (1890):167–72.
"A Few Words About Cholera." *Nation* 1 (1865):306–8.

"A Few Words About the Nerves. I. The Brain and Spinal Cord. II. The Sympathetic System and the Emotions. III. Nervous People." *Galaxy* 6 (1868):41–46, 181–86, 493–99.

"How Shall Women Dress?" *North American Review* 140 (1885):565–68.

"How to Rest." *North American Review* 153 (1891):215–19.

"The Humors of the Anthropologists." *Nation* 1 (1865):141–43.

"The Hygienic Relations of Celibacy." *Nation* 5 (1867):357–58.

"Insomnia and Recent Hypnotics." *North American Review* 156 (1893):18–26.

"Is Drunkenness Curable?" *North American Review* 153 (1891):346–52.

"Madness and Murder." *North American Review* 147 (1888):626–37.

"Men's and Women's Brains." *Popular Science Monthly* 31 (1887):554–58.

"The Mischievous Ice-Pitcher." *North American Review* 148 (1889):738–42.

"Mysterious Disappearances." *Forum* 3 (1887):69–76.

"Perceptional Insanities." *Popular Science Monthly* 22 (1882–83):760–67.

"The Physics and Physiology of Spiritualism." *North American Review* 110 (1870):233–60.

"Poisoning as a Science." *Nation* 1 (1865):242–43.

Preface to *Notes on Epidemics for the Use of the Public,* by Francis E. Anstie. 1st American ed. Philadelphia: Lippincott, 1866.

Preliminary essay in *The Trial of Daniel McFarland for the Shooting of Albert D. Richardson, the Alleged Seducer of His Wife. By a practical law reporter.* New York: New York News Company [1870].

"A Problem for Sociologists." *North American Review* 135 (1882):422–32.

"The Punishability of the Insane." *International Review,* n.s., 11 (1881):440–50.

"Recollections of General Nathaniel Lyon." *Annals of Iowa,* 3d ser., 4 (1899–1901):415–36.

"The Relations Between the Mind and the Nervous System." *Popular Science Monthly* 26 (1884):1–20. Also published in Lehigh University, *Exercises at the Celebration of the Founder's Day, Thursday, October 9, 1884.* Bethlehem, Pa.: Klose, 1884.

"The Sanitary and Physiological Relations of Tobacco." *North American Review* 108 (1869):499–516.

"The Scientific Relations of Modern Miracles." *International Review* 10 (1881):225–42.

"Self-Control in Curing Insanity." *North American Review* 152 (1891):311–18.

"Slaughter-Houses and Health." *Nation* 3 (1866):273–74.

"Society versus Insanity." *Putnam's Magazine* 16 (1870):326–36.

"Stammering. A Few Practical Remarks, Showing How Self-Treatment May Be Employed." *The Voice* 1 (1879):31.

"Sumptuary Laws and Their Social Influence." *Popular Science Monthly* 37 (1890):33–40.

"The Surgical Treatment of President Garfield." *North American Review* 133 (1881):578–87.

"The Treatment of the Insane." *International Review* 8 (1880):225–41.

"What Should a Doctor Be Paid?" *North American Review* 158 (1894):660–67.

"Woman in Politics." *North American Review* 137 (1883):137–46.

FICTION

Hammond's novels are available on microfilm in the Wright American Fiction series.

Doctor Grattan; a Novel. New York: Appleton, 1885. London: Bentley, 1885.
Lal; a Novel. New York: Appleton, 1884.
Mr. Oldmixon; a Novel. New York: Appleton, 1885.
A Mysterious Life; a Four-Act Drama. New York: Swayne, 1901.
On the Susquehanna. New York: Appleton, 1887.
Robert Severne, His Friends and His Enemies. Philadelphia: Lippincott, 1867.
The Son of Perdition. Chicago and New York: Stone, 1898.
A Strong-Minded Woman; or, Two Years After. New York: Appleton, 1885.
With Clara Hammond Lanza. *Tales of Eccentric Life.* New York: Appleton, 1886.

Index

Abbott, R. O., 68
Académie de Médecine, 139
Academy of Natural Sciences of Philadelphia, 7, 32, 34, 44, 47, 48
Agassiz, Louis, 88, 89
Agnew, Cornelius R., 85, 88
alcohol and tobacco, 40–1
American Medical Association, 4, 229
American Neurological Association, 11,
15, 111, 131, 200
animal extracts, 12, 125, 204; advertising
of, 223, 227; chemistry of, 213–14, 217;
physiology of, 211–12; production of,
221–2, 224; profitability of, 222; recep-
tion of, 207–9; scientific basis of, 211;
and self-experiments of WAH, 206; tests
of, 209–10; therapeutic uses of, 209–11
anthropology, 9, 22
aphasia, 134, 138–44; and cerebral localization, 138–41; forms of, 139; and
lateralization, 141–2; pathology of, 139–
40; social implications of, 141
Association of Medical Superintendents of
American Institutions for the Insane,
110, 171
Astor, John Jacob, 9
asylums for the insane, see hospitals, psychiatric
Atlee, Walter F., 64, 201
Aulde, John, 212, 213, 217
Azpell, T. R., 77

Bache, Alexander Dallas, 92
Bailey, W. W., 25
Bain, Alexander, 164
Baird, Spencer Fullerton, 33, 94
Baltimore Infirmary, 51, 53
Baltimore Medical Association, 85
Barker, Fordyce, 128
Barnes, Joseph K., 71
Barthez, A.-C.-E., 135

Bartholow, Roberts, 80
Bastian, Henry Charleton, 148
Bateman, Frederick, 143
Beard, George M., 11, 97, 128, 130, 160,
166–7, 175
Beaumont, William, 18
Becquerel, Henri, 128
Bell, Clark, 112, 113
Bellevue Hospital, 71, 96; Medical Col-
lege, 96, 98; O.AE. Society, 11
Bellows, Henry W., 54, 61, 73, 88
Bernard, Claude, 50
Bingham, John A., 90, 91
Blake, Lillie Devereaux, 193
Blandford, Fielding, 97
Blumenbach, Johann, 145, 146, 149
Borchard, Albert, 82
botanic medicine, 82
Bouillaud, Jean-Baptiste, 139
brain: chemistry of, 147; congestion of,
144; lateralization of, 141–2; and lo-
calization, 138–9, 169, 203–4; metabo-
lism of, 145; sex differences in, 191,
192, 194–6; surgery on, 203–4; weight
of, 191, 194; see also aphasia
Brann, Henry A., 199
Brinton, John H., 80
Broca, Paul, 139
Broker, Thomas, 22
Brown, Bedford, 145
Brown-Séquard, Charles Edouard, 23, 70,
96, 204–9
Browne, Crichton, 166–7
Brucke, Ernst von, 4
Bucknill, John C., 166, 167, 171

Cabanis, Pierre, 165
"calomel order," 84–6, 123, 219
Cameron, Simon, 55
Charcot, J. M., 109, 167, 190
chemistry, 4; medical, 25, 45, 52; in medi-

cine, 5, 21, 213–16; physiological, 31, 48
chiropodists, 82
Civil War battles: Antietam, 73; Shiloh, 61; Virginia Peninsular campaign, 60
code of ethics, 220, 221, 223, 227–8
Coggeshall, Frederic, 209
College of Physicians and Surgeons (New York), 96
College of Physicians of Philadelphia, 92
Collins, William T., 81
Colman, G., 135
Colorado, Mangus, 19
Columbia Chemical Company, 210, 220–1, 223–4
Conkling, Roscoe, 114
Cook, W. H., 82
Coolidge, Richard H., 25, 45–6, 80, 83
Cooper, George E., 63, 72, 91
Corning, J. Leonard, 148
Coues, Elliot, 72
Cross, T. M. B., 97, 98
Cuyler, John M., 71
Czermak, Joseph N., 196

DaCosta, J. M., 70
Dalton, John C., 1, 140, 141
Dana, Charles Loomis, 97, 102, 226
Darrach, William, 64
d'Arsonval, Arsène, 204
Darwin, Charles, 164
Davis, Jefferson, 27
de Vesey, Louis, *see* Xántus, John
Delafontaine, M., 210
DePew, Chauncey, 15
Desault, Pierre, 18
Dewey, John, 195
Dickson, Samuel Henry, 149
Digby, Sir Kenelm, 204
diseases: contagious, 75; scurvy, 20, 21; venereal, 51
diseases, neurological: anorexia nervosa, 197; athetosis, 120–1; case histories of, 153, 158–9; cerebrospinal, 151; chorea, 151; classification of, 151; diagnoses of, 117–19, 121, 153; ecstasy, 199; epilepsy, 197, 203, 209; functional, 151; hypochondria, 126; hysteria, 159, 192, 194, 197–8, 209; locomotor ataxia, 123–4; merycism, 203, myxedema, 205; neurasthenia, 70, 153, 163; and pathology, 152; prognoses of, 121, 153; spinal irritation, 127; treatment of, 121–7, 153, 159; *see also* aphasia; hyperaemia (cerebral); poliomyelitis
diseases, psychiatric (*see also* insanity): aboulomania, 184; dipsomania, 189;

kleptomania, 189; monomania, 183; mysophobia, 185
Dix, Dorothea, 67, 68
Donders, Franz Cornelius, 147
Donkin, H., 167
Doremus, R. Ogden, 113
Douglas, J. H., 9
Draper, John William, 4–5, 146
Du Bois-Reymond, Emil, 4
Duchenne, G.-B.-A., 128, 135, 137
Dupuytren, Guillaume, 6
Durham, Arthur E., 70, 145–6

Echeverria, M. Gonzalez, 95, 136, 188
education (medical), 3, 96, 98, 216; post graduate, 98–105, 174; reform of, 100; in U.S. Army, 80
Edwards, L. A., 64, 77, 83
electrology, 130–1
Electrotherapeutical Society of New York, 130
electrotherapeutics, 82, 119, 127–9, 131, 136
Elliot, L., 220
Elliott, Charles W., 106
Ellis, Thomas T., 73
endocrinology, 205
ethnology, 35, 48, 71, 72
evolution, 192; concepts of, 31–2; human, 231; of language, 143–4; "Vestiges of Creation," 32
examinations (physicians' qualifying), 18, 76–9

fiction (by WAH): *Doctor Grattan*, 183; *Lal*, 28, 32, 191, 194–5; *A Mysterious Life*, 142–3, 229–30; *On the Susquehanna*, 2, 195, 199, 228; *Robert Severne*, 9, 93, 154, 183, 189; *The Son of Perdition*, 199, 230; *A Strong-Minded Woman*, 191, 194–5, 228; *Tales of Eccentric Life*, 16
Finley, Clement A., 53
Fleming, Alexander, 145
Flexner, Abraham, 103
Flint, Austin, Sr., 107
Forsha, Dr., 82
Foster, Frank, 113
Fothergill, J. Milner, 148
free trade, 194, 228
Freeman, George L., 208
French, William G., 179
Frerichs, Friedrich Theodore von, 46, 150
Freud, Sigmund, 110
Frick, Professor, 51

Gaillard, E. S., 112, 126
Gardener, Helen, 196
Garfield, James A., 186

Garrod, Alfred, 21
Georgetown Medical College, 201
Gerhard, W. W., 6
Gibbs, Wolcott, 57
Gibson, George, 36
Gillete, W. R., 96
Gosling, Abraham, 177–8
Gowers, William R., 97
Gray, John P., 99, 110, 171, 172, 173
Gray, Landon Carter, 125, 161, 177, 178
Grier, Judge, 57
Griesinger, Wilhelm, 97, 109, 169
Griffith, Dr., 77
Grissom, Eugene, 172, 173
Gross, Samuel D., 69
Guiteau, Charles J., 112, 186

Hallack, General, 91
Hallowell, Edward, 34
Halpine, Charles G., 88
Hamilton, Allen McLane, 98
Hammond, Esther D. Chapin, 12, 221, 229
Hammond, Graeme M., 15, 46, 102, 112, 144, 230
Hammond, Helen, 15, 236
Hammond, Helen Nisbet, 6, 15, 26, 37, 88, 236
Hammond, John Wesley, 2, 55
Hammond, Jonathan Pinckney, 15
Hammond, Nathaniel Hobart, 15
Hammond, Sarah Pinckney, 2
Hammond, Somerville Pinckney, 37
Hammond, William, Jr., 15
Hammond, William A.: appointment as surgeon general, 55, 57–8; as scientist, 32, 34, 36–8, 40, 44–6, 52, 69, 95, 152; business and financial affairs, 8, 9, 26, 28, 50, 184 (*see also* Columbia Chemical Company; Hammond Animal Extract Company; Hammond Sanitarium; Hammond Sanitarium Company); court martial, 8, 86, 91; death, 230; education, 3–5, 25, 39, 45; family, 2, 7, 15, 37, 46; illnesses and injuries, 23–5, 46, 53, 89; military career, 7, 19, 23, 25, 39–40, 46, 50–1, 53, 55; personality, 12–13, 15, 16, 43, 231; philosophical views, 41, 45; physical description, 12, 43; political and social views, 27–8, 31, 41, 53, 184, 187, 195, 199, 228; religious views, 31, 41, 67, 164, 173, 182, 197–8, 200, 203; social status, 94; vindication of, 8, 92–3, 112–14, 173; *see also* fiction; monographs
Hammond Animal Extract Company, 210, 224

Hammond General Hospital (Point Lookout, Maryland), 74
Hammond Sanitarium, 12; and animal extracts, 205, 206; construction of, 201; facilities of, 202; management of, 203; site of, 201; therapeutic experiments at, 203; use of animal extracts in, 224
Hammond Sanitarium Company, 221, 223–6
Harris, Elisha, 83
Hart, Ernest, 221
Hartshorne, Henry, 7, 57
Harvard University, 95
Harwood, E. C., 112
Hawley, Joseph R., 218
Haydon, James, 220
Hayes, J. J., 63, 65
Hayes, Rutherford B., 114
Head, Henry, 140, 141
Heine, Jacob von, 135
Helmholtz, Hermann von, 4
Hendee, H. S., 84
Hennen, John, 18
Henry, Joseph, 92
Hermann, Dr., 212
homeopathy, 80–1, 194, 207, 212, 218, 228; veterinary, 144
Hopkins, J. G., 158
hospitals (general): administration of, 63; construction of, 56, 175; medical control of, 75; research in, 69
hospitals, military, 63; conditions in, 56; construction of, 56, 61, 73; model for, 63; organization of, 54, 66; physicians in, 66; politics of, 65; research in, 71; sites for, 63; and specialization, 70, 71
hospitals, psychiatric, 172, 173, 175; abuses in, 178, 179; reform of, 172–3, 175–7, 179
Howard, J. M., 81
Hughes, Charles H., 190
Hun, Henry, 211, 218
Hutchinson, Mahlon, 223, 225–6
hydropathy, 40, 82
hyperaemia (cerebral), 41, 154–63, 219; diagnosis of, 156, 161, 162; pathology of, 157; treatment of, 158
hypnotism, 166–7, 183, 197, 215

insanity: classification of, 169–70; clinic for, 97; definition of, 168; medicolegal issues and, 182–8, 190; moral, 183; perceptional, 168; prevalence of, 181–2, 187; treatment of, 176
insomnia, 154–5, 183, 206, 209; treatment of, 149
instruments (medical), 72, 118–19, 127,

131, 137, 156, 189, 215;
ophthalmoscope, 118–19; sphygmograph, 209; surgical, 83
isopathy, 205, 212, 217–19

Jackson, John Hughlings, 97, 140, 141
Jackson, Samuel, 91
Jacob, Sarah, 197
Jacobi, Abraham, 136
Janeway, Edward, 99
Jewell, J. S., 175
Johnston, James C., 182
Johnston, William, 6
Jones, Handfield, 96
journals, medical, 136; *Journal of Nervous
and Mental Diseases,* 111; *Journal of Psy-
chological Medicine,* 108, 110; *Neurological
Contributions,* 112, 176; *The Psychological
and Medico-Legal Journal,* 110–11; *Quar-
terly Journal of Psychological Medicine and
Medical Jurisprudence,* 107

Kearny, Stephen W., 19
Keen, W. W., 70
Kennerly, Dr., 22, 33
King, Dr., 65
Koch, Robert, 212
Kussmaul, Adolf, 143, 150

laboratories, 43, 104; pharmaceutical, 83
Langdon, Eugene, 9
language, evolution of, 143–4
Lanza, Clara Hammond, 16, 46, 108, 142,
144
Lanza, Manfredi, 16, 221, 224
Larrey, Dominique-Jean, 18, 93
LeConte, John (senior), 34
LeConte, John L. (junior), 33, 36, 47, 57
Leidy, Joseph, 7, 33, 34, 35, 47
Letterman, Jonathan, 62, 75
Liebig, Justus von, 1, 4, 39
Lincoln, Abraham, 57, 82, 91, 93
Lippincott, J. B., 9
Long, J. H., 210
Loomis, Henry P., 207
Louis, Pierre, 6
Lozier, Clemence Sophia, 193, 194
Ludwig, Carl, 4
Lum, Sherman B., 82
Luys, J., 170
Lyon, Nathaniel, 27, 31, 36, 41

McCall, George A., 19, 68
McClellan, George B., 60, 81
McClurg, John B., 85
McCrary, 114
McCready, B. F., 98

McDougall, Charles, 60
Magendie, François, 6
Mahan, C. L., 81
Marsh, E. J., 68
Mason, John J., 97
materia medica: antitoxins, 218; Army
supply table, 83, 84, 85; pharmaceutical
manufacturers, 209–10; potash, 21; specific remedies, 82, 83
materialism (philosophical), 196, 197, 200,
233, 234
Maudsley, Henry, 96, 165
*Medical and Surgical History of the War of the
Rebellion,* 71, 73
Medical and Surgical Society (New York),
10
Medical Journal Association (New York),
10
medicalization, 185
medicine (as profession), 10, 79, 86, 101,
227–8
medicine, psychological, 166, 176
Meigs, Montgomery C., 62
Meltzer, S. J., 218
mental illness, *see* diseases, psychiatric;
hospitals, psychiatric; insanity
Merlin, 197
Meyer, Moritz, 97, 129
Meylert, A. P., 78
Michigan Homeopathic Institute, 81
microscopes and microscopy, 25, 39, 48,
51, 72, 137
Mill, John Stuart, 164
mind and body, 4, 41, 44, 157, 160–1,
165, 168, 181, 191, 192 (*see also* materialism [philosophical])
Mitchell, Alice, 190
Mitchell, S. Weir, 1, 7, 47, 49, 57, 69–70,
75, 86, 97, 145, 175
monographs (by WAH): *Cerebral Hyperaemia,* 155–6; *Fasting Girls,* 197; *On
Wakefulness; with an Introductory Chapter
on the Physiology of Sleep,* 155; *The Phys-
ics and Physiology of Spiritualism,* 197;
Physiological Memoirs, 39; *Sleep and Its
Derangements,* 155; *Treatise on Hygiene
With Special Reference to the Military Ser-
vice,* 73; *Treatise on Insanity,* 168, 171,
181; *Treatise on the Diseases of the Ner-
vous System,* 96, 115, 123–6, 151–2,
155, 168, 171, 215–17, 230
Montgomery, William, 26, 27
Moore, George B., 92
Morais, Nina, 193
Morehouse, George Read, 49, 70, 72
Morgan, Charles F., 129
Morris, J. Cheston, 47

Morton, W. J., 112, 177
Mott, Lucretia D., 67
Mott, Valentine, 3
Muir, Sir William, 73
Murray, G. R., 207
Murray, Robert, 91

National Academy of Science, 89–90, 106
National Association for the Protection of
the Insane and the Prevention of Insanity, 177, 179
National Hospital for the Paralyzed and
Epileptic (London), 97
National Institute of Letters, Arts and Sci-
ences, 13, 106, 111
Neftel, W. B., 140
neurology, 118, 126–30, 132; instruction
in, 97; and psychiatry, 108–10, 171–80;
and psychotherapeutics, 159–61; as spe-
cialty, 11–12, 70, 75, 94, 112, 117, 163,
185, 194, 200, 226; surgical, 124, 203–4;
see also diseases, neurological
New York Academy of Medicine, 10
New York College of Veterinary Sur-
geons, 144
New York Commission of Charities and
Corrections, 71
New York County Medical Society, 139
New York Medico-Legal Society, 11, 112–
13, 167
New York Neurological Society, 11, 15,
98, 110, 130; Committee on Asylum
Abuses, 172–3, 176, 178
New York Post-Graduate Medical School,
see education (medical), post graduate
New York Society of Medical Jurispru-
dence, 113, 227
New York Society of Neurology and
Electrology, 111, 130–1
New York State Hospital for Diseases of
the Nervous System, 97, 111, 115
Newberry, Captain, 81
Norris, George W., 6
Northrup, Calvin M., 183
nurses, 66; Catholic sisters as, 64, 67;
female, 54, 67, 68; male, 63

Ohio State Medical Society, 76, 85
Olmsted, Edward, 9
Olmsted, Frederick Law, 54, 59, 60, 61,
88
ophthalmology, 127, 189
organopathy, 208, 212
ornithology, 33

Paine, Martyn, 4, 5
Pasteur, Louis, 212

patients, 126; in animal extract experiments, 206–7; clinic, 103, 115–16; neurological, 69, 115–17, 151–3; private,
116; psychiatric, 174–5, 177–8, 182,
184, 194
Paul, J. M., 135
Pavy, Frederick W., 70
Pawnee (Kansas) Town Association, 26
Peirce, Benjamin, 88, 89
Pennsylvania Hospital (Philadelphia), 6,
18, 53
Pepper, William, 6
Philadelphia Biological Society, 7, 48, 49,
64, 70, 71
poliomyelitis, 135–8; clinical description
of, 135; diagnosis of, 137; pathology of,
135–8; treatment of, 136
Porter, William Henry, 213, 214, 215, 216,
217
positivism, 165, 234
psychiatry: outpatient, 173–4; as specialty,
108, 171, 173–4; *see also* diseases, psychiatric; hospitals, psychiatric; insanity
psychology: animal, 144; medical, 177;
philosophical, 146, 164–5; physiological, 45, 146, 164–71; scientific, 181
psychotherapeutics, 159–61

quacks and quackery, 82, 129, 206, 218,
221, 225

race and racism, 28, 35, 79, 192
Ramsay, Samuel, 59
Ranney, Ambrose, 102
Reber, Charles R., 77
Reeder, Andrew H., 26–8, 87, 90, 91
reform: educational, 195; health, 40; medi-
cal, 75; in medical education, 4; psychi-
atric, 173, 175–9; in psychiatry, 172
Reid, Whitelaw, 181, 190
religion: and anti-Catholic prejudice, 67;
history of, 198, 199; *see also* Hammond,
William A., religious views
Remak, Robert, 128
Reynolds, John, 188
Richardson, Benjamin Ward, 149
Rilliet, Frederic, 135
Roberts, B. F., 218
Roberts, Edmund W., 3
Rockwell, A. D., 128
Roosa, Daniel B. St. John, 75, 99, 189
Ropes, Hannah, 68–9

Satterlee, Richard, 54, 55, 83
Sayre, Lewis, 207
science (in medicine), 5, 16, 105–6
Seguin, Edward C., 149, 175, 176, 178

Semmola, Professor, 217
sexuality: homosexuality, 190; impotence, 205, 207; "mujerados," 22
Shaler, Nathaniel, 146, 148
Shoemaker, John V., 218
Shrady, George, 227
Sidell, J. J., 80
Simons, James, 35
Sims, J. Marion, 126
sleep, 144–9; causes of, 148–9; cycle of, 147; distinguished from stupor, 145; Monro-Kellie doctrine, 144, 149; physiology of, 52, 134, 144, 146, 154; *see also* insomnia
Smith, Aubry, 57
Smith, H. H., 65
Smith, J. D. S., 131
Smith, Joseph R., 59, 65, 77, 81, 91
Smithsonian Institution, 7, 32
Solis-Cohen, Solomon, 218, 219
Spanish-American War, 229
specialties (medical), 11, 46, 71, 75, 95, 116, 121, 126–7, 131, 134, 136, 150, 217, 231; instruction in, 4; *see also names of particular specialties*
Spencer, Herbert, 164
spiritualism, 161, 182, 194, 196, 197
Spitzka, Edward C., 11, 142, 172, 173, 175, 177–9, 196
Springer, William P., 224
Squibb, E. R., 227, 228
Stanton, Edwin, 8, 57–9, 69, 80, 86–9, 91
Steiner, Lewis H., 53
Stockwell, G. Archie, 209
Stone, Robert King, 57
Strong, George Templeton, 55, 62, 86–90
Suckley, George, 76
surgery: and antisepsis, 82, 204; and asepsis, 123; military, 18; neurological, 124, 204; trephination, 203
Swetland, Silas H., 87

Tanner, Dr., 197
Taylor, Charles F., 136
Taylor, Zachary, 6, 19
therapeutics, 126; cardiac, 205; heroic, 123, 162; mental, 159–61, 207, 215; neurological, 122–5, 127; organotherapy, 205, 207, 211, 218; skepticism about, 123; *see also* electrotherapeutics
Thomas, William, 80
Tod, David, 77, 85
Todd, Robert Bentley, 96
Tompkins, E. L., 124
toxicology, 9, 50, 51, 183

Trall, R. T., 82
Tripler, Charles S., 54, 60, 61
Trousseau, A., 139
Turner's Lane Hospital (Philadelphia), 69, 70, 71, 72

Underwood, Michael, 135
Underwood, Sara A., 193–4
University Medical College (New York), 3, 95, 99
University of Maryland, 50, 51; Medical School, 7
University of the City of New York, Alumni Association of the Medical Department, 11
U.S. Army Medical Museum, 71, 80
U.S. Army military posts: Cebolleta (New Mexico), 19–20; Fort Mackinac (Michigan), 51; Fort Meade (Florida), 24; Fort Riley (Kansas), 26, 32, 35, 38; Fort Webster (New Mexico), 23; Laguna (New Mexico), 22; West Point, 25
U.S. Sanitary Commission, 8, 9, 54, 56–7, 60–1, 65, 73, 75, 88, 92
Utica (New York) Asylum, 172

Van Buren, William H., 3, 6, 10, 54, 55, 75, 85, 88
Vance, Reuben A., 98
Vanderpoel, S. Oakley, 66
Variot, G., 206
Velpeau, A.-A.-L.-M., 6
Verein für die gemeinschaftlichen Arbeiten für Förderung der wissenschaftliche Heilkunde, 38, 48
Virchow, Rudolf, 46
Voisin, A., 170

Weber, Dr., 85
Webster, Warren, 83
Wernicke, Carl, 141
Whybrew, C. T., 98
Wigan, A. L., 142
Williams, A., 82
Willis, Benjamin A., 114
Wilson, Henry, 54, 57
Wilson, Robert, 26
women: and feminism and antifeminism, 190–1, 193–6; as hysterics, 192; and lesbianism, 190; as nurses, 68; as physicians, 79, 195; in politics, 191, 194; as professionals, 190, 191; status of, 68, 182, 190, 192, 193; as students, 157, 195; suffrage for, 193
Wood, Robert, 55, 57, 59
Wood, Wallace, 209

Woodward, Joseph J., 49, 72, 80
Woolsey sisters, 68
Wurts, Charles S., 47
Wurtz, Henry, 148
Wyman, Jeffries, 2

Xántus, John, 33, 36, 37, 38

Yates, Richard, 81

Zacharias, I., 82

Printed in the United States
By Bookmasters